Molecular Diagnostics of Cancer

Edited by Pier Paolo Piccaluga

Published in London, United Kingdom

Molecular Diagnostics of Cancer
http://dx.doi.org/10.5772/intechopen.111118
Edited by Pier Paolo Piccaluga

Contributors
Adrian Zety, Ajaykumar Chittipolu, Akbar Pasha, Alexandra Roi, Alexandra Traverse-Glehen, Alexandro Floares, Anna Gazzola, Carmen Floares, Ciprian Ioan Roi, Claudia Mannu, Codruţa Victoria Tigmeanu, Doneti Ravinder, Eduardo Kreutz, Elena Aleksandrovna Kudinova, Fabio Alves, Fernando Roncolato, Florin Manolache, George Calin, Julita Machlowska, Laura-Cristina Rusu, Lavinia Cosmina Ardelean, Mahalakshmi Gunasekaran, Maria Jose Serrano, Marie Donzel, Maryam Etebari, Masahide Takahashi, Mircea Riviş, Mohammad Nurul Amin, Mohsen Navari, Pamela Cruz, Pier Paolo Piccaluga, Rajesh Ranjit, Riccardo Donelli, Roberta Cardim Lessa, Ryszard Maciejewski, Valeria Denninghoff, Vladimir Kanstantinovich Bozhenko, Yong-Yu Liu

First published in London, United Kingdom, 2024 by IntechOpen
IntechOpen is the global imprint of INTECHOPEN LIMITED, registered in England and Wales, registration number: 11086078, 5 Princes Gate Court, London, SW7 2QJ, United Kingdom

British Library Cataloguing-in-Publication Data
A catalogue record for this book is available from the British Library

Additional hard and PDF copies can be obtained from orders@intechopen.com

Molecular Diagnostics of Cancer
Edited by Pier Paolo Piccaluga
p. cm.
Print ISBN 978-1-83769-434-1
Online ISBN 978-1-83769-433-4
eBook (PDF) ISBN 978-1-83769-435-8

For EU product safety concerns:
IN TECH d.o.o., Prolaz Marije Krucifikse Kozulić 3, 51000 Rijeka, Croatia,
info@intechopen.com or visit our website at intechopen.com.

Meet the editor

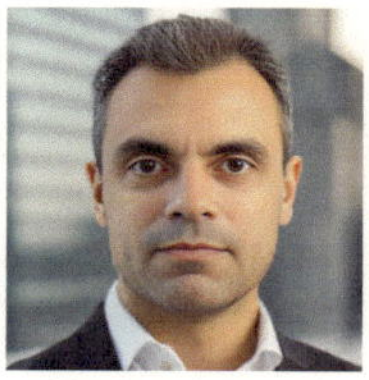

Pier Paolo Piccaluga is an Associate Professor of Pathology in the Department of Medical and Surgical Sciences, Bologna University School of Medicine, Italy. He is also a co-founder and executive physician at the Biobank of Research, IRCCS S. Orsola-Malpighi Hospital, Italy. He has been responsible for the Molecular Pathology Laboratory for many years. In 2018, Dr. Piccaluga was appointed to teach at Queen Mary University of London, UK, and Jomo Kenyatta University of Agriculture and Technology, Kenya. He has taught at the University of Nairobi and the University of Botswana since 2023. He is the author of several international publications and presentations at national and international conferences. He has been involved in several clinical trials as coordinator or sub-investigator and as principal investigator for several research projects. He is the winner of numerous prizes for study and research. Dr. Piccaluga is editor-in-chief for the *World Journal of Hematology, Digital Medicine and Healthcare Technology,* and *Advances in Precision Medicine*.

Contents

Preface

Molecular pathology is a branch of laboratory medicine that uses the analysis of molecules such as DNA, RNA, proteins, and metabolites for the detection and characterization of diseases, including cancer (molecular oncology).

Molecular diagnostics for cancer plays a crucial role in several aspects of cancer care:

- *Early Detection*: Molecular diagnostics can help in the early detection of cancer by identifying specific genetic or molecular alterations associated with the disease. Early detection often leads to more effective treatment outcomes.

- *Personalized Medicine*: Each cancer is unique, and molecular diagnostics can help identify specific genetic mutations or alterations that drive the growth of cancer cells. This information is crucial for tailoring treatments to individual patients, a concept known as personalized or precision medicine.

- *Prognosis*: Molecular diagnostics can provide valuable information about the aggressiveness of a cancer and the likelihood of its recurrence. This information helps clinicians and patients make informed decisions about treatment options and follow-up care.

- *Monitoring Treatment Response*: By analyzing molecular changes during and after treatment, healthcare providers can assess how well a patient is responding to therapy. This allows for timely adjustments to treatment plans if necessary.

- *Targeted Therapies*: Molecular diagnostics guide the use of targeted therapies, which are drugs designed to specifically target the molecular abnormalities driving cancer growth. This approach often results in more effective treatments with fewer side effects compared to traditional chemotherapy.

- *Minimal Residual Disease Monitoring*: After treatment, molecular diagnostics can be used to detect minimal residual disease – small amounts of cancer cells that may remain after treatment. Monitoring for residual disease helps in evaluating the success of treatment and making decisions about additional therapy.

- *Screening for Hereditary Cancer Syndromes*: Molecular testing can identify hereditary mutations that increase the risk of developing certain types of cancer. This information is valuable for identifying individuals who may benefit from early and intensive screening or preventive measures.

Overall, molecular diagnostics has revolutionized cancer diagnosis and management, leading to more precise and personalized approaches to treatment. It enables a deeper understanding of the underlying molecular mechanisms of cancer and helps healthcare professionals make more informed decisions for better patient outcomes.

Pier Paolo Piccaluga
Department of Medical and Surgical Sciences,
Bologna University School of Medicine,
Bologna, Italy

Biobank of Research,
IRCCS Azienda Opedaliera-Universitaria di Bologna,
Bologna, Italy

Section 1

General Features of Molecular Diagnostic in Cancer

Chapter 1

Introductory Chapter: Molecular Diagnostic in Cancer

Pier Paolo Piccaluga

1. Introduction

The Genomic Era in cancer medicine started after the completion of the first human genome study in 2003. Modern pathology and cancer diagnostics now rely on molecular testing to identify genetic alterations that inform diagnosis, prognosis, and treatment decisions. Targeted therapy, immunotherapy, and genomic medicine have become crucial in cancer management. In this introductory chapter, we elucidate the past, present, and potential future of molecular diagnostics to provide a comprehensive overview of molecular diagnostic technologies, testing platforms, and their applications in the treatment of cancer [1].

The term "molecular diagnostics" refers to a group of methods that can be used to identify genetic variations, help in cancer classification and progression prediction, and track therapy efficacy [2].

The earliest molecular diagnostics methods were created in research laboratories in the middle of the previous century. In the early stages of molecular diagnosis, methods, such as recombinant DNA and complementary DNA (cDNA) cloning, were applied to investigate gene sequences [3]. Sanger sequencing was first introduced in 1977 and, for many years, it was the global standard for gene sequencing in clinical laboratories. Polymerase chain reaction (PCR) was later established, and numerous related techniques were subsequently created. In 2000, the first next-generation sequencing (NGS) technology was launched [3], whereas the introduction of the Illumina HiSeq and ThermoFisher Ion Torrent sequencers in 2010 completely paved the way for massively parallel DNA sequencing. Long-read sequencing, also referred to as third-generation sequencing, was the subject of further innovation. The nanopore sequencer is an example of a third-generation sequencer that has the potential to drastically alter the field of molecular diagnostics and nucleic acid sequencing in the near future [4].

2. Modern molecular diagnostic techniques

2.1 Sanger sequencing

Modern molecular diagnostic techniques involve, first of all, a variety of sequencing methods, including Sanger sequencing. Also known as chain termination sequencing, it was once the most widely used sequencing technique and is still considered the gold standard. Frederick Sanger, who received the 1980 Nobel Prize in Chemistry, invented this method for nucleic acid sequencing. The sequencing reaction involves DNA polymerase, primers, deoxynucleic acid, and dideoxy nucleic acid. During sequence extension, the incorporation of dideoxy nucleic acid randomly causes the process to end. After capillary electrophoresis, the collection of fragments of different lengths is analyzed to determine the bases using signals from dideoxy nucleic acid fluorescence [4–6].

Sanger sequencing is a method used to identify single-gene or single-locus mutations quickly. For instance, *EGFR* and *KRAS* mutations in lung cancer, *BCR::ABL1* mutations in chronic myeloid leukemia, and *KIT* and *PDGFRA* mutations in gastrointestinal stromal tumors can be detected using this method. However, the process is slow and takes a long time. Furthermore, the sensitivity is low; the sensitivity of detection for Sanger sequencing is commonly acknowledged to be around 15–20% mutant allele frequency. This implies that in order to achieve reliable detection, approximately 15–20% of the DNA molecules being sequenced must carry the mutation. To prevent the sequencing of wild-type fragments, locked nucleic acid probes can be used, which can raise the limit of detection to 1% or even lower [7].

2.2 Polymerase chain reaction (PCR)

In 1983, Dr. Mullis created a revolutionary technique called the polymerase chain reaction (PCR), which earned him the 1993 Nobel Prize in Chemistry [8]. The reaction involves several components, including DNA polymerase, primers, nucleotides, and a double-stranded DNA template. After denaturation of the template, primers bind to it and extend from the 5′ to the 3′ end, the newly formed DNA copies serve as templates for further replication, leading to exponential amplification of the original template in a chain reaction. The amplified product can be directly observed using gel electrophoresis and subjected to various analyses, such as melting curve analysis, fragment analysis, and restriction fragment length polymorphism (RFLP) analyses based on the size of PCR fragments [9]; or subjected to melting curve analysis based on its dissociation properties [10].

Sanger sequencing, pyrosequencing, single-base extension, and NGS are further methods for sequencing the PCR results. The majority of these techniques include fluorescent tags in the PCR product that allow optical equipment to spot genomic alterations.

Restriction fragment length polymorphism and fragment analysis are both versions of the same method. Both procedures include amplification of a template by PCR using fluorescently labeled primers and sorting of the PCR products by fragment size (length) using capillary electrophoresis [3].

Small and medium-sized insertions and deletions (50 bases to hundreds of bases long) can be quickly found using fragment analysis, some of which may be difficult to find using other technologies or may be easily missed by huge parallel sequencing.

Restriction fragment length polymorphism is also a cost-effective, fast, and easy technique for detecting whether a given location has single-nucleotide variations or methylation, by using sequence-specific restriction enzymes that separate PCR fragments based on the presence of particular palindromic sequences.

This technique has been used in various cancer molecular diagnostics, including clonality studies of lymphomas, and identification of *NPM1* and *FLT3* mutations in acute myeloid leukemia [3].

2.3 Quantitative PCR (qPCR)

The development of quantitative real-time PCR (qPCR) was a significant improvement over traditional PCR. Unlike PCR, which measures the result of amplification, qPCR examines the number of DNA copies during the exponential phase of the reaction, giving a more accurate reflection of the initial template amount [11]. In qRt-PCR, reverse transcription (RT) of RNA to complementary DNA (cDNA) and quantitative detection are two commonly combined techniques for gene expression analysis [12]. These techniques employ fluorescent dye-tipped probes that are examined by an optical system, and the number of copies in the starting material is then determined using standard curves or comparison thresholds. qRT-PCR is widely used for minimal disease detection in chronic myeloid leukemia to monitor the *BCR::ABL1* fusion, in acute myeloid leukemia for *NPM1* mutation, *RUNX1::RUNX1T1* and *PML::RARA* fusions [3].

2.4 Digital PCR (dPCR)

Digital PCR (dPCR) is a relatively new technology that allows for the direct quantification of amplified nucleic acid. Unlike traditional PCR, which amplifies the entire sample in a single reaction, dPCR amplifies thousands or millions of partitions from a single sample [13]. This means that the competitive inhibition, which can be a limiting factor in traditional PCR, has less of an impact on the results, resulting in increased sensitivity of detection [3, 13]. dPCR is commonly used in gene expression analysis, absolute quantification, copy number variation (CNV) detection, and mutation identification. It is also useful for examining liquid biopsy samples due to its high sensitivity.

2.5 Next-generation sequencing

Over a decade ago, next-generation sequencing (NGS), also (probably more properly) named massive parallel sequencing, was developed aiming at enhancing simultaneous detection and capturing all genomic alterations. Recently, it has gained increasing use in clinical practice [14]. The most widespread sequencing platforms are currently the ones employed by Illumina and Ion Torrent [15].

Different chemistries distinguish these two sequencers. Ion Torrent measures changes in electric current as variations in pH, while Illumina detects fluorescence signals. Four fluorescently tagged deoxyribonucleotide triphosphates (dNTPs) of various colors are used to copy the templates on a flow cell during Illumina sequencing. Only the base that is complementary to the template is integrated into the expanding chain or sequencing primer during one reaction round. A laser excites the fluorescent base, and the integrated camera records this distinctive emission spectrum. The template's sequence is identified by analyzing readout of the signals that appear at the same point in sequential photographs.

The Ion Torrent platform uses current, instead of light, as a signal to read DNA fragments. To clonally amplify the DNA library fragments, a bead's surface is utilized. During the sequence reading of each fragment in the bead, the deoxyribonucleotide triphosphate is incorporated into the template DNA by a semiconductor chip with micromachined wells. This chip has an ion-sensitive layer and an ion sensor that detects the hydrogen ions generated during the process.

Enrichment techniques like hybrid capture and amplicon capture are employed by clinical laboratories to select regions of interest for targeted sequencing. These methods have proven to be more cost-effective and time-saving than single-gene tests while also improving assay sensitivity and providing better support for therapeutic decision-making and patient management [16]. Targeted NGS tests have become crucial for identifying cancer driver mutations, assessing microsatellite instability, and determining tumor mutation load.

2.5.1 RNA sequencing

Next-generation sequencing is a powerful tool that can identify gene fusions and evaluate gene expression through the RNA sequencing (RNA-seq) method. Gene fusions are mutations that drive many cancer types, especially those involving the tyrosine kinase domain of growth factors [17]. These mutations can be predictive (being targets), diagnostic, or both [18, 19]. However, targeted DNA sequencing (DNA-seq) has limitations for clinical applications as it cannot detect all structural variants since they often involve long introns that are difficult to map or have repetitive elements. RNA-seq, on the other hand, offers a simple and effective method to identify fusions by capturing the junction of exons from the two fusion partner genes. In order to further improve the detection sensitivity of targeted RNA-seq, sequence-specific primers are often used for known partner genes and universal primers for unknown genes [19].

2.5.2 Nanopore sequencing

Technology for nanopore sequencing was created in 2014. It is now involved in academic research. Nanopore sequencing, in contrast to other sequencing technologies that were already accessible in clinical laboratories, does not call for PCR amplification, may yield long reads (10–100 kb), lower costs, and amplification mistakes, and enhance the quality of *de novo* assembly and mapping. Portable, quick, and inexpensive nanopore sequencing equipment is available [20]. Future developments in virology, gene fusion testing, and germline mutation identification are anticipated as a result of the clinical application of this approach. Additionally, it is anticipated that this technique will be applied at the point of care in the field because these devices are portable. However, the precision and accuracy of nanopore sequencing are still comparatively poor, and efforts are being made to improve them before commercial use [21].

2.5.3 Single-cell sequencing

The use of single-cell sequencing technology is also expanding. Single-cell DNA sequencing analyzes DNA sequences and genomic mutations at the level of individual cells, collects data on temporal and spatial heterogeneity within a particular tumor, and offers details on the development, recurrence, and metastasis of the tumor [22]. By providing details on gene and protein expression, single-cell sequencing of RNA or epigenetic modifications helps to explain phenotypic changes in greater detail [23]. Targeted molecular techniques in cancer therapy are increasingly built on genomic, transcriptomic, and epigenetic data gathered at the level of the individual cell.

Single-cell sequencing has the drawback of requiring fresh or frozen tumor samples to separate individual tumor cells. Through the use of flow cytometry cell sorting, its application to hematological malignancies, particularly myeloid malignancies, is more extensive and easier [24, 25].

2.6 Liquid biopsy/cell-free DNA (cfDNA) assay

A cell-free DNA (cfDNA) assay, sometimes referred to as a liquid biopsy, identifies circulating tumor DNA (ctDNA) in the blood. This method has been recently

Molecular techniques	Variant types				Sensitivity (%)
	SNVs	Small indels	CNV	SVs	
Sanger sequencing	✓	✓			25
Fragment analysis and RFLP	±	✓			5
Allele-specific PCR	✓				1–5
qPCR	✓	±		±	<1
qRT-PCR			✓	✓	0.001
dPCR	✓			±	<1
NGS-Amplicon capture	✓	✓	±	✓	5–10
NGS-Hybridization capture	✓	✓	✓	✓	2–5
NGS-liquid biopsy	✓	✓	±	✓	<1
NGS-RNA sequencing	✓	±		✓	5

± = means may or may not be able to detect those variant types; or with limited ability of detection, CNV = copy number variation, NGS = next-generation sequencing, RFLP = restriction fragment length polymorphism, SNV = single-nucleotide variant, SV = structural variant (Adapted from Jinjuan Yao, Qihui (Jim) Zhai. A narrative review of cancer molecular diagnostics: past, present, and future [J] J Bio-X Res, 2022,05(4): 145–150 [3]).

Table 1.
Schematic comparison of the most common molecular techniques.

developed for utilization in cancer monitoring, drug response assessment, diagnosis, and even early detection. Liquid biopsy offers a thorough examination of genetic changes in the main tumor and any distant metastases [26]. Samples can be taken more frequently and more easier during the course of the disease than with tissue biopsy, giving an evolving overview of changes in genetic cancer alternation.

Liquid biopsy is a diagnostic test that can involve examining either a single gene, or a small or large panel of genes. The purpose of this test is to detect single-nucleotide changes, tiny insertions and deletions, structural variants, and microsatellite instability. The ratio of total cfDNA to ctDNA in the blood of cancer patients can vary significantly based on the type, stage, and size of the tumor. Different types of tumors shed cells at varying rates. Typically, the concentration of ctDNA in the blood increases with the later stage and size of the tumor. Apart from blood, cfDNA can also be obtained from urine, cerebrospinal fluid (CSF), and other bodily fluids.

The main characteristics of the molecular diagnostic technologies described above are summarized in **Table 1**.

3. Clustered regularly interspaced short palindromic repeat (CRISPR) technology

Clustered regularly interspaced short palindromic repeat (CRISPR) is considered as a new approach for identifying cancer mutations by using gene editing technology. CRISPR-associated protein 12 (CAS12) and CRISPR-associated protein 13 (CAS13) caspases, along with the detector and Sherlock technologies ltd, are used to identify genetic changes at the DNA and RNA levels [27–29]. When combined with amplification and NGS, CRISPR technology can be used to selectively enhance the mutant allele by shearing wild-type alleles. This increases the detection sensitivity for low-frequency mutations [3].

CRISPR's readings, stability, mobility, and low cost will make it a useful adjunct to clinical molecular diagnostics.

4. Machine learning (ML) and artificial intelligence (AL)

Large-panel gene expression profile data, sequencing data, including hotspot mutations, insertions, and deletions, focal or genome-wide copy number alterations, structural variants, mutational signatures, and clinical parameters, have been used to develop machine learning (ML) and artificial intelligence (AI) approaches to infer tumor origin.

Researchers from Memorial Sloan Kettering Cancer Center (MSK) have developed an algorithmic classifier using comprehensive genomic profiling data from 7791 tumors that represent 22 different types of cancer. They found that the classifier accurately predicted the type of tumor in 74.1% of an independent cohort of 11,644 patients and in 73.8% of the training set of 7791 patients. This study shows the potential of using machine learning algorithms to improve cancer diagnosis and treatment. In plasma cell-free DNA, the rate of accurate prediction was 75.0%. These results suggest that AI technology can provide additional information on tumor origin, which can further increase the utility of molecular testing, particularly in tumors that have been labeled as cancers of unknown primary type based on histologic and immunophenotypic characteristics [30, 31].

5. Biomarkers' analysis in cancer diagnostics

The detection of cancer biomarkers and the emergence of associated therapies have led to changes in the fundamentals of molecular testing for solid tumors.

The first targeted medication to be licensed by the Food and Drug Administration (FDA) was trastuzumab, which was used to treat human epidermal growth factor receptor 2 (HER2)-positive metastatic breast cancer in 1998 [32]. It was reported in 2004 that gefitinib and erlotinib were used in the treatment of lung adenocarcinomas with activating mutations in *EGFR* [33–35]. Since then, new genetic mutations that are unique to tumors have been discovered and given the green light, including the *KRAS*-resistant mutation and cetuximab in colorectal cancer [36] and the *BRAF* V600E mutant and vemurafenib in melanoma and hairy cell leukemia [37]. Additionally, there are other biomarkers such as mutations in *ALK*, *ROS1*, *KRAS*, *BRAF*, *RET*, and many more in lung adenocarcinoma [38].

Over 20 years ago, single-gene, single-platform testing was the foundation of molecular diagnostics [39]. Traditional low-throughput testing methods, however, are unable to collect all pertinent biomarkers from the small number of tissue samples needed for clinical care and the expansion of cancer biomarkers and targeted medicines. To record all clinically indicated mutations, molecular diagnostics laboratories have had to create more comprehensive platforms. Large, focused NGS panels, such as Foundation One and MSK-IMPACT (Integrated Mutation Profiling of Actionable Cancer Targets), were introduced in 2011 and 2014, respectively. These two panels use the pan-cancer method, screening all solid tumors regardless of tumor type or whether the tumor has known biomarkers for a broad panel of cancer genes. Many people with various cancer kinds have been discovered using this type of technique who may profit from clinical trials settings.

Molecular laboratories face the challenge of developing a range of testing platforms to meet clinical demands for both speed and thoroughness. Neither single-gene testing nor cancer panel testing alone can fulfill these requirements. As a result, an algorithm is sometimes necessary for testing stratification, particularly in tumor types with multiple targets. For example, in lung adenocarcinoma, single-gene testing is performed to detect epidermal growth factor receptor (EGFR), anaplastic lymphoma kinase (ALK), or Kirsten rat sarcoma viral oncogene homolog (KRAS) alterations. This is followed by NGS testing to identify mutations, copy number, and structural variants in other driver genes, as well as to assess microsatellite instability and tumor mutation burden to complete the biomarker identification process.

6. Conclusions: the future of molecular diagnostics

The field of molecular diagnostics has experienced significant and rapid expansion in recent years and is expected to continue to do so. With the help of precise, sensitive, and rapid detection, initial diagnosis and monitoring of diseases will become easier. Molecular diagnostics advancements in early detection have the potential to shape the future of cancer management.

Acknowledgements

The author is grateful to Dr. Shaymaa Khattab for editing assistance, and to Elvira Baumgartner and the IntechOpen Editorial Team for the precious assistance.

Conflict of interest

"The authors declare no conflict of interest."

Notes

This book is dedicated to the memory of *Prof. Alessandro Piccaluga* (1927–1995). Prof. Piccaluga was emeritus Professor of Pathology at Bologna University, where he directed the Institute of Pathologic Anatomy and founded the School of Pathologic Anatomy. He dedicated his career to diagnosis, teaching, and scientific research, giving a substantial contribution to the advancement of lung and kidney pathology.

Author details

Pier Paolo Piccaluga[1,2]

1 Biobank of Research, IRCCS Azienda Opedaliera-Universitaria di Bologna, Bologna, Italy

2 Department of Medical and Surgical Sciences, Bologna University School of Medicine, Bologna, Italy

*Address all correspondence to: pierpaolo.piccaluga@unibo.it

References

[1] Collins FS, Morgan M, Patrinos A. The human genome project: Lessons from large-scale biology. Science. 2003;**300**:286-290

[2] Netto GJ, Saad RD, Dysert PA 2nd. Diagnostic molecular pathology: Current techniques and clinical applications, part I. Proceedings (Baylor University. Medical Center). 2003;**16**:379-383

[3] Yao J, Qihui (Jim) Zhai. A narrative review of cancer molecular diagnostics: Past, present, and future. Journal of Bio-X Research. 2022;**05**(4):145-150

[4] Heather JM, Chain B. The sequence of sequencers: The history of sequencing DNA. Genomics. 2016;**107**:1-8

[5] Shampo MA, Kyle RA. Walter Gilbert—1980 Nobel Prize for Chemistry. Mayo Clinic Proceedings. 2003;**78**:588

[6] Sanger F, Nicklen S, Coulson AR. DNA sequencing with chain-terminating inhibitors. Proceedings of the National Academy of Sciences of the United States of America. 1977;**74**:5463-5467

[7] Ishige T, Itoga S, Matsushita K, et al. Locked nucleic acid probe enhances Sanger sequencing sensitivity and improves diagnostic accuracy of high-resolution melting-based KRAS mutational analysis. Clinica Chimica Acta. 2016;**457**:75-80

[8] Mullis KB, Faloona FA. Specific synthesis of DNA in vitro via a polymerase- catalyzed chain reaction. Methods in Enzymology. 1987;**155**:335-350

[9] Jarcho J. Restriction fragment length polymorphism analysis. Current Protocols in Human Genetics. PubMed. May 2001;Chapter 2:Unit 2.7. DOI: 10.1002/0471142905.hg0207s01. PMID: 18428271

[10] Pryor RJ, Wittwer CT. Real-time polymerase chain reaction and melting curve analysis. Methods in Molecular Biology. 2006;**336**:19-32

[11] Hirakawa Y, Medh RD, Metzenberg S. Quantitative polymerase chain reaction analysis by deconvolution of internal standard. BMC Molecular Biology. 2010;**11**:30

[12] Gadkar V, Filion M. New developments in quantitative real-time polymerase chain reaction technology. Current Issues in Molecular Biology. 2014;**16**:1-6

[13] Taylor SC, Laperriere G, Germain H. Droplet digital PCR versus qPCR for gene expression analysis with low abundant targets: From variable nonsense to publication quality data. Scientific Reports. 2017;**7**:2409

[14] Slatko BE, Gardner AF, Ausubel FM. Overview of next-generation sequencing technologies. Current Protocols in Molecular Biology. 2018;**122**:e59

[15] McCombie WR, McPherson JD, Mardis ER. Next-generation sequencing technologies. Cold Spring Harbor Perspectives in Medicine. 2019;**9**: a036798

[16] Mamanova L, Coffey AJ, Scott CE, et al. Target-enrichment strategies for next-generation sequencing. Nature Methods. 2010;**7**:111-118

[17] Heyer EE, Deveson IW, Wooi D, et al. Diagnosis of fusion genes using

targeted RNA sequencing. Nature Communications. 2019;**10**:1388

[18] Stransky N, Cerami E, Schalm S, et al. The landscape of kinase fusions in cancer. Nature Communications. 2014;**5**:4846

[19] Benayed R, Offin M, Mullaney K, et al. High yield of RNA sequencing for targetable kinase fusions in lung adenocarcinomas with no mitogenic driver alteration detected by DNA sequencing and low tumor mutation burden. Clinical Cancer Research. 2019;**25**:4712-4722

[20] Branton D, Deamer DW, Marziali A, et al. The potential and challenges of nanopore sequencing. Nature Biotechnology. 2008;**26**:1146-1153

[21] Bowden R, Davies RW, Heger A, et al. Sequencing of human genomes with nanopore technology. Nature Communications. 2019;**10**:1869

[22] Baslan T, Hicks J. Unravelling biology and shifting paradigms in cancer with single-cell sequencing. Nature Reviews. Cancer. 2017;**17**:557-569

[23] Clark SJ, Lee HJ, Smallwood SA, et al. Single-cell epigenomics: Powerful new methods for understanding gene regulation and cell identity. Genome Biology. 2016;**17**:72

[24] Brierley CK, Mead AJ. Single-cell sequencing in hematology. Current Opinion in Oncology. 2020;**32**:139-145

[25] Paguirigan AL, Smith J, Meshinchi S, et al. Single-cell genotyping demonstrates complex clonal diversity in acute myeloid leukemia. Science Translational Medicine. 2015;7:281re-281r2

[26] Stewart CM, Kothari PD, Mouliere F, et al. The value of cell-free DNA for molecular pathology. The Journal of Pathology. 2018;**244**:616-627

[27] Mintz RL, Gao MA, Lo K, et al. CRISPR technology for breast cancer: Diagnostics, modeling, and therapy. Advanced Biosystems. 2018;**2**:1800132

[28] Yan F, Wang W, Zhang J. CRISPR-Cas12 and Cas13: The lesser known siblings of CRISPR-Cas9. Cell Biology and Toxicology. 2019;**35**:489-492

[29] Shmakov SA, Sitnik V, Makarova KS, et al. The CRISPR spacer space is dominated by sequences from species-specific mobilomes. MBio. 2017;**8**(5):e01397-e01317

[30] Kleppe A, Skrede OJ, De Raedt S, et al. Designing deep learning studies in cancer diagnostics. Nature Reviews. Cancer. 2021;**21**:199-211

[31] Penson A, Camacho N, Zheng Y, et al. Development of genome-derived tumor type prediction to inform clinical cancer care. JAMA Oncology. 2020;**6**:84-91

[32] Thor A. HER2--A discussion of testing approaches in the USA. Annals of Oncology. 2001;**12**(Suppl 1):S101-S107

[33] Pao W, Miller V, Zakowski M, et al. EGF receptor gene mutations are common in lung cancers from "never smokers" and are associated with sensitivity of tumors to gefitinib and erlotinib. Proceedings of the National Academy of Sciences of the United States of America. 2004;**101**:13306-13311

[34] Paez JG, Jänne PA, Lee JC, et al. EGFR mutations in lung cancer: Correlation with clinical response to gefitinib therapy. Science. 2004;**304**:1497-1500

[35] Lynch TJ, Bell DW, Sordella R, et al. Activating mutations in the epidermal

growth factor receptor underlying responsiveness of non-small-cell lung cancer to gefitinib. The New England Journal of Medicine. 2004;**350**:2129-2139

[36] Lièvre A, Bachet JB, Le Corre D, et al. KRAS mutation status is predictive of response to cetuximab therapy in colorectal cancer. Cancer Research. 2006;**66**:3992-3995

[37] Chapman PB, Hauschild A, Robert C, et al. BRIM-3 study group. Improved survival with vemurafenib in melanoma with BRAF V600E mutation. The New England Journal of Medicine. 2011;**364**:2507-2516

[38] Lindeman NI, Cagle PT, Aisner DL, et al. Updated molecular testing guideline for the selection of lung cancer patients for treatment with targeted tyrosine kinase inhibitors: Guideline from the College of American Pathologists, the International Association for the Study of Lung Cancer, and the Association for Molecular Pathology. Journal of Thoracic Oncology. 2018;**13**:323-358

[39] Sobel ME, Bagg A, Caliendo AM, et al. The evolution of molecular genetic pathology: Advancing 20th-century diagnostic methods into potent tools for the new millennium. The Journal of Molecular Diagnostics. 2008;**10**:480-483

Chapter 2

The Importance of Molecular Diagnostic Techniques on Evaluation of Cancers

Ajaykumar Chittipolu, Akbar Pasha and Doneti Ravinder

Abstract

Cancer is caused by genetic changes controlling cell progression and differentiation. These changes are unregulated when tumours advance and acquire invasive and metastatic capacities due to the innate biologic characteristics of the cancer cell. In vivo and in vitro models show that these molecular changes are crucial for tumour development and survival. These molecular changes can be used to develop pristine cancer treatments. New methodological molecules are being developed to identify cancer-specific modifications in proteins, DNA, and RNA, as well as molecular distinctions between healthy and cancer cells. This approach enables effective early detection, precise diagnosis, and quick cancer therapy. DNA microarray techniques have been developed for identifying cancer-associated mutations and gene profiles. Molecular cancer diagnostics need improvement alongside advances in genomics, precision medicine, and immunotherapy. This chapter discusses different molecular diagnostics in the evaluation of cancers.

Keywords: cancer, molecular diagnosis, cancer detection, genetic modifications, prognosis of cancer

1. Introduction

Cancer therapies are secure and reliable. Each patient would only get a therapy if necessary, and it would be tailored to their cancer. The therapy would not impact other bodily tissues, minimising any potential adverse effects. In other words, the approach would be exact. While there is no perfect cure, molecular diagnostics (in conjunction with targeted medicines) bring us closer to this ideal. The "precision" or "personalised" medical revolution in healthcare includes molecular diagnostics. The capacity to provide personalised medicine, which has been a goal of physicians for centuries, is getting increasingly precise because to advancements in diagnostic and treatment equipment. Currently, the phrase "precision medicine" is used to describe a relatively young and developing discipline that offers crucial information that may be utilised to choose the most effective course of therapy for each patient. Precision medicine uses data from DNA, RNA, proteins, or other similar substances. Molecular diagnostics are essential to precision medicine since they are the tests that find these molecules [1]. There are aspects related to cancer therapy where molecular diagnostics shows significant contribution.

Molecular diagnostics may also be used in differential diagnosis to aid in the cancer diagnosis process. They may assist in distinguishing between cancer and benign tumours. Even classifying distinct cancer subtypes that affect the same tissue may be done with the use of molecular diagnostics. These findings might be used to calculate the aggressiveness of cancer. Blood malignancies, for instance, come in a variety of forms. Subtypes of blood cancer are often identified using molecular diagnostics [2]. AML, or acute myelogenous leukaemia, is one kind of blood cancer that is categorised into poor, moderate, or favourable risk groups based on chromosomal analysis. When an illness is deemed to be of intermediate risk, patients are subjected to molecular testing for a variety of mutations. Other molecular diagnostics are used to identify other AML subtypes, such as acute promyelocytic leukaemia. Treatment options may be affected by the cancer's molecular subtype. Prognosis A prognosis is a prediction of the consequences of medical therapy or the natural course of disease in the absence of treatment. Knowing that certain tumours are more aggressive by nature than others may assist patients and doctors in choosing the best course of action [3]. The gene FLT3 serves as an example. In persons with AML, changes in this gene are a sign of an aggressive malignancy. It is noteworthy that during the last several years, researchers have created drugs intended to block FLT3, and some are now undergoing clinical trials. If these drugs are effective, the existence of FLT3 changes, as identified by a molecular diagnostic, may help predict how well a patient would respond to therapy [4]. Another component of prognosis that molecular diagnostics may assess is the probability that cancer will return after therapy. For women with early-stage, node-negative, oestrogen receptor-positive, invasive breast cancer who will receive hormone treatment, several molecular diagnostics are available to forecast the chance of breast cancer recurrence. Multiple genes are examined by these procedures in cells taken from a breast tumour sample. Prediction of Treatment Response As previously mentioned, molecular diagnostics may assist in determining how patients will react to cancer therapy. A test for HER2/neu gene overexpression in a person's breast cancer tumour tissue is one such. Human epidermal growth factor receptor 2 (HER2) is a protein that is produced by cells when the HER2/neu gene is present [5]. This gene is overexpressed in around one-fourth of all breast tumours, resulting in an excessive amount of the protein being generated. Cells develop and divide more quickly due to the additional protein. Treatment for breast tumours with overexpression of HER2/neu may include the use of a medication called trastuzumab, which blocks the function of the HER2 protein. Because the findings of the test may also be used to evaluate the prognosis (i.e., the aggressiveness of the cancer), testing for HER2/neu is another example of a molecular diagnostic with several clinical applications.

2. Role of pharmacokinetics in cancer therapy

Pharmacokinetics is the study of how medications are absorbed, distributed, broken down, and eliminated. Pharmacokinetics When you ingest a tablet, the drug must be absorbed and dispersed throughout the body to reach the site of action—in this example, the malignant tissue—where it will have the desired effect. After some time, the drug is broken down and eliminated by the body, necessitating the need for further treatment. Genetics is only one of many variables that affect these processes' pace of progression. Genetic variations cause some individuals to metabolise medications more quickly than others, which has significant consequences for several cancer therapies [6]. One example of this is the drug irinotecan, which is used to treat colon cancer. Irinotecan is metabolised more slowly by individuals with the genetic sequence UGT1A1*28 than by those without it. These people need to get a lesser dosage of the medicine than usual to avoid drug accumulation in the body. Monitoring therapy Response Naturally, both patients and medical professionals want to know right once if a therapy is effective. For colon and numerous other malignancies, simple blood tests and other molecular diagnostics have been developed to assess therapy response throughout the course of treatment [7, 8]. As in the instance of the blood cancer chronic myelogenous leukaemia, certain malignancies may become drug resistant. Imatinib, a drug that blocks a protein produced by an aberrant combination of genes, is often used to treat this malignancy. Years of imatinib treatment may be necessary for those with chronic myelogenous leukaemia, and in some individuals, the genetic makeup might alter with time. Reduced pharmaceutical efficacy might result from this adjustment. Therefore, molecular diagnostic testing may be used on individuals who no longer react to imatinib to evaluate whether the gene has altered. Patients with cancer who have had effective treatment are often followed up on a regular basis to look for symptoms of recurrence. When it comes to some malignancies, molecular diagnostics may help in figuring out if the disease has returned. It is debatable whether people without cancer symptoms should be monitored for recurrence of breast, prostate, and ovarian cancers using molecular diagnostics. Future research is anticipated to result in improved molecular diagnostics that can more precisely track disease recurrence in people who have had effective treatment [9].

3. Role of molecular biomarker in diagnosis

A cancer biomarker is a trait that may be used to predict a patient's prognosis, cancer risk, or incidence. These traits could be cellular, molecular, physiologic, or image based. The emphasis of the current review is on cellular and molecular cancer biomarkers. These biomolecules, which are present or created by cancer cells or healthy cells in response to cancer, may be discovered in tissues or bodily fluids. In order to find changes in nucleic acid, amino acids and other related components, or other biomolecules that may be used for cancer prognosis, diagnosis, cancer therapy, predicting drug response, or cancer monitoring, biomarker testing in cancer entails profiling tumours or bodily fluids. As opposed to cancer biomarker testing, genetic testing is used to find germline genetic changes linked to cancer susceptibility, hereditary cancer, or syndromes associated with cancer. Germline genetic markers may supply valuable information about therapy alternatives in addition to information on cancer risk. In a larger sense, they may also be thought of as cancer biomarkers [10].

Molecular Alterations Can be Inherited or Acquired. A genetic change's ability to be handed down from one generation to the next relies on the kind of cell it occurs. Germ cells and somatic cells both have the potential to experience genetic changes. The reproductive cells in humans are called germ cells. Somatic cells are all other cell types often known as nonreproductive cells. Mutations are often used to describe changes in DNA. DNA alterations that have detrimental effects on health though not always referred to as mutations [11]. However, occasionally DNA alterations that are "good" for the organism are referred to as mutations, such as when DNA alterations help plants or living things to adapt to their surroundings more effectively. Consequently, the meaning of the term "mutation" is ambiguous. Hereditary mutations or germline mutations refer to mutations that take place in germ cells. Only mutations in these cells can be passed on to the next generation since only eggs and sperm can produce embryos. Increased vulnerability to an illness or a change in how the body metabolises a medicine are both consequences of germline mutations. On the other hand, mutations that take place in somatic cells are referred to as somatic mutations and may result from environmental exposure or spontaneous cellular processes. When cells do their regular tasks, including creating new cells and repairing DNA damage, spontaneous mutations might happen. Somatic mutations occur in healthy tissue, which subsequently progresses to cancer. Even though they happen in the same gene, somatic and germline mutations might have distinct effects on health. One such gene is P53, which has been linked to cancer [12].

3.1 Chromosomal modifications as cancer biomarkers

Biomarkers for cancer may be specific chromosomal abnormalities. Typically, the chromosomal mutation is both a biomarker and the primary driver of the malignancy. One instance of a targeted treatment is imatinib. Treatments for cancer that explicitly target chemicals involved in the development, spread, and advancement of cancer cells are known as targeted cancer treatments. These medications work to stop the reproduction or proliferation of cancer cells. Different chromosomal irregularities chromosomal translocations, such as the one that results in the Philadelphia chromosome, are typical in many different cancer types [13]. Most of the time, this translocation produces fusion proteins that are unable to turn off by themselves; in fact, more than 200 such proteins have been discovered. The anaplastic lymphoma kinase (ALK) gene is another example regulate the cell growth is often regulated by the ALK gene. About 3–5% of persons with non-small-cell lung cancer have this gene mutation in their tumour tissue, which plays a crucial role in various malignancies. People with non-small cell lung cancer whose tumour is positive for the ALK fusion gene may benefit from a targeted medication called crizotinib, which has been created to suppress the extra protein generated by ALK overactivity [14]. Chromosome inversion, or the end-to-end swapping of a section of DNA inside the same chromosome, is another chromosomal defect that sometimes manifests in cancer. Copy number variation is the name given to a third kind of chromosomal abnormality. This comprises chromosomal deletions (where a portion is lost) and amplifications (where a portion of the chromosome is duplicated). Gene duplication and gene amplification are additional terms used to describe chromosomal duplication. In this instance, a DNA fragment is improperly copied once or more. Overproduction of the protein may result from gene duplication in some regions, which may then lead to overactivity [15]. Human epidermal growth factor receptor 2 (HER2), a protein, is the case for certain breast tumours that are referred to as being "HER positive." Typically, this protein aids in cell growth. This gene causes malignancies to develop quickly and invade other tissues when they have an excessive number of copies. To check for this mutation, there are molecular diagnostic techniques available. Trastuzumab (Herceptin®), a medication that renders the HER2 protein inactive, was created because of the finding that HER2 was linked to breast tumours that grew more quickly [16]. Another medication called lapatinib (Tykerb®) prevents some proteins, including HER2, from doing their job. We all have genetic variances, in other words. Some of these variances are passed down via our families, while others are picked up during our lifetimes. Generic variation may take many distinct forms. Single nucleotide polymorphisms are variations in the DNA sequence that occur in at least 1% of the population yet vary from everyone else by one nucleotide base pair. SNPs are responsible for 90% of all DNA variation in humans. SNPs may be either good or negative; some can be helpful, while others might be detrimental, and yet others might have no discernible impact at all. There are several distinct kinds of mutations that may take place. Point mutations are changes in a single nucleotide base to a different base, whereas insertions and deletions are changes in new nucleotide bases introduced into the sequence. In DNA, insertions and deletions are collectively known as indels. By counting the amount of DNA bases involved, they are arbitrarily separated from chromosomal deletions and amplifications. In accordance with current use, indel is used to describe deletions or insertions that include 1 to 50 nucleotides or less, while copy number variation is used to explain bigger deletions and insertions that generally involve more than 100 nucleotides [17].

3.2 Cancer biomarkers using proteins

The sort of biomarker that is being assessed by molecular diagnostics most often is protein biomarkers. Some proteins are released by tumours and reach the circulation. After that, these proteins may be assessed using a blood sample and a molecular diagnostic test. HER2 protein, which is the protein produced by the HER2/neu gene, and oestrogen receptor levels in breast tumours are two additional proteins that may be detected in tissue. An example of a protein biomarker is carcinoembryonic antigen (CEA) [18]. Patients who have previously been diagnosed with cancers of the rectum, thyroid, lung, breast, liver, pancreas, stomach, and ovaries have their blood levels of this protein monitored rather than utilised for diagnosis. In certain cases, a CEA test is carried out before to therapy and then repeatedly carried out during therapy to assess the efficacy of the treatment and look for cancer development or recurrence. The CEA levels may potentially affect the stage and prognosis of certain cancers. In certain cases of malignancies, the CEA test is only useful in individuals whose cancer has metastasised (spread outside of the initial area) and is used in combination with other biomarkers and clinical testing [19].

4. Partner diagnostics

There is a rising tendency towards employing molecular diagnostics to identify people with a specific biomarker that might be targeted with a specific treatment as our understanding of the biology of cancer advances. Since they enable focused therapy, molecular diagnostics are often referred to as companion diagnostics.

4.1 Genomics

The Human Genome Project, a major undertaking that resulted in the sequencing of all 3 billion nucleotide bases in human DNA, was completed in 2003. The study of how several genes interact to carry out a certain function is known as genomics, and this endeavour contributed to the emergence of this field. Because they lacked the tools to examine several genes at once in the past, researchers tended to concentrate on single genes. The laboratory techniques and advanced computer technologies needed for this kind of investigation have only recently become accessible [20]. It has become clear thanks to genomics that alterations in several genes and proteins are often linked to cancer. Consequently, molecular diagnostics, or assessments of several genes at once, have been developed to study gene profiles. For instance, OncotypeDX® Breast Cancer Assay is one of the most popular and well-researched gene profile or genomic assays. This investigation analyses a panel of 21 genes that provides information about breast cancer. It is designed to be used by female patients with early-stage (Stage I or II), node-negative, invasive breast cancer that is positive for the oestrogen receptor and who will undergo hormone therapy. The result of this test is a score that represents the likelihood of a recurrence of breast cancer; the higher the score, the more likely the tumour will come back. This test may also determine if chemotherapy added to a woman's hormone treatment (also known as adjuvant therapy) will be beneficial in the case of early stages [21].

4.2 Proteomics

Multiple proteins may be found simultaneously using proteomic molecular diagnostics. It is challenging and hard for researchers to create proteomic tests that are effective for cancer since cells produce so many distinct proteins (one gene might produce many proteins). It is anticipated that breakthroughs would result from the collection of enormous datasets, or data listing protein levels in hundreds of thousands of individuals with varied health issues who participated in several research. Researchers will examine these datasets when more of them become accessible to identify protein patterns that could be connected to tumours in the hopes of developing helpful proteomic-based molecular diagnostics [22, 23].

5. Aspects of molecular diagnosis methods

Today, polymerase chain reaction (PCR) is a crucial technique in molecular diagnostics that allow medical professionals to "see" changes in our DNA that may be the underlying cause of medical issues and that may aid in the identification of novel biomarkers that can be specifically targeted by precision medications. They are often referred to as "diagnosis in vitro" or "in vitro diagnostics." The Latin phrase "in vitro," meaning "in glass," refers to the initial experiments conducted using glass test tubes. The distinction can be made between "in vivo diagnostics," which are conducted on a living human subject and provide visual information, and "in vitro diagnostics," which are presently conducted on bodily samples such as blood, saliva, or cancer cells. X-ray imaging, ultrasound imaging, and computed tomography (CT) scanning are often employed techniques for in vivo diagnostic purposes [24, 25]. Molecular diagnostics is sometimes referred to as "in vitro diagnostics" since all current molecular diagnostics are performed in vitro. Diagnostic techniques that combine in vitro and in vivo research are now widely used. For example, certain body molecules are marked with substances that make them visible using imaging technology when radioactive oestrogen is supplied to a person and imaging is utilised to examine oestrogen receptors in the living body. Obtaining a test specimen or a sample of tissue is the first step in a molecular diagnostic. According to the objective and kind of test, many procedures are employed to obtain tissue samples. Blood samples are often drawn from veins in the arm. Urine and mouth-saliva samples may both be examined. Skin samples may be taken after local anaesthesia [26]. When samples need to be collected from a solid tissue abnormality or tumour, a fine needle biopsy is the easiest and least invasive procedure. This includes inserting a thin needle into the tissue and aspirating cells. A core needle biopsy may be used if a larger amount of tissue is needed to extract cells and a small amount of surrounding tissue. Excisional and incisional biopsies, which each remove a portion of the anomaly or tumour, may also be used during surgery to remove more tissue. To collect cells, it is also possible to scrape tissues naturally exposed to the environment, such as the cervix and face. Another method involves inserting an endoscope—a bendable, lighted device—through one of the body's natural holes. Small bits of tissue may be removed by the doctor using the endoscope to evaluate any anomalies on the organ's lining.

5.1 Maintaining tissues

Any tissue that is not immediately subjected to molecular diagnostic tests may be processed and kept for later use. Using formalin and wax to embed the tissue sample is one method of tissue preservation. Snap-freezing the tissue and keeping it at 80°C is another option. The vitality of the tissue for molecular diagnostic testing may be impacted by tissue type, collecting techniques, and storage techniques. Tissue banks are often used to store tissue that will likely not be used for many years, such as for research. DNA, protein, and RNA may all be preserved snap-frozen and kept at a temperature of 80°C for long periods of time [27].

5.2 DNA detection techniques

The direct identification of the nucleotide bases present in DNA is known as DNA sequencing. This technique, often called the Sanger method, was created for the first time by Fred Sanger. The DNA is initially split into two strands using the Sanger technique. One strand is then repeatedly replicated using chemicals that halt the copying process at various points along the DNA strand. Numerous shorter DNA strands of various lengths are produced because of this process. The chemicals employed to halt the replicating process have allowed the researchers to determine which nucleotide is at the end of each fragment. As a result, they can put together the DNA fragments to show the original DNA strand's sequence [28].

Today, it is possible to sequence DNA in a much quicker and less costly manner. Next-generation sequencing, or NGS, is the technique that is now most widely employed. Using a slide, the size of a Band-Aid®, this approach allows for the simultaneous operation of 500 million different sequencing processes. The slide is then placed into a device that examines each response independently and records the DNA sequences in a computer. It is a copying process comparable to the Sanger technique; however, it does not call for the use of modified nucleotide bases [29].

5.2.1 Probes of DNA

In many molecular diagnostic procedures, DNA probes are a crucial tool for identifying the presence of certain DNA sequences. The fact that each nucleotide base in DNA can only connect to one other base is used to the benefit of DNA probes. Building a DNA probe involves connecting nucleotide bases that complement the desired DNA sequence. For instance, you might create a probe using the sequence GGGAA if you were attempting to detect the sequence CCCTT. The appropriate circumstances would allow this probe to connect to CCCTT but no other DNA sequences [30]. DNA probes are much longer than just a few nucleotides; they are then combined with tissue samples that have been prepared for the test. After allowing the probes to bind to or hybridise with tissue DNA, they are removed by washing. The probe will adhere to a complimentary DNA sequence it detects if it matches one and will not wash away. Then, a fluorescent signal that indicates the existence of the sequence in a person's DNA may be seen. The DNA probes will wash off, and no fluorescence will be seen if the subject's DNA does not contain the problematic DNA sequence [31, 32].

5.2.2 Genomic microarrays

The capability of DNA microarrays to simultaneously identify hundreds of genes is crucial to the science of genomics. In DNA microarrays, DNA probes with specific DNA sequences are "arrayed" or "spotted" in a grid pattern on a very thin glass surface. Thousands of tiny dots aligned in exact rows and columns make up the DNA microarray. A single DNA probe, like the one previously mentioned, is included in each dot and is intended to hybridise with the corresponding DNA sequence present in the tissue sample. Numerous probe sites enable simultaneous detection of a wide variety of DNA sequences. Thus-called "high throughput," or the simultaneous examination of several DNA sequences, is made possible by this. An analysis sample comprising the subject's DNA is created once the DNA probes have been positioned in the microarray [33]. The sample's double-stranded DNA has undergone denaturement or been split into two complimentary single strands. After being divided into smaller pieces, the strands are then covered with fluorescent pigment. The chip is filled with the sample's labelled DNA, which is then given time to combine with the DNA probes. After washing the microarray, DNA that has not yet hybridised will come off, while DNA that has will not. Fluorescence is then used to identify bound and unbound DNA. If the DNA probe and the sample DNA have successfully hybridised, that area of the array will light up. Computers have information on which place corresponds to DNA sequence and can determine whether that sequence is present in the sample [34]. The array's detecting strategy may employ one to four colours, depending on the technology. Other names for DNA microarrays include genome chip, GeneChip® (a trademark for a particular device), and gene array. Bead, capillary, and well arrays all function similarly and may be used to mount microarrays on surfaces than glass. In other words, DNA probes are connected to the surface of the array (whose sequence is obviously known since you put them in), enabling thousands of genes or even the whole genome to be studied in a single experiment. Different gene variants are sometimes found through microarray analysis. The BRCA1 gene, for instance, has more than 800 mutations, which raises the risk of breast and several other cancers. These differences can all be discovered using a single microarray [35].

5.2.3 Cytogenetic evaluation

Examining the number and makeup of chromosomes is a component of cytogenetic testing. Dr. Janet Rowling, who made the important discovery that chromosomal aberrations might result in cancer in the 1970s, founded this discipline. While some do not classify cytogenetic testing as a "molecular diagnostic" since it does not include the detection of molecules like DNA, we will discuss it here so that it may be contrasted with more contemporary techniques [36]. Traditional cytogenetic tests include collecting cells from a specific region of the body and cultivating them for at least one day in a test tube. The cells that are dividing are then halted or, to put it another way, "frozen" in the act of dividing. Because only at this stage can the chromosomes be seen under a standard microscope, it is crucial that the cells actively dividing. On a microscope slide, the dividing cells are next put. A standard microscope is used to examine each chromosome in several cells (often at least 20). This kind of test is often used to identify Down syndrome, a condition in which the afflicted person has an extra copy of chromosome 21. By just counting the chromosomes, this genetic condition may be identified. Blood malignancies like leukaemia may also be classified using cytogenetics.

5.2.4 Fluorescence in situ hybridisation (FISH)

FISH, commonly referred to as molecular cytogenetic testing, is a technique for identifying and mapping genetic material, including genes or DNA sequences within genes. FISH is a technique for examining individual DNA segments under a fluorescence microscope to determine their existence, absence, relative location, and/or quantity. FISH is more adaptable than traditional cytogenetic methods since it may be used on cells that are not actively dividing. FISH is extremely useful for locating copy number alterations, notably translocations and amplifications, which typically occur with HER2 in breast and gastric malignancies. FISH makes use of fluorescent dye-coated DNA probes. The double strands of DNA in the chromosomes are split apart by special processing. For the DNA probe to connect to complementary DNA sequences in the chromosomal sample, it is then inserted. Following sufficient time for hybridisation, the probes are examined under a fluorescence microscope. Under the fluorescence microscope, hybridisation of the DNA probes with the chromosomal DNA may be seen [37, 38].

5.2.5 Primers

DNA primers are DNA sequences that act as the basis for DNA replication. DNA polymerases, the proteins that aid in DNA replication, are unable to start the process of creating new DNA from scratch. They are limited to adding nucleotide bases to an already-existing strand. Primers play an important role in this process since they start it off, while DNA polymerases finish it off. The laboratory technique known as polymerase chain reaction (PCR) amplifies little quantities of DNA to make it easier to detect and analyse. To separate the strands, heated double-stranded DNA is first used. After that, the temperature is decreased, and primers attach to the DNA's single strands. Then, the DNA copying enzyme (DNA polymerase, represented by the letter 'P' in PCR) replicates each individual strand. After heating the material, the procedure is repeated to separate the freshly formed double strands. The quantity of DNA strands doubles with each cycle of the procedure. The DNA sequence may be produced in a billion copies by PCR in a matter of hours [39, 40].

5.2.6 In-the-moment PCR

Like ordinary PCR, real-time PCR also detects or quantifies the DNA during the same process in addition to copying it. In typical PCR, the final product is examined once the reaction is finished. Real-time PCR is utilised in a variety of companion diagnostics to assess the likelihood that malignancies may react to certain therapy. Reverse-transcription PCR, or RT-PCR for short, is a PCR method that is covered in the next section. Most experts concur that real-time PCR, which is distinct from reverse-transcription PCR, should not be shortened to RT-PCR. To prevent misunderstanding, reverse-transcription PCR should only be referred to by the acronym RT-PCR.

5.3 RNA detection techniques

Many of the techniques just discussed for DNA detection have been modified to detect RNA. Since RNA tests can tell us if the DNA is actively being converted into proteins, they are helpful for assessing the level of gene expression.

5.3.1 Phosphorylation-dependent PCR

Reverse-transcription (RT)-PCR is comparable to PCR; however, it detects RNA rather than DNA. The chemical intermediary known as RNA is responsible for copying and translating the DNA code into proteins. In RT-PCR, the same procedures as in PCR are used, but instead of DNA, a form of RNA is used in the sample, which might be taken from a tumour, blood, urine, etc. A key advancement in research and medical technology is the capacity of RT-PCR to identify expressed genes as opposed to those that are just present. It is possible to utilise RT-PCR to evaluate if cancer has spread to other areas since it may identify even very low amounts of active genes.

5.3.2 MicroRNAs

MicroRNAs, which were first identified in 1993, are a class of RNA rather than a technique. Small, single-stranded RNA molecules called microRNAs, sometimes known as miRNAs, have a length of 19 to 25 nucleotides and attach to certain regions of bigger RNA molecules to stop them from synthesising proteins. MicroRNAs interfere with gene expression in this manner. Quantitative real-time, reverse-transcription polymerase chain reaction (PCR) is used in several microRNA testing [41].

5.4 Techniques for protein detection

Instead of the DNA that encodes them, proteins may be directly detected by molecular diagnostics. Immunohistochemistry is one of the most widely utilised strategies for protein detection. This procedure uses antibodies, a mechanism our immune systems use to get rid of foreign proteins from the body. In immunohistochemistry, a sample in which a target protein is to be identified is combined with antibodies that bind to the target protein. The antibodies are already marked with a marker of some kind, often a fluorescent one visible under a fluorescence microscope. In a test tube, the sample is combined with the antibodies, and they are given time to bind. Once removed, the sample is washed. The antibodies will bind to the protein of interest if it is present in the sample, which will result in a visible coloured label that can be viewed under a microscope. Antibodies not bound will wash away. Both qualitative and quantitative immunohistochemistry is possible. Oestrogen receptors are often found using immunohistochemistry [42, 43].

6. Other techniques in molecular diagnosis

6.1 Next-generation sequencing

NGS, technologies, and advances in sequencing technology are relatively affordable clinical testing platforms. These platforms enable multiple gene targets anywhere between a few and several hundred nanograms of DNA. Cost, projected test volume, intended genomic target breadth, and required sensitivity will all be taken into consideration when deciding which NGS platform to use. The depth of sequencing that is necessary depends on the latter variable. The price increases as the number of targets increases (e.g., entire genome > whole exome > tailored exome) [44].

Through operating additional instances concurrently (batching), it is possible to reduce the cost of reagents like chips for library preparation and flow cells for sequencing. Batching is made simpler by labelling individual samples with molecular barcodes to enable sample deconvolution during bioinformatic processing. The sorts of modifications that may be identified depend on the platform that is used. Hybrid capture sequencing is the favoured method when breadth is required (whole exome, whole genome, focused panels), while amplicon sequencing is recommended for targeted panels that are optimised for read depth and test sensitivity. Hybrid capture sequencing is often used for this purpose, particularly when more comprehensive copy change information is sought. Furthermore, when translocation detection is required, the hybrid capture strategy should be used since DNA-based rearrangement detection necessitates the assay's ability to capture significant amounts of intronic sequence, which is where breakpoints are most often found. For the detection of translocations, hybrid capture sequencing is sensitive and specific when the breakpoints and partner genes for a given target are known with confidence. For specimens with a low tumour concentration in comparison to the typical contaminating stromal cells, the sensitivity of this method can occasionally be constrained. The ability of algorithms to distinguish between reads with poor mapping that indicate rearrangement and reads with poor sequencing quality determines their sensitivity, specificity, and, ultimately the dependability of the sequencing-based approach to rearrangement detection. False negative and positive findings may also occur with copy number calls, which are determined by comparing the read depth at a specific locus in the sample to a known diploid normal sample. The former happens when there is little tumour present, whereas the later might happen if there has been significant DNA degradation. Given these restrictions, parallel techniques like FISH should be accessible to validate or disprove unexpected or subpar results, or to be used in specimens with tumour content too low to reliably produce a translocation or copy number result by sequencing. When accessible, IHC for protein overexpression may also aid in validating the importance of new rearrangement breakpoints or partners. For translocation identification, laboratories may also think about using RNA-based sequencing techniques. The substantial technological advancements, such as the development of anchored multiplex PCR, it is now possible to identify fusion sequences from the short RNA fragments seen in formalin-fixed tissues.

The read "pileups" may be immediately visualised, and unusual occurrences can be readily noticed using any of the several publicly accessible genomes viewing tools (Integrated Genome Viewer; Genome Viewer, both from the Broad Institute, Cambridge, MA, USA). The potential of misinterpreting extremely low-level mutational events as clinically relevant when they may really be technical artefacts is evident when the data may be visualised. To optimise the assay sensitivity and specificity within the constraints of the specific sequencing technology, bioinformatics workflows should be used to create automated calls. Laboratories should use care while manually reviewing NGS data and refrain from enthusiastically endorsing low-level readings that are below the limit of assay detection established during validation [45].

6.2 Liquid biopsy

The term "liquid biopsy" describes the process of identifying tumour components in body fluids. These components might be tumour DNA or living cells (circulating tumour cells, or ctDNA), cerebrospinal fluid, blood, saliva, and urine specimens are among the fluids that may include these components. In contrast to invasive tissue biopsies, cell-free circulating tumour DNA (ctDNA) may serve as a non-invasive cancer biomarker. To identify ctDNA from tumours, translational cancer researchers are examining the use of liquid biopsies. In the future, ctDNA could be used as a non-invasive method for selecting therapeutic candidates and real-time monitoring of treatment response. All people have measurable levels of cfDNA in their plasma, which is a by-product of normal cell death, which releases DNA fragments with a nucleosome-bound length of around 160 base pairs into the bloodstream. Additionally, tumour cells discharge their contents into the bloodstream, and the quantity of ctDNA that can be detected varies according to the severity of the illness. Most presently accessible technologies often fail to identify ctDNA in patients with early illness. In general, lung cancer-related ctDNA release may be seen at concentrations between 0.1% and 5% of total cfDNA. Therefore, to identify tumour-specific abnormalities in the plasma in most patients, extremely sensitive approaches are required. The ctDNA analysis focused on EGFR mutations and T790M mutations that confer TKI resistance [46]. Activating hotspot mutations and the T790M mutation that causes TKI resistance have received the most attention in published methodologies for ctDNA analysis in lung cancer. Techniques including real-time PCR, ddPCR, and NGS are often used. The patients who tested negative for these mutations in the plasma undertook routine biopsies and repeat testing on the tumour tissue. Detecting EGFR mutations in plasma similarly predicts how patients will react to EGFR TKIs as detecting mutations in tissue.

An unfavourable outcome is linked to the inability to eradicate the EGFR mutation in the blood after 8 weeks of combination platinum-based therapy and erlotinib treatment. Third-generation inhibitors can detect changes in the plasma levels of the T790M mutation in the relapse situation, and these changes often reflect the clinical state as determined by conventional radiographic staging. There have been cases when the plasma levels of T790M drop, yet the patient continues to advance radiographically. This might be an indication of the diversity of resistance mechanisms. Given that plasma-based testing is less sensitive than tissue-based testing, plasma genotyping assays should be designed to have the highest possible positive predictive value. This strategy will lessen the possibility of false positive outcomes, which might erode confidence in a finding and impair a clinician's ability to choose a course of treatment. However, if a plasma assay is negative, tissue biopsy or further plasma testing should be done to learn more about the tumour's genotype [47]. When performed on plasma samples, single gene tests are effective because they may quickly and confidently provide answers to clinical issues in a group with a high pre-test probability. Numerous interesting academic and commercial assays have been produced because of efforts to create NGS-based methods from plasma. To maximise test sensitivity and clinical actionability, these assays are often designed to maximise depth rather than breadth of sequencing. Improvements to NGS design for use in plasma specimens, focused bait design, adjustments to the library preparation chemistry, sequencing to thousands-fold depth of coverage, and molecular barcoding to identify and suppress PCR mistakes have all been proposed. Given the right setup, translocations and copy number changes may also be found in plasma [47, 48].

7. Validation on molecular diagnosis

This real-world instance highlights a significant flaw in molecular diagnostics: their inconsistency. The PSA test, which analyses PSA blood levels, is non-specific and often results in overdiagnosis and over-treatment [49].

7.1 Validity of analysis

For molecular diagnostics to be effective, it must have both analytical and clinical validity. Analytical validity is the main topic of this part, whereas clinical validity is covered in the next section. A test's analytical validity relates to how effectively it captures the intended outcome. For instance, a test intended to find a mutation linked to melanoma should not provide a positive result for a completely unrelated mutation linked to diabetes.

7.2 Specificity

Specificity and sensitivity are two independent but related features of validity that excellent tests must demonstrate. These ideas may be used for both the clinical validity of the biomarker and the analytical validity of the molecular diagnostic test. Let us start with specificity. The test's specificity determines how well it can recognise people without the biomarker or disease. In other words, a particular test only returns a positive result when the biomarker or disease is present. Referring to our PSA example, 80% of men with positive PSA results do not have prostate cancer. This is since elevated PSA levels are not just related to prostate cancer; they are also linked to benign prostatic hypertrophy, or prostate enlargement, which is a rather common medical issue in older men. As a result, one of the issues with the PSA test as a tool for prostate cancer screening is that it lacks specificity. Analytical validity is a need for specificity. A specimen in which the true biomarker does not exist may test positive for an imperfectly repeatable or erroneous test. It also relies on the context of usage. It may have to do with the distinction between cancer and other diseases, between tumours, etc. The difficulty with a lack of specificity is that it may lead to emotional distress and force patients to seek risky follow-up tests and therapies. For instance, Men may get a needle biopsy if their PSA levels are high and/or they have abnormal results on a digital rectal exam. Such biopsies may be financially burdensome and might lead to worry and anxiety. Although prostate needle biopsies are generally safe, they may also lead to incontinence and erectile dysfunction in 1% of patients and serious bleeding or infections of the prostate gland or urinary system. Considering the dangers and downsides associated with these tests, it is important to limit the number of patients who undergo them needlessly, as is the case with any medical procedures. It is important to note that among men who have previously received a diagnosis for prostate cancer, the PSA test is still utilised to monitor recurrence. This demonstrates a crucial issue regarding molecular diagnostics: they may have several clinical applications, and the therapeutic value of those uses may change [50].

7.3 Sensitivity

One may think of sensitivity as specificity's antithesis. Sensitivity is the test's capacity to accurately identify patients who have the biomarker or disease; in other words, it should accurately identify everyone who has the biomarker or ailment. If the test is sensitive, you may reasonably expect to have a positive result if you have the biomarker or illness.

8. Positive and negative aspects

The outcomes of molecular diagnostics, like any testing, may be categorised as right or erroneous. A test is considered to have produced a genuine positive result when it accurately identifies a person as having a certain biomarker or disease.

A test is considered to have produced a genuine negative result when it accurately ascertains that a subject does not possess a certain biomarker or disease. We always want the test findings to be accurate or truthful; thus, this is the perfect scenario. The findings are considered false when a test yields inaccurate results. False positive results occur when a test declares someone to have a biomarker or ailment when they do not.

Tests that are reliable and effective have high rates of true positives and true negatives and low percentages of false positives and false negatives. In a perfect world, the test would not only show who has the biomarker or disease but would also show who does not have the biomarker or condition. Very few molecular diagnostics in practice come close to achieving this objective. The phrases positive and negative predictive values (PPV and NPV) are often used in molecular diagnostic testing. A highly specific test will have a high positive predictive value, meaning that if it comes back positive in a patient, it is almost certain that the patient has the ailment. In other words, if a patient's test results are negative, it is exceedingly improbable that the patient really has the ailment. A highly sensitive test will have a high negative predictive value. No exam, however, is flawless. It may be preferable to have a larger positive predictive value or negative predictive value depending on the situation.

Three factors determine the predictive values, both positive and negative:

- The condition's frequency in the general population
- The test's level of sensitivity
- The test's granularity

If the prevalence in the case were far greater, let us say 50%, happening in half of the 100,000 persons, we would have spotted 45,000 real positives but still had 10,000 false positives. The positive predictive value would have been 82% in this instance as 45,000 of the 55,000 positives were genuine positives. The significance of the usage context and analytical validity for a particular molecular diagnostic is brought out by these factors.

8.1 Reliable testing

Test reliability is an additional component of analytical validity. The capacity to repeat test findings is referred to as test reliability. If a molecular diagnostic is done on Monday and shows that a tumour is positive for a certain gene, it ought to show the same thing on Tuesday. Unreliable tests are obviously useless for determining diagnoses or appropriate treatments. HER2 Molecular Diagnostics Reliability There is a problem with the tests that are used to find HER2 overexpression in breast cancer. A gene called HER2/neu is overexpressed in around one-fourth of breast tumours, as was previously explained. A surplus of HER2 protein is produced by cells because of this overexpression. Because the HER2 protein is important in cell growth and replication, cells with excess HER2 experience an excess of signals directing them to proliferate and divide. Trastuzumab is a drug that prevents the HER2 protein from functioning. However, this drug can only be used to treat malignancies that have HER2/neu overexpression, which can only be identified with a test (a companion diagnostic). For this aim, two separate test types are available: one based on immunohistochemistry and the other based on FISH. Even though many women get trustworthy and accurate findings from these tests, according to the American Society for Clinical Oncology (ASCO) and College of American Pathologists (CAP) recommendations, 20% of HER2 testing performed today may be false. These diagnostics may reveal overexpression of HER2/neu in certain tumours that first test negative and vice versa. These dependability issues are significant since the tests are used to guide therapy. A woman may not get the therapy she needs if a test result is falsely negative (i.e. if a tumour overexpresses HER2/neu, but the test results are negative). In contrast, a woman may get a therapy that is less likely to be helpful to her if a test result is false positive (that is, if the tumour does not overexpress HER2/neu but the test yields a positive result). Lack of standardisation in molecular diagnostics is one factor contributing to the sometimes-inaccurate nature of the tests for HER2/neu overexpression. In a perfect world, molecular diagnostics would be standardised, which would imply that every time they were done, they would be done in the same manner, on the same machinery, with the same chemicals. This is often not the case, however. Reliability may be challenging to get in molecular diagnostics since many of them need exact measurements, complex machinery, and/or various chemical mixes. The methods used to collect, prepare for analysis and keep tissue samples, or so-called pre-analytic variables, may all affect how consistently findings from a molecular diagnostic are obtained. The molecular makeup and consistency of the tissue may be significantly changed by these variables. Therefore, the collection, processing, and storage methods used for a tissue sample that is assessed using the same molecular diagnostic might affect the outcomes. This may be seen, for instance, in the difference between tissue samples that are fixed with formalin and embedded in paraffin and those that are frozen. Scientific investigations using molecular diagnostics may vary depending on pre-analytical conditions as well. Although standardisation of the pre-analytic parameters is preferred, it is still crucial that they be consistently reported. On Biospecimen Reporting for Improved Study Quality (BRISQ), experts released guidelines in 2011. When using human biospecimens, it is required to provide some pre-analytical information that is utilised to assess, interpret, compare, and repeat the findings of the experiment. These recommendations define these pre-analytical data.

ASCO-CAP advises labs to follow stringent tissue sample handling practises, among other things, to counteract the unreliability of molecular diagnoses. According to these standards, new HER-2 tests should also demonstrate 95% agreement with an existing HER-2 reference test that has been clinically validated (i.e., the reference test forecasts clinical outcome). Along with proficiency testing and competence evaluations, strict laboratory accreditation criteria are advised. It is crucial to standardise procedures so that findings from various patients and labs can be compared and so that anybody undergoing pathology testing may be sure that their results are correct. A test sample with a specific, known quantity of the biomarker being identified may sometimes be included in the kits of tests offered by the manufacturer. After that, the test may be calibrated using this standard. An internal standard, such as 100 micrograms of a protein, could be included in a test kit, as an example. They should also discover that the reference sample has 100 micrograms when they run it via other labs. By doing this, labs may confirm that their test produces accurate findings and that its results are like those of other laboratories. By mandating proficiency testing for labs, it may be possible to standardise laboratory tests. For instance, blood samples may be submitted to involved labs for the analysis of the relevant drug. The capacity of each participating laboratory to provide reliable findings determines whether it will get certification, which is determined by the evaluation of all the participating labs' results at a single location. Some businesses have developed molecular diagnostics that need to send test samples to the business's own laboratory to solve the dependability issue. In this situation, the test may be conducted in the same manner each time, and the business has control over the accuracy of the findings. This is true for the test Oncotype® DX, which aids in determining the probability of benefit from further (adjuvant) treatment and the recurrence of breast cancer. Healthcare experts collect breast tumour samples for this test, which are then sent to the company's laboratory for examination. Clinical Validity The term "clinical validity" describes a test's capacity to provide data that is clinically relevant. The biomarker's tight relationship to a clinically significant outcome, such as a patient's reaction to treatment or the cancer's aggressiveness, is what determines the biomarker's clinical validity. According to our earlier illustration, the PSA test's lack of clinical validity—that is, the fact that regular PSA testing does not lengthen a man's life—is one reason it is ineffective as a prostate cancer screening tool. Clinical usefulness, which is discussed in greater detail in the section after this one, is connected to the idea of clinical validity. According to some experts, clinical utility is the capacity of a test to offer information that is clinically relevant—the same definition as clinical validity. Other specialists, on the other hand, think that clinical utility is a more comprehensive idea that includes a usefulness in the clinic's practical aspects. Clinical validity is seen by many experts, including a committee of the Institute of Medicine, as a measurement of whether the test accurately separates one population into two or more with various biological or clinical features or outcomes. Even though the difference is statistically significant, if it is not significant enough to warrant treating the two groups differently ot if understanding the difference is not linked to a therapeutic option for one group but not the other that enhances clinical outcomes, it is not clinically useful. It is noteworthy that several tests or assays may exist for a particular biomarker. They might vary in their therapeutic utility and analytical and clinical validity. Prior to being suggested to guide treatment in a particular use context, as indicated above, for patient care, each must be evaluated independently.

9. Conclusion

In conclusion, there has been a paradigm change in cancer diagnosis. Cancer is no longer simply identified based on morphological factors. Molecular changes at the DNA, mRNA, miRNA, and proteome levels and immunohistochemistry changes are increasingly supporting the diagnostic criteria. Advanced technology with high throughput and several platforms makes it possible to analyse all these as well as the whole genome more quickly and affordably. Precision medicine based on pharmacogenomics is being developed because of this, which is having a big influence on how medicine is now practised. It is now understood that a tumour may not be identified by a single gene modification but rather by a panel of genomic abnormalities that are "signature," allowing for focused treatment approaches and monitoring based on the tumour-specific alterations. The aim of cancer diagnosis in personalised medicine is to establish the proper prognosis and direct the course of treatment so that every patient receives precision medicine, which is the appropriate medication at the right dosage.

Author details

Ajaykumar Chittipolu[1], Akbar Pasha[2] and Doneti Ravinder[2]*

1 Department of Medicinal Chemistry, Vision College of Pharmaceutical Sciences and Research, Bodduppal, Hyderabad, India

2 Department of Genetics, Osmania University, Hyderabad, Telangana, India

*Address all correspondence to: ravi4bios@gmail.com

References

[1] Zhao K, Hu Y. Microbiome harbored within tumors: A new chance to revisit our understanding of cancer pathogenesis and treatment. Signal Transduction and Targeted Therapy. 2020;**5**(1):136

[2] Ng KL, Rajandram R, Morais C, Yap NY, Samaratunga H, Gobe GC, et al. Differentiation of oncocytoma from chromophobe renal cell carcinoma (RCC): Can novel molecular biomarkers help solve an old problem? Journal of Clinical Pathology. 2014;**67**(2):97-104

[3] Khwaja A, Bjorkholm M, Gale RE, Levine RL, Jordan CT, Ehninger G, et al. Acute myeloid leukaemia. Nature Reviews Disease Primers. 2016;**2**(1):1-22

[4] Knight TE, Edwards H, Meshinchi S, Taub JW, Ge Y. "FLipping" the story: FLT3-mutated acute myeloid Leukemia and the evolving role of FLT3 inhibitors. Cancers. 2022;**14**(14):3398

[5] Salvo EM, Ramirez AO, Cueto J, Law EH, Situ A, Cameron C, et al. Risk of recurrence among patients with HR-positive, HER2-negative, early breast cancer receiving adjuvant endocrine therapy: A systematic review and meta-analysis. The Breast. 2021;**57**:5-17

[6] Relling MV, Evans WE. Pharmacogenomics in the clinic. Nature. 2015;**526**(7573):343-350

[7] Fatunde OA, Brown SA. The role of CYP450 drug metabolism in precision cardio-oncology. International Journal of Molecular Sciences. 2020;**21**(2):604

[8] Wen H, Jung H, Li X. Drug delivery approaches in addressing clinical pharmacology-related issues: Opportunities and challenges. The AAPS journal. 2015;**17**:1327-1340

[9] Poudel G, Tolland MG, Hughes TP, Pagani IS. Mechanisms of resistance and implications for treatment strategies in chronic myeloid leukaemia. Cancers. 2022;**14**(14):3300

[10] Thapa R, Wilson GD. The importance of CD44 as a stem cell biomarker and therapeutic target in cancer. Stem Cells International. 2016;**2016**:15, Article ID 2087204

[11] Heard E, Martienssen RA. Transgenerational epigenetic inheritance: Myths and mechanisms. Cell. 2014;**157**(1):95-109

[12] Mattick J, Amaral P. RNA, the Epicenter of Genetic Information. 1st ed. CRC Press; 2022

[13] Røsland GV, Engelsen AS. Novel points of attack for targeted cancer therapy. Basic & Clinical Pharmacology & Toxicology. 2015;**116**(1):9-18

[14] Roskoski R Jr. Anaplastic lymphoma kinase (ALK) inhibitors in the treatment of ALK-driven lung cancers. Pharmacological Research. 2017;**117**:343-356

[15] Harbers L, Agostini F, Nicos M, Poddighe D, Bienko M, Crosetto N. Somatic copy number alterations in human cancers: An analysis of publicly available data from the cancer genome atlas. Frontiers in Oncology. 2021;**11**:700568

[16] Johnson KB, Wei WQ, Weeraratne D, Frisse ME, Misulis K, Rhee K, et al. Precision Medicine, AI, and the Future of Personalized Health Care. Clinical

and Translational Science. 2021 Jan;**14**(1):86-93

[17] Anzalone AV, Gao XD, Podracky CJ, Nelson AT, Koblan LW, Raguram A, et al. Programmable deletion, replacement, integration and inversion of large DNA sequences with twin prime editing. Nature Biotechnology. 2022;**40**(5):731-740

[18] Al-Shaheri FN, Alhamdani MS, Bauer AS, Giese N, Büchler MW, Hackert T, et al. Blood biomarkers for differential diagnosis and early detection of pancreatic cancer. Cancer Treatment Reviews. 2021;**96**:102193

[19] Linhares P, Carvalho B, Vaz R, Costa BM. Glioblastoma: Is there any blood biomarker with true clinical relevance? International Journal of Molecular Sciences. 2020;**21**(16):5809

[20] Manzoni C, Kia DA, Vandrovcova J, Hardy J, Wood NW, Lewis PA, et al. Genome, transcriptome and proteome: The rise of omics data and their integration in biomedical sciences. Briefings in Bioinformatics. 2018;**19**(2):286-302

[21] Ow TJ, Sandulache VC, Skinner HD, Myers JN. Integration of cancer genomics with treatment selection: From the genome to predictive biomarkers. Cancer. 2013;**119**(22):3914-3928

[22] Ghose A, Gullapalli SV, Chohan N, Bolina A, Moschetta M, Rassy E, et al. Applications of proteomics in ovarian cancer: Dawn of a new era. Proteomes. 2022;**10**(2):16

[23] Rasooly A, Jacobson J. Development of biosensors for cancer clinical testing. Biosensors and Bioelectronics. 2006;**21**(10):1851-1858

[24] Dwivedi S, Purohit P, Misra R, Pareek P, Goel A, Khattri S, et al. Diseases and molecular diagnostics: A step closer to precision medicine. Indian Journal of Clinical Biochemistry. 2017;**32**:374-398

[25] Zhang L, Guo H. Biomarkers of COVID-19 and technologies to combat SARS-CoV-2. Advances in Biomarker Sciences and Technology. 2020;**2**:1-23

[26] Wang X, Ha D, Yoshitake R, Chan YS, Sadava D, Chen S. Exploring the biological activity and mechanism of xenoestrogens and phytoestrogens in cancers: Emerging methods and concepts. International Journal of Molecular Sciences. 2021;**22**(16):8798

[27] Mengel M, Loupy A, Haas M, Roufosse C, Naesens M, Akalin E, et al. Banff 2019 meeting report: Molecular diagnostics in solid organ transplantation–consensus for the Banff human organ transplant (B-HOT) gene panel and open source multicenter validation. American Journal of Transplantation. 2020;**20**(9):2305-2317

[28] Eren K, Taktakoğlu N, Pirim I. DNA Sequencing Methods: From Past to Present. Eurasian J Med. 2022 Dec;**54**(Suppl1):47-56. DOI: 10.5152/eurasianjmed.2022.22280. PMID: 36655445.

[29] Gupta N, Verma VK. Next-generation sequencing and its application: Empowering in public health beyond reality. Microbial Technology for the Welfare of Society. Sep 13 2019;**17**:313-341

[30] Köbel M, Kang EY. The evolution of ovarian carcinoma subclassification. Cancers (Basel). Jan 14 2022;**14**(2):416

[31] Lopez A, Liu J. Covalent and noncovalent functionalization of graphene oxide with DNA for smart

sensing. Advanced Intelligent Systems. 2020;**2**(11):2000123

[32] Turner MB, Cizmic JM, Rosansky DB, Ceja J, Patterson M, Kilcoyne S, Thurber K, Kim G, Dwyer TJ, Purse BW. Sequence-Specific Fluorescence Turn-On Sensing of RNA by DNA Probes Incorporating the Tricyclic Cytidine Analogue DEAtC. Bioconjugate Chemistry. 2023 Jun 21;**34**(6):1061-1071

[33] Jonczyk R, Kurth T, Lavrentieva A, Walter JG, Scheper T, Stahl F. Living cell microarrays: An overview of concepts. Microarrays. 2016;**5**(2):11

[34] Mosolygó T, Laczi K, Spengler G, Burián K. A practical approach for quantitative polymerase chain reaction, the gold standard in microbiological diagnosis. Sci. 2022;**4**(1):4

[35] Zou S, He HJ, Zong Y, Shi L, Wang L. DNA Microarrays: Applications, Future Trends, and the Need for Standardization. Springer Series on Fluorescence. Vol. 6. Berlin, Heidelberg: Springer; 2008. DOI: 10.1007/4243_2008_036

[36] Zizak Z, Klaus A, Kozarski M, Vunduk J, Niksic M, Juranic Z. 137: Antitumor activities of some macrofungi extracts. European Journal of Cancer. 2014;**50**:S30-S31

[37] Shakoori AR. Fluorescence in situ hybridization (FISH) and its applications. Chromosome Structure and Aberrations. 2017:343-367

[38] Montazerinezhad S, Emamjomeh A, Hajieghrari B. Chromosomal abnormality, laboratory techniques, tools and databases in molecular cytogenetics. Molecular Biology Reports. 2020;**47**:9055-9073

[39] Hoose A, Vellacott R, Storch M, Freemont PS, Ryadnov MG. DNA synthesis technologies to close the gene writing gap. Nature Reviews Chemistry. 2023;**7**(3):144-161

[40] O'Donnell M, Langston L, Stillman B. Principles and concepts of DNA replication in bacteria, archaea, and eukarya. Cold Spring Harbor perspectives in biology. 2013;**5**(7):a010108

[41] Kuo MC, Liu SC, Hsu YF, Wu RM. The role of noncoding RNAs in Parkinson's disease: Biomarkers and associations with pathogenic pathways. Journal of Biomedical Science. 2021;**28**(1):1-28

[42] Karagoz A, Tombuloglu H, Alsaeed M, Tombuloglu G, AlRubaish AA, Mahmoud A, Smajlović S, Ćordić S, Rabaan AA, Alsuhaimi E. Monkeypox (mpox) virus: Classification, origin, transmission, genome organization, antiviral drugs, and molecular diagnosis. Journal of Infection and Public Health. Feb 9 2023;**16**(4):531-541. ISSN 1876-0341

[43] Labib M, Kelley SO. Single-cell analysis targeting the proteome. Nature Reviews Chemistry. 2020;**4**(3):143-158

[44] Safiabadi Tali SH, LeBlanc JJ, Sadiq Z, Oyewunmi OD, Camargo C, Nikpour B, et al. Tools and techniques for severe acute respiratory syndrome coronavirus 2 (SARS-CoV-2)/COVID-19 detection. Clinical Microbiology Reviews. 2021;**34**(3):e00228-e00220

[45] Bates MF, Sorensen MJ. Genetic testing for adrenal Tumors—What the contemporary surgeon should know. Surgical Oncology Clinics. 2023;**32**(2):303-313

[46] Leung E, Han K, Zou J, Zhao Z, Zheng Y, Wang TT, et al. HPV sequencing facilitates ultrasensitive detection of HPV circulating tumor DNA. Clinical Cancer Research. 2021;**27**(21):5857-5868

[47] Bulbul A, Leal A, Husain H. Applications of cell-free circulating tumor DNA detection in EGFR mutant lung cancer. Journal of thoracic disease. 2020;**12**(5):2877

[48] Ku BM, Kim YJ, Park D, Lee SH, Ahn JS, Park K, et al. Role of circulating tumor DNA profiling in patients with non-small cell lung cancer treated with EGFR inhibitor. Oncology. 2022;**100**(4):228-237

[49] Ilic D, Djulbegovic M, Jung JH, Hwang EC, Zhou Q, Cleves A, et al. Prostate cancer screening with prostate-specific antigen (PSA) test: A systematic review and meta-analysis. BMJ. 2018;**362**

[50] Hanin A, Cespedes J, Pulluru Y, Gopaul M, Aronica E, Decampo D, Helbig I, Howe CL, Huttner A, Koh S, Navarro V. Review and standard operating procedures for collection of biospecimens and analysis of biomarkers in new onset refractory status epilepticus. Epilepsia. Apr 11 2023;**64**(6):1444-1457

Section 2

Oncogenes and Oncosuppressor Genes

Chapter 3

RET Proto-Oncogene

Masahide Takahashi

Abstract

The rearranged during transfection (*RET*) proto-oncogene encodes a transmembrane receptor tyrosine kinase and its alterations cause various cancers and developmental disorders. Gain-of-function mutations caused by gene rearrangements have been found in papillary thyroid carcinoma, non-small-cell lung carcinoma, and other cancers, while point mutations are responsible for hereditary cancer syndrome, multiple endocrine neoplasia type 2, and sporadic medullary thyroid carcinoma. Loss-of-function point mutations or deletions lead to Hirschsprung disease, a developmental disorder associated with aganglionosis of the intestinal tract. RET is also involved in various physiological and developmental functions through activation by glial cell line-derived neurotrophic factor (GDNF) family ligands (GFLs). Gene knockout studies have revealed that GDNF-RET signaling plays an essential role in the development of the enteric nervous system, kidney, and urinary tract, as well as in the self-renewal of spermatogonial stem cells. Moreover, recent progress in developing RET-selective inhibitors has significantly contributed to treating patients with *RET*-altered cancers. This chapter describes and discusses the functions associated with disease and physiology.

Keywords: *RET* proto-oncogene, glial cell line-derived neurotrophic factor, thyroid cancer, non-small-cell lung cancer, Hirschsprung's disease

1. Introduction

The rearranged during transfection (*RET*) oncogene was identified as a new transforming gene by the transfection of NIH3T3 cells with human lymphoma DNA in 1985 [1]. The transforming gene was generated by recombining two unlinked human DNA sequences that most likely occurred during transfection. Hence, the term *RET* stems for "*RE*arranged during *T*ransfection." The active *RET* transforming gene encodes a fusion protein comprising a carboxy-terminal tyrosine kinase domain and an amino-terminal dimerizing domain, fused by rearrangement [2]. The dimerizing domain is necessary for tyrosine kinase activation. Subsequently, the name *RET* was retained to designate the carboxy-terminal of the gene as a tyrosine kinase domain (*RET* proto-oncogene).

Alterations in the *RET* proto-oncogene have been found in various human cancers and developmental disorders, including thyroid cancer, non-small cell lung cancer, multiple endocrine neoplasia type 2 (MEN2), and Hirschsprung disease (HSCR) [3]. In addition, next-generation DNA and RNA sequencing approaches have identified less frequent *RET* rearrangements and mutations in various cancers, including colon and breast cancers. The mechanisms by which these mutations lead to RET activation or inactivation have been extensively studied [4, 5]. Ongoing clinical trials on RET-selective inhibitors have demonstrated remarkable efficacy and continue to improve the outcomes of patients with *RET* alterations without increased toxicity [6].

2. Structure and expression of *RET* proto-oncogene

The *RET* proto-oncogene encodes a receptor tyrosine kinase with a unique extracellular domain that consists of four cadherin-like domains and a cysteine-rich region with 16 cysteine residues in a stretch of 120 amino acids (**Figure 1**) [3, 7–9]. Alternative 3′ splicing produces three different isoforms (1072, 1106, and 1114 amino acids) with short (9 amino acids, referred to as RET9), intermediate (43 amino acids, RET43), and long (51 amino acids, RET51) carboxy-terminal tails. RET9 and RET51 are two major isoforms highly conserved among various species [4, 5]. The human *RET* proto-oncogene is located on chromosome 10q11.2 and comprises 21 exons.

RET expression is observed in the developing excretory and nervous systems during the embryogenesis of mice and rats [10, 11]. It is highly expressed in the nephric duct, ureteric bud, and collecting ducts of developing kidneys. RET is also expressed in enteric neural crest-derived cells, the autonomic and dorsal root ganglia of the peripheral nervous system, the neuroepithelial cells of the ventral neural tube, and several cranial ganglia in the central nervous system. In agreement with this expression

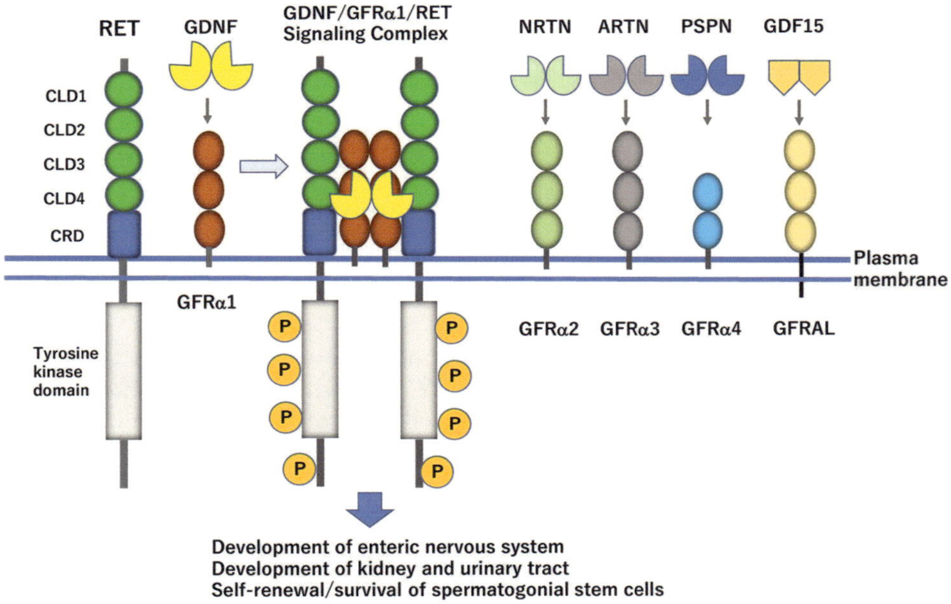

Figure 1.
RET activation by GDNF family ligands (GFLs). GDNF, NRTN, ARTN, and PSPN preferentially bind to GFRα1, GFRα2, GFRα3, and GFRα4, respectively, and activate RET. GDNF/GFRα1/RET signaling complex is essential for developing the enteric nervous system, kidney, and urinary tract and for self-renewal/survival of spermatogonial stem cells. GDF15 is a stress response cytokine. GDF15 binds to GFRAL and activates RET, as observed for GFLs. GDNF, glial cell line-derived neurotrophic factor; NRTN, neurturin; ARTN, artemin; PSPN, persephin; GDF15, growth differentiation factor-15; GFRAL, GDNF family receptor α-like; CLD, cadherin-like domain; CRD, cysteine-rich domain.

pattern, *Ret*-deficient mice exhibit a lack of enteric neurons in the entire gastrointestinal tract and kidney agenesis or severe dysgenesis, elucidating the pivotal roles of RET in development [3]. After birth, various peripheral and central nervous system neurons continue to express RET, whereas their expression disappears in adult kidneys.

3. Activation of RET by glial cell line-derived neurotrophic factor (GDNF)-family ligands

In 1993, GDNF was purified and cloned as a neurotrophic factor that enhances the survival of midbrain dopaminergic neurons [12]. GDNF has also been shown to be a potent trophic factor for spinal motor and central noradrenergic neurons. Additionally, GDNF is essential for the survival and differentiation of peripheral sympathetic, parasympathetic, sensory, and enteric neurons. GDNF is structurally related to the transforming growth factor (TGF)-β and contains seven cysteine residues called cysteine knot motifs. Furthermore, three other proteins of the GDNF family ligands (GFLs), including neurturin (NRTN), artemin (ARTN), and persephin (PSPN), were identified, sharing approximately 40% amino acid identity with each other and possessing neurotrophic effects on various neurons [3].

Physiologically, RET is activated by GFLs through a unique multicomponent receptor complex consisting of a glycosylphosphatidylinositol-anchored co-receptor (GDNF family receptor α 1–4, GFRα1–4) as a ligand-binding component and RET tyrosine kinase as a signaling component (**Figure 1**). The formation of the GFL-GFRα-RET 2:2:2 ternary complex results in the activation of various intracellular signaling pathways necessary for physiological function [13–15]. GDNF, NRTN, ARTN, and PSPN use GFRα1, GFRα2, GFRα3, and GFRα4, respectively, as their preferred ligand-binding receptors (**Figure 1**), although crosstalk occurs between the ligand and co-receptor pairs to a certain extent [16, 17]. Despite the crosstalk demonstrated *in vitro*, knockout mouse studies have exhibited specific roles for each GFL-GFRα-RET complex. For example, *Gdnf-, Gfrα1-,* and *Ret*-deficient mice share phenotypes characterized by a lack of enteric neurons in the entire gastrointestinal tract, kidney agenesis, and severe dysgenesis [18–20]. Both *Nrtn*- and *Gfrα2*- deficient mice showed a reduced number of myenteric neurons in the intestine and a drastic reduction in cholinergic innervation in the lacrimal and salivary glands, indicating that the preferred GFL-GFRα-RET complex plays specific roles *in vivo* [16].

More recently, another ligand of the TGF-β superfamily, growth differentiation factor 15 (GDF15), has been shown to bind to GFRα-like (GFRAL) and activate RET (**Figure 1**), regulating food intake and body weight [21–24]. GDF15 is a stress-induced hormone, and its plasma levels are markedly increased in various human diseases, including cardiovascular and chronic kidney diseases, diabetes, advanced cancer, and serious infections. Co-expression of GFRAL and RET was detected in neurons of the hindbrain area postrema and the nucleus of the solitary tract, where RET activation by GDF15 plays a pivotal role in body weight control.

4. Activation of RET intracellular signaling pathways by GFLs and their roles in the development

Following RET activation by GFLs, many tyrosine residues in the intracellular region are phosphorylated, activating various signaling pathways. The intracellular region of RET contains 18 tyrosine residues, two of which are in the juxtamembrane domain, 11 in the kinase domain, and five in the C-terminal region. Of the five tyrosine residues in the C-terminus, three (Y1015, Y1029, and Y1062) were common between RET9 and RET51, and two (Y1096 and Y1102) were present only in RET51. Each phosphorylated tyrosine interacts with specific adaptor proteins. For example, phosphorylated Y981, Y1015, Y1062, and Y1096 represent binding sites for SRC, phospholipase Cγ (PLCγ), SHC/FRS2/DOK1–6/IRS1–2, and GRB2, respectively (**Figure 2**). The signal transducer and activator of transcription 3 (STAT3) bind to phosphorylate Y752 and Y928 [3, 17]. As a result, the RAS/mitogen-activated protein kinase and/or phosphatidylinositol-3 kinase pathways were activated through the phosphorylation of Y1062 or Y1096 (**Figure 2**). Activation of the PLCγ pathway through phosphorylated Y1015 regulates protein kinase C activity and Ca^{2+} release from the endoplasmic reticulum, increasing intracellular Ca^{2+} levels and inducing Ca signaling.

The importance of each intracellular signaling pathway has been demonstrated in mouse gene-targeting studies. *Ret* mutant mice in which tyrosine 1062 was replaced with phenylalanine (Y1062F) exhibited severe defects in enteric neurons in the intestinal tract, small kidneys, and a lack of spermatogonial stem cells, indicating a crucial role for Y1062 signaling in development [25–27]. *Ret* Y1015F mutant mice show abnormalities in the kidney and ureter, such as multicystic kidneys and megaureters, but produce only minor abnormalities in the enteric nervous system [28]. The PLCγ

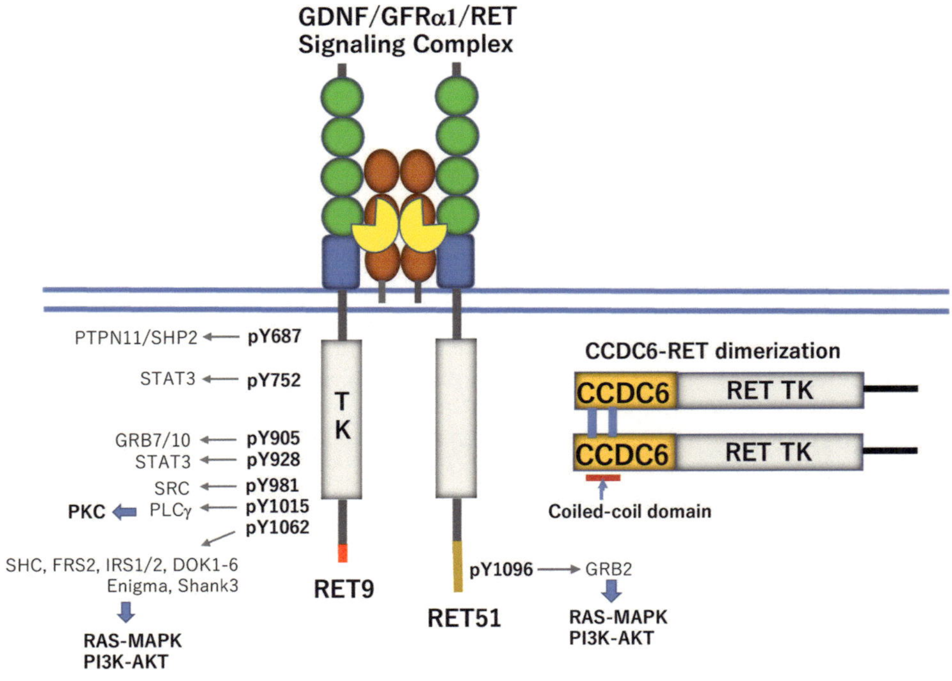

Figure 2.
RET activates intracellular signaling pathways via phosphotyrosines and CCDC6-RET fusion. Phosphorylated tyrosines in RET intracellular domain interact with a wide range of adaptor proteins, activating downstream signaling pathways, including the RAS/MAPK, PI3K-AKT, and PLCγ-PKC pathways. For example, phosphotyrosine 1062 represents a multifunctional docking site for SHC, FRS2, and DOK family proteins. CCDC6-RET fusion identified in human cancers dimerizes via the coiled-coil domain present in the amino terminus of CCDC6.

pathway is critical for upper and lower urinary tract development, and mutations that abrogate this pathway generate features reminiscent of congenital anomalies of the kidneys or urinary tract (CAKUT).

HSCR is a relatively common congenital malformation associated with aganglionosis of the gastrointestinal tract (prevalence: one in 5000 live births). The disease is characterized by the absence of the intramural nervous plexuses, myenteric plexus (Auerbach plexus), and submucosal plexus (Meissner plexus). *RET* is a major causative gene of HSCR in which various mutations, including missense, nonsense, and frameshift mutations or partial/complete deletions, have been detected [29, 30]. *RET* mutations are found in approximately 50% of patients with familial HSCR and 10–20% of sporadic cases. These mutations inactivate and abrogate RET signaling, which is responsible for the migration and proliferation of enteric neural crest-derived cells during embryogenesis. Since HSCR mutations have been identified along the entire coding sequence, various mechanisms that perturb RET intracellular signaling have been demonstrated [3, 31]. For example, most mutations identified in the extracellular domains impair RET cell surface expression, most likely because of protein misfolding. Mutations in the kinase domain result in complete or partial impairment of kinase activity. Some mutations in the C-terminal tail impair intracellular signaling due to decreased binding of adaptor proteins such as SHC.

5. *RET* rearrangement in human cancer

In human cancers, *RET* rearrangement or fusion was first identified in papillary thyroid carcinoma (PTC) at a relatively high frequency (~25%) [32]. Subsequently, an extensive series of studies by the same group, including 177 papillary thyroid carcinomas, 37 follicular carcinomas, 15 anaplastic carcinomas, 18 medullary thyroid carcinomas, and 34 benign adenomas by Southern blot analysis, revealed rearrangements in 19% of papillary thyroid carcinomas, but not in other malignant and benign tumors [33]. However, at a lower frequency, RET rearrangements have been reported in other types of cancers such as follicular, anaplastic, and medullary thyroid carcinomas, as well as in benign thyroid lesions, such as follicular adenoma, at variable frequencies [34]. Somatic rearrangements involve the 3′ sequence of *RET* with a tyrosine kinase domain and the 5′ sequence of partner genes with a dimerizing domain such as the coiled-coil domain. *RET* breakpoints often occur within intron 11 and less frequently within introns 7, 10, and others [3].

Further studies reported that the prevalence of *RET* rearrangements in PTC varies significantly in different geographic regions, ranging from 3% in Saudi Arabia to 85% in Australia [34]; this may be because of racial differences in genetic backgrounds, environmental factors, or variations in screening techniques such as Southern blot analysis, reverse transcription polymerase chain reaction, and *in situ* hybridization. Integrated multi-platform analyses performed using The Cancer Genome Atlas network yielded *RET* rearrangements in 6.8% of PTC samples (33/484 cases) [35]. In addition, it is notable that *BRAF* mutations (prevalence: approximately 60%) and *RET* fusions are largely mutually exclusive in PTCs.

The most prevalent fusion genes were coiled-coil domain containing 6 (*CCDC6*)-*RET* (named *RET/PTC1*) (**Figure 2**) and nuclear receptor coactivator 4 (*NCOA4*)-*RET* (named *RET/PTC3*), which accounted for >90% of all *RET* rearrangement-positive PTCs (**Table 1**) [36]. Since *CCDC6* and *NCOA4* are located on chromosome 10q, as observed for *RET*, both *RET/PTC1* and *RET/PTC3* are created by

Cancer	Prevalence	*RET* fusions
Papillary thyroid carcinoma in general population	5–20%	*CCDC6-RET* *NCOA4-RET*
Papillary thyroid carcinoma after Chernobyl reactor accident	50–80%	*NCOA4-RET* *CCDC6-RET*
Non-small cell lung carcinoma	1–2%	*KIF5B-RET* *CCDC6-RET*
Colon carcinoma	~0.2%	*CCDC6-RET* *NCOA4-RET*
Salivary intraductal carcinoma	~40%	*NCOA4-RET* *TRIM27-RET*

Table 1.
Prevalence of RET fusions in human cancer.

paracentric inversion of this chromosome. Other partner genes, including *PRKAR1A (RET/PTC2)*, *GOLGA5, TRIM24, TRIM27, TRIM33, KTN1, RFG9, ELKS, PCM1,* and *HOOK3,* and *RET* fusions with these genes are created by intrachromosomal translocation. There are at least 19 different 5′ partner genes for *RET* fusion in PTC [34, 37].

The prevalence of *RET* rearrangement is much higher (49–87%) in radiation-induced PTCs following the Chernobyl nuclear accident or the atomic bomb in Japan (**Table 1**). The highest frequency was observed in post-Chernobyl children [34]. Interestingly, in post-Chernobyl PTCs that developed less than 10 years after the accident, *RET/PTC3* was most frequently detected, whereas tumors found after a longer latency preferentially carried *RET/PTC1.* In the case of PTC patients exposed to radiation from the atomic bomb, *RET* fusions occurred at a higher frequency of 50% in patients with high doses (>0.5 Gy) [38]. In patients with thyroid tumors (benign or malignant) who received external therapeutic radiation, the prevalence of *RET/PTC* was reported to be high (52–84%). In contrast, the prevalence of *BRAF* mutations was low in patients with radiation-induced PTCs.

RET rearrangement is also found in a portion (1–2%) of non-small-cell lung carcinomas (NSCLC) (**Table 1**) [39–41]. The most common *RET* fusions in lung cancer are kinesin family member 5B (*KIF5B*)*-RET* (~80%) and *CCDC6-RET* (~15%), followed by fusions such as *NCOA4-RET, TRIM33-RET,* and *CUX1-RET* [36]. *KIF5B* is located on the short arm of chromosome 10, and the pericentric inversion of this chromosome creates the *KIF5B-RET* fusion. Patients with *RET* fusion-positive NSCLCs show unique clinicopathological characteristics: relatively young (<60 years old), female, and nonsmokers.

Next-generation DNA and RNA sequencing technologies have identified less frequent *RET* fusions in various cancers. These include colorectal, breast, ovarian, salivary gland intraductal carcinomas, chronic myelomonocytic leukemia, and spitzoid tumors. Large-scale analyses have revealed that *RET* fusions can be detected in 0.2% of colorectal cancers (6/3117 cases) [42] and 0.1% of breast cancers (8/9693 cases) [43]. The *CCDC6-RET* and *NCOA4-RET* fusion genes were identified in both tumors. Interestingly, a high frequency (>40%) of *RET* fusions, including *NCOA4-RET* and *TRIM27-RET*, was detected in salivary intraductal carcinoma but not in salivary duct carcinoma (**Table 1**) [44]. In addition, new *RET* fusions *ETV6-RET* and *VIM-RET* were identified in 16% (8/49 cases) and 2% (1/49 cases) of secretory carcinomas of the salivary gland [45]. These findings suggest that detecting specific RET fusions helps in diagnosing specific salivary gland carcinomas.

6. *RET* mutations in MEN2 and sporadic cancer

Medullary thyroid carcinoma (MTC) is a malignant tumor of the neural crest-derived parafollicular C cells that produce calcitonin. MTC develops either sporadically (~75% of cases) or as a component of the hereditary cancer syndrome MEN2 (~25% of cases). MEN2 is an autosomal-dominant cancer syndrome characterized by the development of MTC and pheochromocytoma derived from adrenal chromaffin cells. Based on clinical phenotypes, MEN2 is classified into three subtypes: MEN2A, MEN2B, and familial medullary thyroid carcinoma (FMTC). The affected family members by MEN2A develop MTC (~100% of cases), pheochromocytoma (~50% of cases), and parathyroid hyperplasia/adenoma (hyperparathyroidism, ~20% of cases). Lichen amyloidosis is occasionally observed in MEN2A patients. MEN2B is a more aggressive subtype with early onset of MTC (~100%) and pheochromocytoma (~50%). In addition, MEN2B patients display a more complex phenotype, including mucosal neuroma, hyperganglionosis of the intestine, medullated corneal nerve, and marfanoid habitus, but not hyperparathyroidism. FMTC is characterized by MTC, which usually develops later in life and is now considered an indolent subtype of MEN2A.

Germline *RET* mutations are responsible for MEN2 syndrome [46–49]. The majority of *MEN2A* mutations (>95%) have been identified in one of six cysteine residues (codons 609, 611, 618, and 620 in exon 10 and codons 630 and 634 in exon 11) in the cysteine-rich region of the RET extracellular domain (**Figure 3A**). Among them, approximately 85% of *MEN2A* mutations affect codon 634. The same cysteine mutations were also found in FMTC, with a high frequency of ~60% for codon 609, 611, 618, 620, or 630 substitutions

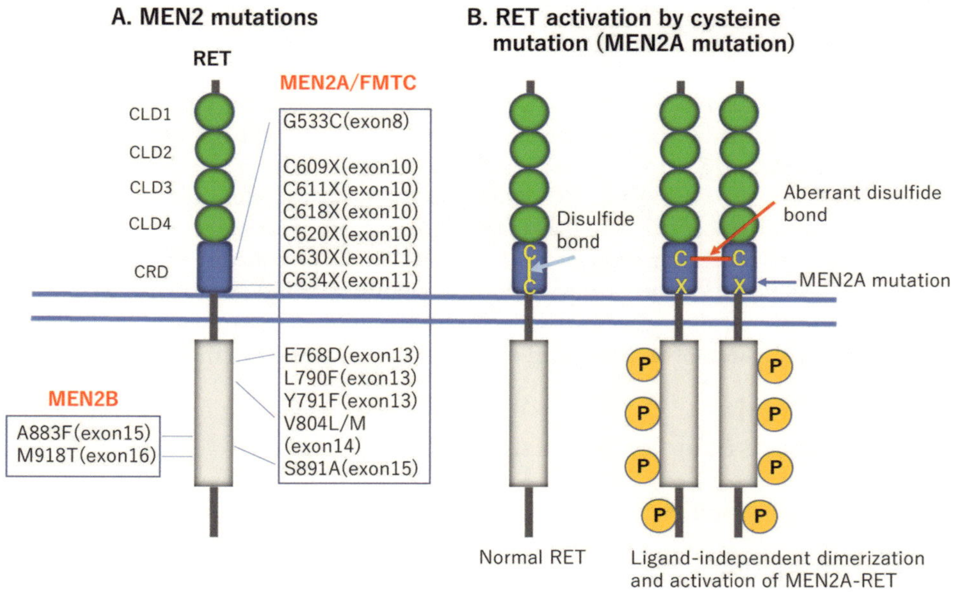

Figure 3.
Germline RET mutations in MEN2. A. the majority of MEN2A mutations (>95%) are identified in one of six cysteine residues (codons 609, 611, 618, and 620 in exon 10 and codons 630 and 634 in exon 11) in the cysteine-rich domain (CRD) of the RET extracellular region. In addition to cysteine substitutions, MEN2A/FMTC mutations are less frequently found at non-cysteine residues in both the extracellular and intracellular regions. The M918 mutation is detected in >95% of MEN2B patients. B. Mechanism of RET activation by cysteine mutations. When a cysteine residue is replaced with another amino acid (designated X) in MEN2A/FMTC, mutant RET proteins form aberrant ligand-independent dimerization, resulting in constitutive activation.

and a low frequency of ~30% for codon 634. In addition, other point mutations, including Gly533Cys (G533C) (exon 8 in the extracellular domain), Glu768Asp (E768D), Leu790Phe (L790F), Tyr791Phe (Y791F), Val804Met/Leu (V804M/L), and Ser891Ala (S891A) substitutions (exons 13–15 in the kinase domain), have been reported in some FMTC and/or MEN2A families (**Figure 3A**) [3, 31]. Moreover, a 9- or 12-base pair duplication in exon 11 and a 9-base pair duplication in exon 8, which creates an additional cysteine residue, have been reported in two MEN2A families and one FMTC family, respectively [5].

We and others have demonstrated that cysteine mutations in MEN2A or FMTC result in ligand-independent constitutive activation (dimerization) of mutant RET by forming aberrant intermolecular disulfide bonds (**Figure 3B**). Cysteine residues are thought to form the intramolecular disulfide bonds necessary for the appropriate tertiary structure of the RET protein. The hypothesis is that when a cysteine residue is replaced with a non-cysteine residue by *MEN2A* mutations, the partner cysteine involved in the disulfide bond becomes free and forms an aberrant intermolecular disulfide bond with mutant RET, leading to constitutive activation (dimerization) (**Figure 3B**) [50, 51].

Two specific missense mutations, Met918Thr (M918T) and Ala883Phe (A883F), were associated with the development of MEN2B (**Figure 3A**). The M918T mutation accounts for more than 95% of MEN2B patients, while fewer than 4% are accounted for by the A883F mutation [3, 31]. In addition, double germline mutations at codons 804 and 806 (V804M and Y806C) were found in a Japanese patient with clinical features characteristic of MEN2B [52]. *MEN2B* mutations identified in the tyrosine kinase domain appear to activate RET in a monomeric form, probably because of a conformational change in the catalytic core of the kinase domain. Some reports have suggested that *MEN2B* mutations alter the substrate specificity of RET [3], although the signaling pathway crucial for developing MEN2B clinical phenotypes remains elusive.

According to data published in a public database in 2015 (COSMIC; Catalog of Somatic Mutations in Cancer), somatic *RET* mutations have been identified at a high frequency (>40%; 667/1662 cases) in sporadic MTC patients. M918T mutations were the most frequent in these patients, and cysteine mutations (C634, C630, C620, C618, and C611) and E768D, A883F, and S891A mutations in the kinase domain have also been observed in sporadic MTC [36, 37]. Oncogenic *RET* mutations have also been detected in 0.5% (8/1489 cases) of colorectal cancer [42] and 0.2% (16/9693 cases) of breast cancers [43]. Moreover, studies using next-generation sequencing have revealed the presence of RET mutations in a variety of cancers at a low frequency, including endometrial and ovarian cancer, hepatoma, skin melanoma, glioblastoma multiforme, meningioma, gastrointestinal stromal tumor, Merkel cell carcinoma, paraganglioma, and atypical lung carcinoid [53].

7. *RET* mutations in molecular diagnostic

RET genetic screening using next-generation sequencing is essential for the diagnosis of patients with MTC. The majority of MEN2 mutations are found in exons 10-11 and exons 13-16 of the *RET* proto-oncogene (**Figure 3**). After diagnosis, annual screening for MTC and pheochromocytoma should be carried out and prophylactic thyroidectomy for preventing metastasized MTC is recommended. The timing of prophylactic thyroidectomy is based on risk stratification of the *RET* mutation proposed by the American Thyroid Association (ATA). The revised ATA guidelines use 'highest risk' (HST), 'high risk' (H), and 'moderate risk' (MOD) that are associated with aggressiveness [54]. The ATA-HST category incudes patients with MEN2B and *RET* M918T mutation, and the ATA-H category includes patients with *RET* C634 mutations and the *RET*

A883F mutation. The ATA-MOD category includes patients with *RET* mutations other than M918T, C634 and A883F. *RET* genetic screening is beneficial for early diagnosis and optimal treatment of patients with both hereditary and sporadic MTC.

8. *RET* overexpression in breast cancer

RET has been reported to be overexpressed in 40–60% of breast tumors across multiple tumor subtypes [55]. In particular, its expression is common in the estrogen receptor (ER)-positive subtype and is associated with larger tumor size, higher stage, and reduced overall survival. Elevated RET expression was also observed in ER-positive breast cancer cell lines, mirroring observations from patient samples. Treatment with estradiol induced the transcription of RET, GFRα, and ARTN, suggesting a regulatory mechanism for RET function. Multiple estrogen response elements have been identified within the *RET* enhancer region, which is approximately ~50 k bp relative to the *RET* transcriptional start site. *In vitro* study revealed that GDNF stimulation in breast cancer cells induces ER phosphorylation and estrogen-independent activation of the ER pathway, resulting in increased tumor cell proliferation and survival. RET-mediated ER phosphorylation involves the mammalian target of the rapamycin signaling pathway and is correlated with resistance to endocrine therapies such as tamoxifen [56, 57]. In addition, RET overexpression was observed in some human epidermal growth factor receptor 2 (HER2)-positive breast cancers. Using patient-derived xenograft models and cell lines, GDNF has been demonstrated to induce crosstalk between RET and HER2 *via* Src kinase, thereby conferring resistance to HER2-targeting therapy [58]. Thus, RET may be a useful target against endocrine- and trastuzumab-resistant breast cancers.

9. Development of selective RET kinase inhibitors for targeted therapy

Various tyrosine kinase inhibitors (MTKIs) have recently been used to treat *RET*-altered cancers. MTKIs include vandetanib, cabozantinib, sorafenib, sunitinib, ponatinib, lenvatinib, alectinib, and RXDX-105. However, MTKIs have demonstrated limited clinical efficacy, as indicated by their lower objective response ratios (ORRs), shorter progression-free survival rates, and significant off-target adverse effects [36, 59].

The RET-selective TKIs selpercatinib and pralsetinib have been developed to treat *RET*-altered cancers to overcome these problems. In phase1/2 trials, selpercatinib and pralsetinib demonstrated remarkable efficacy in *RET* fusion-positive NSCLC, with ORRs among treatment-naïve and platinum-based chemotherapy-pretreated patients of 85% and 64%, respectively, for selpercatinib, and 70% and 61%, respectively, for pralsetinib. Notably, both inhibitors also exhibited antitumor activity in patients with brain metastasis of NSCLC [36, 60–62].

In *RET*-mutant MTC patients who previously received MTKI treatment (cabozantinib, vandetanib, or both) and patients with treatment-naïve *RET*-mutant MTC, the ORRs were 69 and 73%, respectively, for selpercatinib [63]. In patients with previously treated *RET*-fusion-positive thyroid cancer, the ORR was 79% for selpercatinib. Patients who received pralsetinib also showed similar safety and remarkable efficacy in *RET*-mutant or fusion-positive thyroid cancer [64].

As observed for inhibitors of other tyrosine kinases, resistance to selective RET inhibitors occurs *via* both on-target and off-target mechanisms. After a dramatic initial response, the G810C/R/S and Y806C/N mutations demonstrated acquired resistance to inhibitors [65, 66]. They were detected in the RET tyrosine kinase domain's solvent front and hinge regions. In addition, L730V/I resistance mutations at the roof of the solvent-front site were identified as strongly resistant to pralsetinib, but not to selpercatinib [67]. Novel RET kinase inhibitors have been developed to overcome these mutations. In addition, several reports have shown bypass mechanisms (off-target mechanisms) of resistance, including *MET* or *FGFR1* amplification and *KRAS NRAS* or *BRAF* mutations [66]. Thus, developing multiple therapeutic strategies is necessary to enhance the clinical benefits of selective RET kinase inhibitors.

10. Conclusion

Since the discovery of the *RET* gene in 1985 [1], research on RET function has made significant progress in cancer research, developmental biology, and neuroscience [3]. Many point mutations or rearrangements of the *RET* proto-oncogene have been identified in various hereditary and nonhereditary cancers, and the mechanisms of RET activation have been elucidated. Long-sought RET-selective inhibitors (selpercatinib and pralsetinib) have been developed, significantly increasing the therapeutic efficacy of *RET*-mutant cancers. Further development of new inhibitors is expected to overcome resistance to selective inhibitors.

In developmental biology, RET functions, including intracellular signaling, are being extensively studied to understand the mechanisms underlying the development of the enteric nervous system, kidneys, and spermatogenesis. *RET* is a major causative gene of HSCR, an enteric nervous system developmental disorder. In contrast to the mutations identified in cancers, HSCR mutations are loss-of-function mutations. In addition, the activation of RET by GFLs enhances the survival of dopaminergic, motor, and sensory neurons. Therapeutic strategies targeting RET are expected for treating neurodegenerative diseases such as Parkinson's disease and amyotrophic lateral sclerosis, as well as for nerve pain.

Moreover, recent findings demonstrating the association between RET activation by GDF15 in neurons of the brainstem and a decrease in food intake are opening up a new field of research [21–24]. These findings may advance our understanding of the mechanisms underlying cachexia in patients with cancer. It is expected that future research on the RET function will continue to have a profound impact on life and medical science.

Acknowledgements

The author thanks all laboratory members and research collaborators for insightful discussion. Work at the author's laboratory is partly supported by Grant-in-aid for Scientific Research from the Ministry of Education, Culture, Sports, Science and Technology (MEXT) of Japan. I would like to thank Editage (www.editage.com) for English language editing.

Conflict of interest

The author declares no conflict of interest.

Author details

Masahide Takahashi
International Center for Cell and Gene Therapy, Fujita Health University, Toyoake, Aichi, Japan

*Address all correspondence to: mtakaha@med.nagoya-u.ac.jp; masahide.takahashi@fujita-hu.ac.jp

References

[1] Takahashi M, Ritz J, Cooper GM. Activation of a novel human transforming gene, *ret*, by DNA rearrangement. Cell. 1985;**42**:581-588. DOI: 10.1016/0092-8674(85)90115-1

[2] Takahashi M, Cooper GM. *Ret* transforming gene encodes a fusion protein homologous to tyrosine kinases. Molecular and Cellular Biology. 1987;**7**:1378-1385. DOI: 10.1128/mcb.7.4.1378-1385.1987

[3] Takahashi M. RET receptor signaling: Function in development, metabolic disease, and cancer. Proceedings of the Japan Academy Series B. 2022;**98**:112-125. DOI: 10.2183/pjab.98.008

[4] Takahashi M. The GDNF/RET signaling pathway and human diseases. Cytokine and Growth Factor Reviews. 2001;**12**:361-373. DOI: 10.1016/s1359-6101(01)00012-0

[5] Arighi E, Borrello MG, Sariola H. RET tyrosine kinase signaling in development and cancer. Cytokine and Growth Factor Reviews. 2005;**16**:441-467. DOI: 10.1016/j.cytogfr.2005.05.010

[6] Addeo A, Miranda-Morales E, den Hollander P, et al. RET aberrant cancers and RET inhibitor therapies: Current state-of-the-art and future perspectives. Pharmacology & Therapeutics. 2023;**242**:108344. DOI: 10.1016/j.pharmthera.2023.108344

[7] Takahashi M, Buma Y, Iwamoto T, Inaguma Y, Ikeda H, Hiai H. Cloning and expression of the *ret* proto-oncogene encoding a tyrosine kinase with two potential transmembrane domains. Oncogene. 1988;**3**:571-578

[8] Takahashi M, Buma Y, Hiai H. Isolation of *ret* proto-oncogene cDNA with an amino-terminal signal sequence. Oncogene. 1989;**4**:805-806

[9] Iwamoto T, Taniguchi M, Asai N, Ohkusu K, Nakashima I, Takahashi M. cDNA cloning of mouse *ret* proto-oncogene and its sequence similarity to the cadherin superfamily. Oncogene. 1993;**8**:1087-1091

[10] Pachnis V, Mankoo B, Costantini F. Expression of the c-ret proto-oncogene during mouse embryogenesis. Development. 1993;**119**:1005-1017. DOI: 10.1242/dev.119.4.1005

[11] Tsuzuki T, Takahashi M, Asai N, Iwashita T, Matsuyama M, Asai J. Spatial and temporal expression of the ret proto-oncogene product in embryonic, infant and adult rat tissues. Oncogene. 1995;**10**:191-198

[12] Lin LF, Doherty DH, Lile JD, Bektesh S, Collins F. GDNF: A glial cell line-derived neurotrophic factor for midbrain dopaminergic neurons. Science. 1993;**260**:1130-1132. DOI: 10.1126/science.8493557

[13] Jing S, Wen D, Yu Y, et al. GDNF-induced activation of the ret protein tyrosine kinase is mediated by GDNFR-alpha, a novel receptor for GDNF. Cell. 1996;**85**:1113-1124. DOI: 10.1016/s0092-8674(00)81311-2

[14] Treanor JJ, Goodman L, de Sauvage F, et al. Characterization of a multicomponent receptor for GDNF. Nature. 1996;**382**:80-83. DOI: 10.1038/382080a0

[15] Klein RD, Sherman D, Ho WH, et al. A GPI-linked protein that interacts with ret to form a candidate neurturin receptor. Nature. 1997;**387**:717-721. DOI: 10.1038/42722

[16] Airaksinen MS, Saarma M. The GDNF family: Signalling, biological functions and therapeutic value. Nature Reviews Neuroscience. 2002;**3**:383-394. DOI: 10.1038/nrn812

[17] Kawai K, Takahashi M. Intracellular RET signaling pathways activated by GDNF. Cell and Tissue Research. 2020;**382**:113-123. DOI: 10.1007/s00441-020-03262-1

[18] Schuchardt A, D'Agati V, Larsson-Blomberg L, Costantini F, Pachnis V. Defects in the kidney and enteric nervous system of mice lacking the tyrosine kinase receptor ret. Nature. 1994;**367**:380-383. DOI: 10.1038/367380a0

[19] Sánchez MP, Silos-Santiago I, Frisén J, He B, Lira SA, Barbacid M. Renal agenesis and the absence of enteric neurons in mice lacking GDNF. Nature. 1996;**382**:70-73. DOI: 10.1038/382070a0

[20] Cacalano G, Fariñas I, Wang L-C, et al. GFRα1 is an essential receptor component for GDNF in the developing nervous system and kidney. Neuron. 1998;**21**:53-62. DOI: 10.1016/s0896-6273(00)80514-0

[21] Hsu JY, Crawley S, Chen M, et al. Non-homeostatic body weight regulation through a brainstem-restricted receptor for GDF15. Nature. 2017;**550**:255-259. DOI: 10.1038/nature24042

[22] Mullican SE, Lin-Schmidt X, Chin CN, et al. GFRAL is the receptor for GDF15 and the ligand promotes weight loss in mice and nonhuman primates. Nature Medicine. 2017;**23**:1150-1157. DOI: 10.1038/nm.4392

[23] Yang L, Chang CC, Sun Z, et al. GFRAL is the receptor for GDF15 and is required for the anti-obesity effects of the ligand. Nature Medicine. 2017;**23**:1158-1166. DOI: 10.1038/nm.4394

[24] Emmerson PJ, Wang F, Du Y, et al. The metabolic effects of GDF15 are mediated by the orphan receptor GFRAL. Nature Medicine. 2017;**23**:1215-1219. DOI: 10.1038/nm.4393

[25] Jijiwa M, Fukuda T, Kawai K, et al. A targeting mutation of tyrosine 1062 in ret causes a marked decrease of enteric neurons and renal hypoplasia. Molecular and Cellular Biology. 2004;**24**:8026-8036. DOI: 10.1128/MCB.24.18.8026-8036.2004

[26] Wong A, Bogni S, Kotka P, et al. Phosphotyrosine 1062 is critical for the in vivo activity of the Ret9 receptor tyrosine kinase isoform. Molecular and Cellular Biology. 2005;**25**:9661-9673. DOI: 10.1128/MCB.25.21.9661-9673.2005

[27] Jijiwa M, Kawai K, Fukihara J, et al. GDNF-mediated signaling via RET tyrosine 1062 is essential for maintenance of spermatogonial stem cells. Genes to Cells. 2008;**13**:365-374. DOI: 10.1111/j.1365-2443.2008.01171.x

[28] Jain S, Knoten A, Hoshi M, et al. Organotypic specificity of key RET adaptor-docking sites in the pathogenesis of neurocristopathies and renal malformations in mice. Journal of Clinical Investigation. 2010;**120**:778-790. DOI: 10.1172/JCI41619

[29] Romeo G, Ronchetto P, Luo Y, et al. Point mutations affecting the tyrosine kinase domain of the RET proto-oncogene in Hirschsprung's disease. Nature. 1994;**367**:377-378. DOI: 10.1038/367377a0

[30] Edery P, Lyonnet S, Mulligan LM, et al. Mutations of the RET proto-oncogene in Hirschsprung's disease. Nature. 1994;**367**:378-380. DOI: 10.1038/367378a0

[31] Takahashi M, Kawai K, Asai N. Roles of the RET proto-oncogene in cancer and development. JMA Journal. 2020;**15**:175-181. DOI: 10.31662/jmaj.2020-0021

[32] Grieco M, Santoro M, Berlingieri MT, et al. PTC is a novel rearranged form of the ret proto-oncogene and is frequently detected in vivo in human thyroid papillary carcinomas. Cell. 1990;**60**:557-563. DOI: 10.1016/0092-8674(90)90659-3

[33] Santoro M, Carlomagno F, Hay ID, et al. Ret oncogene activation in human thyroid neoplasms is restricted to the papillary cancer subtype. Journal of Clinical Investigation. 1992;**89**:1517-1522. DOI: 10.1172/JCI115743

[34] Nikiforov YE. RET/PTC rearrangement in thyroid tumors. Endocrine Pathology. 2002;**13**:3-16. DOI: 10.1385/ep:13:1:03

[35] Cancer Genome Atlas Research Network. Integrated genomic characterization of papillary thyroid carcinoma. Cell. 2014;**159**:676-690. DOI: 10.1016/j.cell.2014.09.050

[36] Subbiah V, Yang D, Velcheti V, Drilon A, Meric-Bernstam F. State-of-the-art strategies for targeting RET-dependent cancers. Journal of Clinical Oncology. 2020;**38**:1209-1221. DOI: 10.1200/JCO.19.02551

[37] Romei C, Ciampi R, Elisei R. A comprehensive overview of the role of the RET proto-oncogene in thyroid carcinoma. Nature Reviews Endocrinology. 2016;**12**:192-202. DOI: 10.1038/nrendo.2016.11

[38] Hamatani K, Eguchi H, Ito R, et al. RET/PTC rearrangements preferentially occurred in papillary thyroid cancer among atomic bomb survivors exposed to high radiation dose. Cancer Research. 2008;**68**:7176-7182. DOI: 10.1158/0008-5472.CAN-08-0293

[39] Kohno T, Ichikawa H, Totoki Y, et al. *KIF5B-RET* fusions in lung adenocarcinoma. Nature Medicine. 2012;**18**:375-377. DOI: 10.1038/nm.2644

[40] Takeuchi K, Soda M, Togashi Y, et al. RET, ROS, and ALK fusions in lung cancer. Nature Medicine. 2012;**18**:378-381. DOI: 10.1038/nm.2658

[41] Lipson D, Capelletti M, Yelensky R, et al. Identification of new *ALK* and *RET* gene fusions from colorectal and lung cancer biopsies. Nature Medicine. 2012;**18**:382-384. DOI: 10.1038/nm.2673

[42] Le Rolle AF, Klempner SJ, Garrett CR, et al. Identification of characterization of *RET* fusion in advanced colorectal cancer. Oncotarget. 2015;**6**:28929-28937. DOI: 10.18632/oncotarget.4325

[43] Paratala BS, Chung JH, Williams CB, et al. *RET* rearrangement are actionable alterations in breast cancer. Nature Communications. 2018;**9**:4821. DOI: 10.1038/s41467-018-07341-4

[44] Skálová A, Vanecek T, Uro-Coste E, et al. Molecular pofiling of salivary gland intraductal carcinoma revealed a subset of tumors harboring NCOA4-RET and novel TRIM27-RET fusions: A report of 17 cases. American Journal of Surgical Pathology. 2018;**42**:1445-1455. DOI: 10.1097/PAS.0000000000001133

[45] Skálová A, Banečkova M, Thompson LDR, et al. Expanding the molecular spectrum of secretory carcinoma of salivary glands with a novel VIM-RET fusion. American Journal of Surgical Pathology. 2020;**44**:1295-1307. DOI: 10.1097/PAS.0000000000001

[46] Mulligan LM, Kwok JBJ, Healey CS, et al. Germline mutations of the *RET*

proto-oncogene in multiple endocrine neoplasia type 2A. Nature. 1993;**363**:458-460. DOI: 10.1038/363458a0

[47] Donis-Keller H, Dou S, Chi D, et al. Mutations in the RET proto-oncogene are associated with MEN 2A and FMTC. Human Molecular Genetics. 1993;**2**:851-856. DOI: 10.1093/hmg/2.7.851

[48] Hofstra RM, Landsvater RM, Ceccherini I, et al. A mutation in the RET proto-oncogene associated with multiple endocrine neoplasia type 2B and sporadic medullary thyroid carcinoma. Nature. 1994;**367**:375-376. DOI: 10.1038/367375a0

[49] Carlson KM, Dou S, Chi D, et al. Single missense mutation in the tyrosine kinase catalytic domain of the RET proto-oncogene is associated with multiple endocrine neoplasia type 2B. Proceedings National Academy Science U. S. A. 1994;**91**:1579-1583. DOI: 10.1073/pnas.91.4.1579

[50] Asai N, Iwashita T, Matsuyama M, Takahashi M. Mechanism of activation of the *ret* proto-oncogene by multiple endocrine neoplasia 2A mutations. Molecular and Cellular Biology. 1995;**15**:1613-1619. DOI: 10.1128/MCB.15.3.1613

[51] Santoro M, Carlomagno F, Romano A, et al. Activation of RET as a dominant transforming gene by germline mutations of MEN2A and MEN2B. Science. 1995;**267**:381-383. DOI: 10.1126/science.7824936

[52] Iwashita T, Murakami H, Kurokawa K, et al. A two-hit model for development of multiple endocrine neoplasia type 2B by *RET* mutations. Biochemical Biophysical Research Communications. 2000;**268**:804-808. DOI: 10.1006/bbrc.2000.2227

[53] Kato S, Subbiah V, Marchlik E, Elkin SK, Carter JL, Kurzrock R. *RET* aberrations in diverse cancers: Next-generation sequencing of 4,871 patients. Clinical Cancer Research. 2017;**23**:1988-1997. DOI: 10.1158/1078-0432.CCR-16-1679

[54] Wells SA, Asa SL, Dralle H, et al. Revised American Thyroid Association guidelines for the management of medullary thyroid carcinoma. Thyroid. 2015;**25**:567-610. DOI: 10.1089/thy2014.0335

[55] Morandi A, Plaza-Menacho I, Isacke CM. RET in breast cancer: Functional and therapeutic implications. Trends in Molecular Medicine. 2011;**17**:149-157. DOI: 10.1016/j.molmed.2010.12.007

[56] Morandi A, Martin LA, Gao Q, et al. GDNF-RET signaling in ER-positive breast cancers is a key determinant of response and resistance to aromatase inhibitors. Cancer Research. 2013;**73**:3783-3795. DOI: 10.1158/0008-5472.CAN-12-4265

[57] Plaza-Menacho I, Morandi A, Robertson D, et al. Targeting the receptor tyrosine kinase RET sensitizes breast cancer cells to tamoxifen treatment and reveals a role for RET in endocrine resistance. Oncogene. 2010;**29**:4648-4657. DOI: 10.1038/onc.2010.209

[58] Pecar G, Liu S, Hooda J, Atkinson JM, Oesterreich S, Lee AV. RET signaling in breast cancer therapeutic resistance and metastasis. Breast Cancer Research. 2023;**25**:26. DOI: 10.1186/s13058-023-01622-7

[59] Li AY, McCusker MG, Russo A, et al. RET fusions in solid tumors. Cancer Treat Reviews. 2019;**81**:101911. DOI: 10.1016/j.ctrv.2019.101911

[60] Drilon A, Oxnard GR, Tan DSW, et al. Efficacy of Selpercatinib in

RET fusion-positive non-small-cell lung cancer. New England Journal of Medicine. 2020;**383**:813-824. DOI: 10.1056/NEJMoa2005653

[61] Gainor JF, Curigliano G, Kim DW, et al. Pralsetinib for RET fusion-positive non-small-cell lung cancer (ARROW): A multi-cohort, open-label, phase 1/2 study. The Lancet Oncology. 2021;**22**:959-969. DOI: 10.1016/S1470-2045(21)00247-3

[62] Subbiah V, Gainor JF, Oxnard GR, et al. Intracranial efficacy of Selpercatinib in RET fusion-positive non-small cell lung cancers on the LIBRETTO-001 trial. Clinical Cancer Research. 2021;**27**:4160-4167. DOI: 10.1158/1078-0432.CCR-21-0800

[63] Wirth LJ, Sherman E, Robinson B, et al. Efficacy of Selpercatinib in RET-altered thyroid cancers. New England Journal of Medicine. 2020;**383**:825-835. DOI: 10.1056/NEJMoa2005651

[64] Subbiah V, Hu MI, Wirth LJ, et al. Pralsetinib for patients with advanced or metastatic RET-altered thyroid cancer (ARROW): A multi-cohort, open-label, registrational, phase 1/2 study. Lancet Diabetes Endocrinology. 2021;**9**:491-501. DOI: 10.1016/S2213-8587(21)00120-0

[65] Solomon BJ, Tan L, Lin JJ, et al. RET solvent front mutations mediate acquired resistance to selective RET inhibition in RET-driven malignancies. Journal of Thoracic Oncology. 2020;**15**:541-549. DOI: 10.1016/j.jtho.2020.01.006

[66] Rosen EY, Won HH, Zheng Y, et al. The evolution of RET inhibitor resistance in RET-driven lung and thyroid cancers. Nature Communications. 2022;**13**:1450. DOI: 10.1038/s41467-022-28848-x

[67] Shen T, Hu X, Liu X, Subbiah V, Mooers BHM, Wu J. The L730V/I RET roof mutations display different activities toward pralsetinib and selpercatinib. NPJ Precision Oncology. 2021;**5**:48. DOI: 10.1038/s41698-021-00188-x

Chapter 4

Restoration of Tumor Suppression to Cancer Carrying p53 Mutations

Mohammad Nurul Amin and Yong-Yu Liu

Abstract

Missense mutations of tumor suppressor genes enable cancerous cells generating variable mutant proteins and promote malignant development. These mutant proteins lose the original functions in suppressing tumorous cells but also commit oncogenic activities to tumor progression. Targeting mutants of the p53 tumor suppressor merges a specific approach for cancer treatments. This chapter will highlight the progress from our group and those of others in this filed. We will introduce new concepts and molecular mechanisms underlying the expression of mutant proteins and cancer resistance to conventional treatments. Furthermore, we will introduce the potential agents holding great promises in preclinic studies for cancer treatments.

Keywords: missense mutation, p53 tumor suppressor, cancer stem cells, antitumor immunity, RNA methylation

1. Introduction

The tumor suppressor p53 plays a pivotal role in maintaining genome integrity and protecting the cells from neoplastic transformation. Apart from its well-known function in cell-cycle arrest, DNA repair, apoptosis, and senescence, recent reports show that p53 also regulates the stemness of cells and immune response against tumorigenesis and tumor progression [1–3]. p53 maintains homeostasis between self-renewal and differentiation and prevents either dedifferentiation or reprogramming of somatic cells to cancer stem-like cells [2]. By modulating transcription of genes, those proteins are involved in regulating immune recognition and response, p53 conserves immune surveillance and destruction against cancerous cells.

TP53 gene is frequently mutated in almost of all types of human cancer. The majority of its genetic alterations are missense mutations occurred in the DNA-binding domain (DBD) [4, 5]. p53 hotspot mutations, which are frequently detected missense mutants and located in the DBD, can be categorized into "contact" mutants (R248, R273) and conformational mutants (R175H, G245, R249, and R282) [6, 7]. These mutants not only lose the canonical tumor-suppressive functions of the wild-type p53 (wt-p53) but also commit any gain-of-function (GOF) of mutant p53 (mut-p53) that favors cancerous cell survival and promotes tumor progression [7–9]. mut-p53 proteins primarily execute as transcription factor, regulate the expression of several genes and non-coding RNAs, and confer oncogenic properties, including sustained proliferation, resistance to cell death, replicative immortality, and evading immune destruction [10]. In recent years, novel functions of mut-p53 in promoting dedifferentiation of somatic cells to cancer stem cells (CSCs) and in avoiding antitumor immunity have gathered considerable attention. Cancer cells that carry mut-p53 not only withstand the genomic instability but also adore oncogenic signals to malignant transformation. The correlation of GOF mut-p53 to cancer stemness was realized in the undifferentiated thyroid carcinoma [11] and a poor prognosis of patients with cancers [12]. This was further supported by GOF mut-p53 endorsed tumorigenicity of embryonic stem cells (ESCs) and these mut-p53 dependent ESCs share the gene signature with undifferentiated tumors carrying mut-p53 [2, 13]. GOF mut-p53 can alter the immunogenicity of cancer cells and further confine immune escape [3, 14].

Since p53 missense mutation is the most come genetic alterations in cancers, targeting these GOF mut-p53 holds a great promise for developing selective and effective treatments against cancer. In this chapter, we will briefly review the progress in GOF mupt-p53 and cancer progression and discuss various mechanisms driving alteration of cellular plasticity and the immune response upon mut-p53 and the efforts to delineate novel ways to specifically target CSCs residing in mut-p53 tumors and enhance antitumor immunity.

2. p53 mutations and cancer

2.1 p53 transactivates and regulates the expression of p53-target genes to suppress tumor

Tumor suppressor p53 acts as a central regulator in a myriad of cellular signaling pathways that control the cell cycle and maintain the integrity of the human genome [15]. p53 functions primarily as a transcription factor for modulating the expression of approximately 350 p53-target or responsive genes [5, 16, 17]. p53 protein is biologically active as a homotetramer (4 × 393 amino acid residues) and its domain structure contains a transactivation domain (TA), a proline-rich region (PR), DNA-binding domain (DBD), oligomerization domain (OD), and regulatory domain (Reg), sequentially located from amino terminus to carboxyl terminus (**Figure 1a,c**). The core domain, DBD (residues 94–292) forms a structure, including a central β-sandwich scaffold and additional elements, providing the DNA-binding surface [18, 19]. This p53 core domain has a low thermodynamic stability and it can rapidly unfold at body temperature ($t_{1/2}$, 9 min) [20, 21]. This low stability is linked with the structural plasticity required to facilitate p53 binding to DNA and other proteins, and may have implications with the susceptibility to mutations frequently detected in cancers [5, 22].

2.2 Hotspot mut-p53 in the DBD display oncogenic function

GOF Tumor suppressive function of p53 is inactivated by genetic mutations in approximately 42% of cancers, and its apoptotic pathways are impaired in those of other cancers. Mut-p53 proteins in cancer cells, either homotetramer or heterotetramer, not only lose the tumor suppressor function of wt-p53 but also endow the gain-of-function (GOF) that displays oncogenic activity, contributing to cancer progression (**Figure 1a**) [23]. Mutations in the TAD lead to truncated p53 that can activate apoptotic target genes [24]. However, most mutations occur in DBD and lead to functional inactivation. A majority of *TP53* mutations (~80%) are detected in the

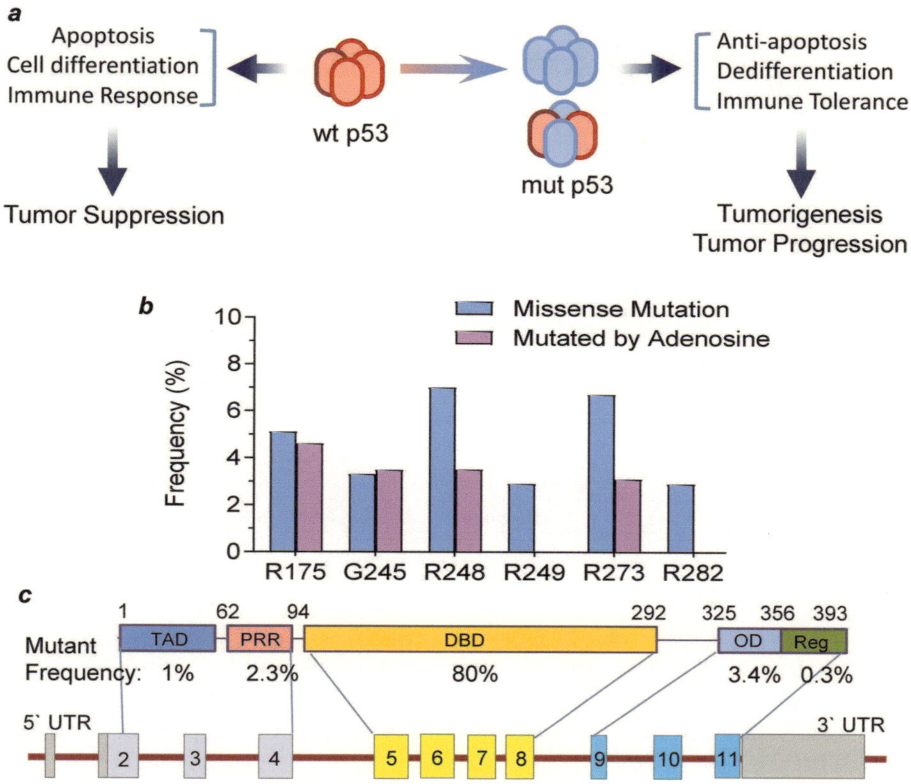

Figure 1.
p53 mutation and cancer development. ***a,*** *p53 mutation turns tumor suppressor into oncogenic factors. Wild-type p53 protein (wt) forms a tetrameric transcription factor and suppresses tumorigenesis and tumor progression via apoptosis, cell differentiation, and immune response. Wt, wild-type of p53; Mut, mutant p53.* ***b,*** *hotspot p53 mutants. Among p53 mutations, all hotspot missense mutations are more commonly detected than others in cancer cases and all are located in the DNA-binding domain (DBD). Further, missense proteins caused by adenosine in each hotspot mutated codon are more common than others.* ***c,*** *p53 domain structure. TAD, transactivation domain; PRR, proline-rich region; DBD, DNA-binding domain; OD, oligomerization domain; Reg, regulatory domain.*

exons 5–8 that encode the DBD of p53 protein (**Figure 1c**) [25]. The main mutant types of *TP53* include missense mutations (~73%), frameshift mutations (~11%), non-sense mutations (~7%), silencing mutations (~5%), and splice mutations (~2%) [6, 26]. Missense mutations of *TP53* result in single amino acid substitutes, which can present GOF activity during tumorigenesis, such as p53 R175H and p53 R273H that promote tumor invasion and migration [27–29]. Splice mutations generate alternative proteins that can also advance tumor development [30]. Among p53 mutants, the most common mutation sites that are called hotspot mutations in cancer cases occur at the codons of R175, G245, R248, R249, R273, and R282 (**Figure 1b**). Based on the COSMIC Database (https://cancer.sanger.ac.uk/signatures/), it has been found that the most substitution mutations among mut-p53 are G to A transitions (G > A, 29.05%), followed by C to T transitions (C > T, 25.90%) [31]. The transited "A" from others (C > A, G > A, T > A) accounts for 34.82% of all p53 missense mutants. Interestingly, G > A (~15% of all) is major transition for R175, G245, R248 and R273 hotspot mutations (**Table 1** and **Figure 1b**). mut-p53 is usually divided into two categories. One category is DNA contact mutations (contact mut-p53), which occur in the amino acids in contact with DNA and cause inability of mut-p53 protein binding

Mutation	Overall Frequency	Wild-Type Codon	Mutant Codon	Class of Activation	GOF
*G > **A** (~14.7%)*					
R175H	4.6%	CGC	CAC	Conformation	GOF
R248Q	3.5%	CGG	CAC/CAA	DNA contact	GOF
R273H	3.1%	CGT	CAT	DNA contact	GOF
R245S	2.8%	GGC	AGC	Conformation	
G245D	0.68%	GGC	GAC	Conformation	
*C > **T** or G > **T***					
G248W	2.8%	CGG	TGG	DNA contact	GOF
R273C	2.7%	CGT	TGT	DNA contact	
R282W	2.4%	CGG	TGG	DNA contact	GOF
R249S	1.8%	AGG	AGT	Conformation	

*G > **A**, guanine transited to adenine; C > **T**, cytosine transited to thymine; G > **T**, guanine transited thymine.*

Table 1.
Hotspot p53 mutations and their codon transitions in human cancer.

to DNA, such as p53 R273H and p53 R248Q. Another category is conformational mutations (conformational mut-p53), which occur in amino acids that maintain the structure and can result in unfolded proteins, such as p53 R175H, p53 Y220C, and p53 R249S [32].

2.3 Mut-p53 is a specific target for cancer treatments

mut-p53 proteins exert oncogenic GOF mainly via altered transcriptional mechanisms. wt-p53 protein recognizes and binds to DNA response elements, then recruits transcription factors, histone acetyltransferases, chromatin remodeling complexes, to form the pre-initiation complex for transcription [31, 33]. It has been reported that mut-p53 cannot bind to the response element for wt-p53, but exerts its GOF activity via different mechanisms. For instance, mut-p53 can bind to diverse transcription factors and cofactors (NF-Y, p73, NRF2, Ets-1), thus altering transcription of target genes [33]. In cancer cells upon DNA damage, mut-p53/NF-Y complex recruits p300 and then binds to NF-Y target promoters, leading to histone acetylation and overexpression of NF-Y target genes permitting tumor progression [34]. In some cases, mut-p53 (G245S) can directly bind to DNA with some specific structures, such as nuclear matrix attachment regions (MARs), and regulate transcriptions [35]. mut-p53 also can interact with other cellular proteins, thereby altering the functions of these proteins. In the knock-in mice, mut-p53 (R270H) antagonized the p63/p73-regulated transcription for tumor suppression via Notch1 pathway, and then promoted tumorigenesis and tumor progression [36]. It is noted that altered cellular localization of particular mut-p53 also contributes to its GOF. p53 E258K, R273H, and R273L mutants, which were located in the cytoplasm, could inhibit autophagy in colon cancer cells [37].

mut-p53 spectrum differs between tumors and is associated with poor prognosis in cancer patients. Frequency of mut-p53 in tumor tissue samples from 10,000 cancer patients is 42% (https://www.cbioportal.org/). However, the frequency is significantly higher in small cell lung cancer (89%) and in colorectal cancer (73%). Strikingly, mut-p53 is highly associated with a poor prognosis in different types of cancers observed. The cBioportal for Cancer Genomics Database revealed that mut-p53 expression is negatively correlated with overall survival of patients with breast cancer, pancreatic cancer, hepatobiliary cancer, bone cancer, non-small cell lung cancer, and thyroid cancer [31]. For example, in breast cancer cases, although mut-p53 is in 30–35% all cases, mut-p53 is often detected in ~80% of triple-negative (TN) breast cancer, which always are poorer in prognosis than any other subtypes of breast cancer [38].

3. p53 mutants promote cancer stemness

The major oncogenic properties of GOF mut-p53, including enhanced metastasis, chemoresistance, and angiogenesis are integral to cancer stem cell (CSC). Indeed, recent studies indicate that GOF mut-p53 (R175H, R248W, R273H) promotes cancer stemness.

3.1 p53 maintains the balance of self-renewal and differentiation for homeostasis

By controlling the proliferation, differentiation, and apoptosis, p53 plays a significant role in ensuring genomic integrity of normal stem cells. Apart from its classical function, p53 also maintains tissue hemostasis between self-renewal and differentiation [1, 39]. p53 acts as a barrier to somatic cells counteracting the reprogramming process [39]. Human somatic cell can be reprogrammed to induced pluripotent stem (iPS) cells by induction of reprogramming factors (Oct4, SOX2, KLF4, and c-MYC) that are highly expressed in ESCs and regulate the signaling required for pluripotency (**Figure 2**) [40]. Silencing p53 expression with siRNA in adult fibroblasts can enhance the efficacy of generating iPS cells up to 110-fold [41]. Conversely, reduction of p53 signaling, by deleting or knocking down p53 or its target gene p21, increases reprogramming efficiency [42]. Moreover, p53 may upregulate miR-199a-3p expression so as in turn impose G1 arrest to decrease reprogramming efficacy [43]. mut-p53 plays a critical role in driving CSC phenotype [29, 44, 45]. GOF mut-p53 proteins lack the DNA-binding ability to p53-target genes, instead, they can piggyback on other transcription factors to regulating expression of a large number of genes and non-coding RNAs for malignant stemness.

3.2 GOF mut-p53 increases cancer stemness

CSC or cancer stem-like cell excuses as seed for tumorigeneses, and further promotes cancer progression as well as resistance to therapies. wt-p53 protein regulates the quantity and quality of adult stem cells to ensure normal tissue development with less tumorigenic risk. However, mut-p53 proteins, which inactivate p53 signaling and display GOF, can disrupt this balance, thereby promoting pluripotency and reprogramming somatic cells, including adult stem cells for initiating tumor [2]. Recent studies indicated that prevalent mut-p53 (R175H, R273, R248W) boosts the stemness properties of cancer cells (**Figure 2**) [29, 46–48]. Either "contact" or "conformation" mut-p53 in DBD execute GOF properties in favor cell survival and promoting tumor progression [8]. The potential role of mut-p53 played in CSC formation was realized from the correlation of undifferentiated tumors to mut-p53 in thyroid cancers [11].

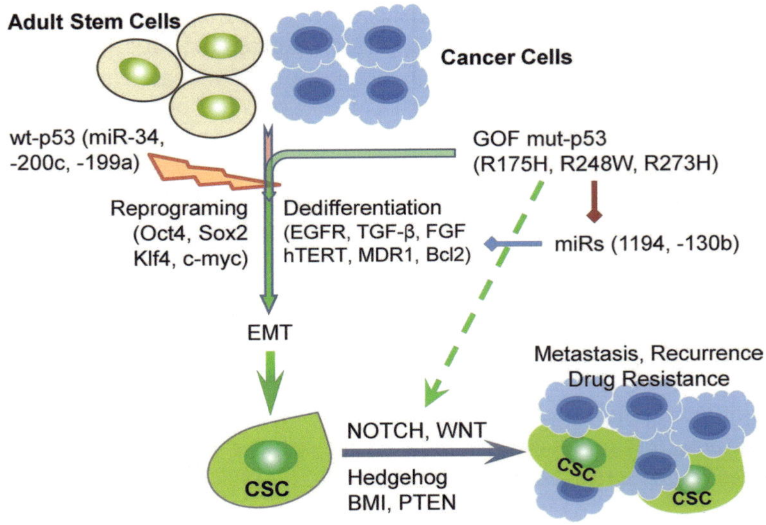

Figure 2.
p53 mutants determinate cancer Stemness. p53 regulates the balance of cell proliferation and differentiations of cell population for homeostasis. Mut-p53 can result in either the reprograming of adult stem cells or dedifferentiating cancer cells to form cancer stem cells. Further, Mut-p53 sustains cancer stemness via enhancing the expression of genes involved in signaling pathways of NOTCH, WNT, hedgehog, BMI, and PTEN, thus promoting tumor metastasis, drug resistance, and even recurrence. Wt, wild-type; CSC, cancer stem cell; miR, microRNA; EMT, epithelial-mesenchymal transition.

Undifferentiated tumors of breast and brain expressed the same gene signature as embryonic stem cells (ESCs) [49]. Further, it has been recognized that the novel property of mut-p53 not only enhances the reprogramming efficiency of somatic cells but also promotes malignant potentials of mouse embryonic fibroblasts (MEFs) [13]. Introducing pluripotent factors (Oct4, Sox2, c-Myc, and KLf4) into adult differentiated cells can reprogram them to their embryonic state or result in dedifferentiation.

3.3 Mut-p53 promotes cell reprogramming/de-differentiation to enrich CSCs

GOF mut-p53 (R172H, corresponding to the R175H in human) enhanced the efficiency of the reprogramming process compared to p53 deficiency in MEFs [13]. Importantly, mut-p53 induced alterations in the reprogrammed cells to malignancy [13]. Although p53-knockout MEFs maintained the pluripotent capacity *in vivo* after the reprogram with Oct4 and Sox2, the mut-p53 cells displayed malignant pluripotency and generated tumors (**Figure 2**) [13]. While reprogrammed cells with p53-deficiency formed differentiated teratomas, mut-p53 reprogrammed MEFs formed undifferentiated malignant tumors [13]. This clearly indicates that GOF mut-p53 not only eliminates cancerous cells by apoptosis but also advances malignant pluripotency. A set of miRNAs has been identified, whose expression is altered (increased miR-15b, decreased miR-155) in a p53-dependent manner during transition of MEFs to induced pluripotent stem cells and these miRNAs may regulate the mut-p53 (R172H)-driven stemness [50]. Our group reported that introducing mut-p53 (R273H) via CRISPR/Cas9 editing into colorectal cancer SW48 cells markedly increased CSC population [29]. These mut-p53 cells that expressed low levels of p21 and PUMA while expressing high levels of Klf4, Oct4, c-Myc, TGF-β, and Zeb1, together promoted cancer cells to EMT and enhanced tumorigenesis *in vitro* and *in vivo* [29]. These indicate that mut-p53 (R273H) can reprogram or dedifferentiate cells to enhance cancer stemness in Colorectal cancer (**Figure 2**). Other reports showed that colorectal cancer SW480 cells (mut-p53 R273, P309S) harbored an increased population of CD44, Lgr5, and ALDH positive CSCs, as mut-p53 transcriptionally upregulates these CSC markers to promote CSC population [45]. Other works revealed that GOF mut-p53 (R175H, R273H) promotes cancer stemness through PI3K/AKT2-mediated integrin and growth factor signaling in cancer cells of glioblastoma and breast cancer [44]. AKT2 can enhance the phosphorylation of WASP interacting protein (WIP) and stabilize YAP/TAZ, thus supporting SCS survival and phenotypic maintenance (**Figure 2**) [44]. Mut-p53 can also induce the nuclear accumulation of YAP/TAZ and the activity via interacting with SREBP transcription and increased geranylgeranyl pyrophosphate from mevalonate biosynthesis for promoting self-renewal of breast cancer cells [51].

CSCs also can be derived from cancer cells. There are two CSC populations existed in tumors: the intrinsic CSCs that are inherently present in the tumor and the induced CSCs that arise from differentiated tumor cells as a consequence of EMT signaling [52]. During cancer development, a small numbers of aggressive cancer cells possessing cellular plasticity undergo reversible transformations, including epithelial to mesenchymal transition as well as mesenchymal to epithelial transition, and migrate to other tissues or organs to form metastasis [53]. Cancerous EMT is different from the embryonic one and requires CSCs being able to intravasate/extravasate and colonize at distant sites. EMT of cancer cells can be triggered by many extracellular signals, including transforming growth factor b (TGF-β), bone morphogenetic proteins (BMPs), Wnt, Notch, epidermal growth factor, fibroblast growth factor, and many others [54]. These signals, via modulating certain transcription factors (TFs) (such as Snail, Twist, Zeb, and others) independently or in combination, suppress epithelial phenotype, and further enhance mesenchymal traits, including enhanced migratory capacity, invasiveness, resistance to apoptosis, and production of extracellular matrix ECM components [55, 56]. These "migratory cells", after EMT, have the ability to form secondary tumors and differentiate into non-stem cancer cells, which are the very traits of self-renewal, and are increased resistance to chemotherapy and highly metastatic [52, 57].

One of the major GOF properties of mutant p53 is invasion and metastasis. Mut-p53-induced EMT triggers stemness properties in cancer cells and enriches CSCs in tumors under treatments [29, 58]. wt-p53 promotes epithelial differentiation through transcriptional activation of miR-200c [59], which inhibits the translation of EMT activator Zeb1/Zeb2 and then represses the expression of self-renewal factors like Bmil and possibly Klf4 and Sox2 [60, 61]. Conversely, loss of p53 in mammary epithelial cells reduces the expression of miR-200c and promotes EMT and stemness properties, thus generating high-grade breast tumors [59]. These findings were corroborated that loss of p53 increased levels of stemness regulators (Bmi1, Klf4, Vimentin) and EMT inducers (Snail, Twist, Zeb1, and Zeb2) in pancreatic acinar cells [62, 63]. p53 has also been implicated in suppressing EMT and the stemness of PC-3 prostate cancer cells by miR-145 [64]. PC3 cancer cells carrying wt-p53 expressed high levels of epithelial marker E-cadherin, while presented reduced levels of mesenchymal markers (fibronectin, vimentin, N-cadherin, and Zeb2) as well as CSC markers (CD44, Oct4, c-Myc, Klf4). Inhibition of miR-145 promoted EMT, as increased mesenchymal markers and CSC markers in those cells [64]. These indicate that wt-53 plays a crucial role in maintaining epithelial phenotype and suppressing pluripotency factors to maintain a differentiated state via miR-145 and p21 [29, 64]. However, loss or inactivation of p53 suppression on pluripotent genes would result in activation of EMT and stemness factors. GOF mut-p53 further promotes EMT and stemness phenotypes by activating genes regulating them. For example, mut-p53 (R175H, R248W, R273H) was found to suppress miR-130b expression by binding to its promoter, thereby upregulating Zeb1 expression and promoting stemness via Zeb1-mediated Bmis expression (**Figure 2**) [48, 65]. miR-194 is another p53-responsive miRNA and represses the expression of Bmi1 oncogene that mediates pluripotency. Mut-p53 suppresses miR-194 and leads endometrial cancer cells to EMT and cancer stemness [64]. It has been found that mut-p53 (R273H) upregulates the expression of lncRNAs (lnc273–31, lnc273–34) and is implicated in EMT and CSC maintenance in colorectal cancer cells [48]. These studies highlight that mut-p53-mediated EMT phenotype confers stemness in different cancer cell lines, however, it is still required to further explore the underlying mechanisms by which mut-p53 regulates EMT genes driving cancer stemness.

3.4 Mut-p53 enhances drug resistance of cancer stem cells

A major GOF endowed by mut-p53 to cancer cells is drug resistance. Mut-p53 restrictively modulates various cellular pathways and advances cell resistance to anticancer drugs. It is more attractive to find out the specific pathways by which mut-p53 enhances the drug resistance of CSCs. For example, CSCs highly express ATP-binding cassette (ABC) transporters, that efflux drugs out of cells and confer cells resistance to chemotherapy [66, 67]. Interestingly, MDR1 (multidrug resistance 1, also named P-glycoprotein) that is the most common protein detected in tumors with drug resistance remains suppressed by wt-p53 in normal cells, but is stimulated by mut-p53 in cancer cells during tumorigenesis and associated with poor progression [68–70]. wt-p53 suppressed the expression of ABCG2 (also named breast cancer resistance protein, BCRP), which highly expresses and protects adult stem cells from drugs or toxins, but through NF-κ B pathway, ABCG2 is expressed in breast cancer cells [67, 71]. Under induced DNA damage, p53 is stabilized by feedback regulation in normal cells and it triggers cell death by apoptosis. However, this regulation mainly via p53/ubiquitin-mediated degradation is completely lost in mut-p53 cancer cells. Under DNA damage conditions, GOF *mut-p53* increases ephrin-B2 expression, which in turn induces *ABCG2* expression [72]. In addition, GOF mut-p53 augments the expression of anti-apoptotic proteins (Bcl-2, Bcl-xL) and represses pro-apoptotic proteins (Bax, Bad, Bid) [73]. Similarly, CSCs suppress the levels and function of Bcl-2 family proteins (Bax, Bad) to attenuate drug-induced cell death [74]. Compared to their lack in somatic cancer cells, CSCs express high levels of DNA repair genes that help them repair DNA damage inflicted by chemotherapeutic drugs [75]. It has been found that murine mesenchymal stem cells (MSCs) with mut-p53 ($R172H^{/+}$), like CSCs, express high levels homologous recombination repair and non-homologous end joining genes and induce malignant tumors in mice [76]. Also, iPS cells expressing mut-p53 (R273H, P309S) induce the expression of CD44, Lgr5, and ALDH and generate tumors [45]. Aldehyde dehydrogenase (ALDH) serves as a main marker for colorectal CSC, and notably, it is a detoxifying enzyme via the $NAD(P)^+$-dependent oxidation and mediates cancer drug resistance [45, 77]. CSC phenotype is extensively driven by epigenetic factors, including miRNAs and even glycosphingolipids [78, 79]. Our recent works showed that suppressing ceramide glycosylation by glucosylceramide synthase, which is one response to cell stress under chemotherapy and generates globotriaosylceramide (Gb3) and other glycosphingolipids, can decrease GOF of mut-p53, cancer stemness, and MDR1-mediated drug resistance [29, 80, 81].

4. p53 mutants and immune evasion

mut-p53 in cancer cells contributes to immune evasion by regulating the expression of immunomodulating molecules and influencing immune cells, particularly natural killer (NK) cells and cytotoxic CD8+ T-cells and immune response in the tumor microenvironment (TME).

4.1 Mut-p53 modulates the expression of immunomodulatory ligands to affect immune response

p53 controls the expression of numerous genes, including TRAIL, DR5, TLRs, Fas, PKR, ULBP1/2, and CCL2 as well as T-cell inhibitory ligand PD-L1, which are involved in the immunological response to cancer [82]. TRAIL is expressed by several immune cells like NK cells, NK T-cells, T-cells macrophages, and dendritic cells (DCs). TRAIL binds to DR5 to cause apoptosis in a wide range of cancer types while maintaining cancer cell specificity, making it an attractive target for combination with immunotherapy [83, 84]. Toll-like receptor (TLR) 3, 5, 7, 8, and 9 play a major role in the innate immune response and stimulate the synthesis of type I interferon (IFN) via IFN regulatory factors (IRFs) [85]. IRF5 and IRF9 can be activated directly by p53 and IRF5 can induce release of cytokines leading cancer cells to apoptosis [86]. The Fas receptor defects can cause loss of immune tolerance, an accumulation of $CD4^{-}CD8^{-}$ T-cells, and production of autoantibodies [87, 88]. Under genotoxic conditions, dsRNA-activated protein kinase (PKR) regulated by p53 contributes to p53-mediated tumor suppression, also mediates inflammatory signals to activate inflammasome and proteins [89, 90]. NK cells have NKG2D receptors, which bind to ULBP1/2 ligands on the surface of tumor cells. Direct p53-target genes are ULBP1/2 ligands that improve NK cell-mediated target cell identification [14, 91]. Chemokine ligand 2 (CCL2, MCP-1) is a potent chemokine for monocytes and other immune cells. Much evidence indicates that CCL2 in the tumor microenvironment (TME) plays an immunosuppressive role [92]. GOF mut-p53 can upregulate the expression of CCL2 and tumor necrosis factor α (TNF-α) via nuclear factor kappa B (NFκB) signaling, consequently increasing microglia and monocyte-derived immune cell infiltration [93]. Several studies exhibit a correlation between mut-p53 and lack or decrease of cytotoxic immune cells.

4.2 Mut-p53 defects immunosurveillance via inactivation of NK cells

p53 maintains the immunosurveillance that recognizes neoplastic cells and initiates immune elimination; however, mut-p53 allows immune evasion and cancer progression [94, 95]. Immunosurveillance, either innate or adaptive immune responses, is composed of and relies on $CD4^{+}$ T helper (Th) cells, $CD8^{+}$ cells, natural killer (NK) cells and, in some cases, neutrophils [96, 97]. Among immune cells, NK cells distinguish tumor cells from normal cells mainly by relying on a balance of inhibitory and activating receptors in these cells. In brief, inhibitory receptors, such as the killer immunoglobulin-like receptors (KIR) of NK cells, recognize the major histocompatibility complex class I (MHC-I) molecules that are highly expressed in normal cells and prevent them from immune attack. Conversely, tumor cells often down-regulated express MHC-I molecules and further induce the engagement of activating receptors of NK cells, including natural cytotoxicity receptors (NCR) and the NK group membrane D (NKG2D) [98]. The cytotoxicity of NK cells is regulated by signals on both the NK cells and the targeted tumor cells. wt-p53 can upregulate the expression of ULBP1 and ULBP2 ligands on cancer cells to activate NK cells via activation of NKG2D receptor and enhance the antitumor functions of NK cells (**Figure 3**) [14, 99, 100]. Murine models showed that the mut-p53 (G242A corresponding to the G245A in human) suppressed the expression of active NKG2D ligand Mult-1 (while increasing the inhibitory ligand H60a) and reduced host NK cell population and activation, allowing breast tumor evade immune attack (**Figure 3**) [14]. Reactivating p53 function with CP31398 in breast cancer cell lines carrying mut-p53 (R280K, L194F, R175H) activated NK cells and killed cancer cells by granzyme B or NK cell-induced apoptosis [101].

4.3 Mut-p53 proteins serve as neoantigens mediating CD8 T-cells

p53 is a tumor antigen that can differentiate cancer cells from normal cells. Recently, numerous studies showed that missense mutations of p53 in cancer cells generate neoantigens that can improve response to immunotherapy [102–104]. Tumors that express immunogenic mut-p53 (Y220C, G245S) peptides have higher expression of programmed cell death ligand 1 (PD-L1) and higher levels of tumor-infiltrating cytotoxic T-cells, as compared to tumors with wt-p53 [104, 105]. The relative contribution of mut-p53 neoantigen and immune suppression to the

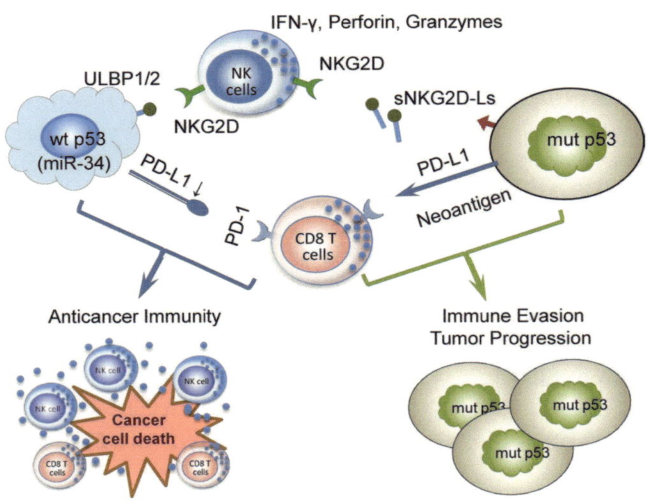

Figure 3.
p53 modulates immune response combating tumor. p53 maintains immune surveillance and immune attack against cancer cells. In addition to the effects of MHC-I molecules, tumor cells expressing wt-p53 can present the ULBP1/2 surface ligands to activate host NK cells via NKG2D receptors. These wt-p53 tumor cells suppress PD-L1 inhibitory ligands, thus MHC-I molecules activate CD8+ T-cells. Activated NK cells and CD8+ T-cells excuse anticancer immunity by cytokines and induced cell death (IFN-γ, perforin, granzymes). Tumor cells expressing Mut-p53 deactivate NK cells by soluble NKG2D ligands (sNKG2D-ls) and deactivate CD8+ T-cells by overexpression of PD-L1 ligand, thus resulting in immune evasion and tumor progression. Neoantigen expressed by Mut-p53 tumor cells is weak immunogenic for activating CD8+ T-cells.

overall state of the TME varies across cancer types. Identifying personalized clinical approaches to targeting mutant p53 to stimulate the immune response requires careful investigation.

Recognition of MHC-I peptides by T-cells receptor (TCR) can primarily activate T-cells and the activated effector T-cells including CD4 or CD8 further upregulate co-inhibitory receptors, such as PD-1 (also known as PDCD1), to keep protective immunity in check [106]. Cancer cells can overexpress co-inhibitory ligands (such as PD-L1) to constrain T-cell activity [107]. PD-L1, an immune checkpoint protein expressed by cancer cells or other host cells binds to the programmed cell death protein 1 (PD-1) on cytotoxic $CD8^+$ T-cells and results in T-cell inactivation [108]. p53 repressed the expression of PD-L1 via miR-34a in non-small cell lung cancer, and loss of p53 activity increases PD-L1 surface expression, which can suppress T-cell function and result in immune evasion (**Figure 3**) [109]. Further, mut-p53 (R172H) correlates with increased PD-L1 expression in lung cancers and that may help to identify patients responsive to checkpoint inhibitors targeting PD-L1 (**Figure 3**) [105, 109–111].

4.4 Activation of p53 reverses immunosuppression within tumor microenvironment (TME)

Regulatory T-cells (Tregs), myeloid-derived suppressor cells (MDSCs), and type 2 macrophages (M2) within the TME sustain pro-tumor inflammation and immunosuppression [112]. Tregs permit tumor growth by suppressing the activity of CD4+ T, CD8+ T, macrophages, and other polymorphonuclear cells (PMNs) [113, 114]. Tregs can promote angiogenesis, metastasis, and immune suppression through modulation of suppressive cytokines and surface ligands [115, 116]. p53 deficiency in prostate, ovarian, and subcutaneous pancreatic cancer can increase Treg cell populations, which are involved in suppressing effector T-cells in tumors and in the periphery [114, 117]. Mutant p53 encourages tumorigenic TGF-β signaling, which influences B cells, T regs, CD8+ and CD4+ T-cells in a variety of ways to stimulate immunosuppression [118, 119]. Activation of p53 can decrease Treg population and enhance T-cell-mediated tumor cell killing [117] and/or reverse an immunosuppressed TME by eliminating MDSCs through triggering cell death and/or reversing their immunosuppressive ability [120]. p53 can also be regulated by cytokine signaling, consistent with the observation that persistent inflammation causes stress that contributes to both tumorigenesis and tumor progression.

5. Restoration of p53 to suppress tumor progression

Mut-p53 promotes tumorigenesis and cancer progression not only because loss of wt-p53 but also the dominant-negative activities of mut-p53, which execute oncogenic GOF [22, 31, 121]. Since mut-p53 occurs in ~50% of human cancers with poor prognosis, barely in normal tissues, it has been emerged a specific therapeutic target. Approaches for directly targeting mut-p53 mainly include: (1) restoration of the DNA-binding conformation; (2) depletion or degradation of mut-p53 proteins; and (3) epigenetic restoring wt-p53 expression. More information regarding clinically available FDA-approved drugs and drugs in clinical trials for targeting mut-p53 or restoring p53 functions can be found in recent reviews [22, 122].

5.1 Reactivation of the transcriptional activity

mut-p53 proteins alter the expression of target genes transcriptionally and the conformation for protein-DNA has been recognized as crucial step [5]. Reactivating the transcriptional activity of mut-p53 is an effective strategy to eradicate cancer in 20 years. Many studies found that small molecule compounds and peptides can induce changes in the spatial conformation and folding pattern of mut-p53, are referred to reactivators (**Table 2, Figure 4**).

Restoring p53 binding: Among small molecules of reactivators, the most representative one is APR-246 (also known as eprenetapopt or PRIMA-1^{MET}), which is involved in more than 13 clinical trials, including phase 3 (**Table 2**). As a novel and more effective reactivator, prodrug APR-246 is converted to a Michael acceptor methylene quinuclidinone (MQ) that binds covalently to the cysteines, leading to refolding protein and restoring the activity in transcription of p53-target genes [123, 124]. Consistent with its capacity of reactivating mut-p53 (R175H, R273H), the anticancer

Regimen	Target spectrum	Indications	Clinical Trials
Res. Transcriptional Activity			
APR-246 alone or plus others (azacitidine, pembrolizumab)	R175H, R273H by the thiol groups binding	Multiple tumors	~ 13 trials in Phases I, I/II, III
ADH-6, ReACp53	R175H, R248, R273 by inhibiting aggregation	Cancer cells	n/a
PC14586	Y220C by	Solid tumors	Phase I/II
Arsenic trioxide (ATO) ATO + decitabine	R175H G245, R249, R282 by rescue functionality	Tumors, AML, MDS MDS, AML	~5 trials Phases I, I/II, III
C-peptide (361–382), pCAPs *N-peptides*	R273H and others Prevent MDM2 binding	Cancer cells	n/a
Degrading mut-p53			
Ganetespib + paclitaxel Ganetespib + docetaxel	R175H, R248Q by HSP90 inhibition	Ovarian cancer NSC lung cancer	Phase I/II Phase III
Vorinostat + MLN9708 Vorinostat + pazopanib	R175H, R273H by HDAC6 inhibition	Solid tumors Advanced cancer	Phase I Phase I
MCB613	R175H by inhibiting deubiquitinase USP15	Ovarian cancer cells	n/a
Restoring p53 expression			
C6-ceramide, Cer-RUB nanomicelles PDMP, Genz667161	Deletion; R273H, R238W by m6A-mediated pre-mRNA splicing	Colon cancer cells Ovarian cancer cells	n/a
Neplanocin A	R273H by m6A inhibition	Colon cancer cells	n/a

PDMP and Genz667161 are GCS inhibitors.

Table 2.
Targeting p53 mutants directly to improve cancer treatments.

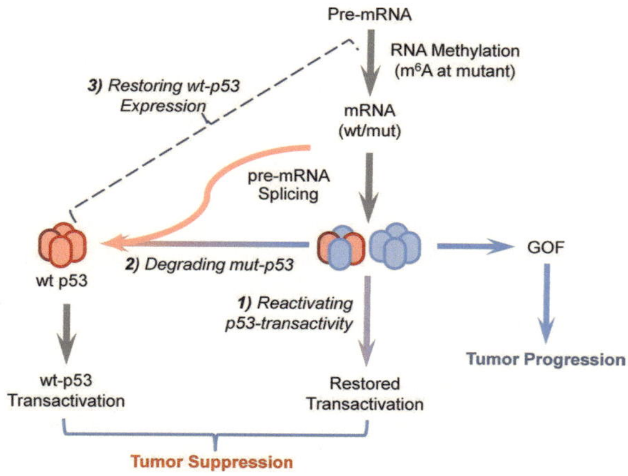

Figure 4.
Restoration of p53 in tumor suppression. Cancer cells dominantly express mutant p53 proteins from mRNA (wt, Mut) and promote tumor progression. The transcriptional activity of mutant p53 in tumor suppression can be restored directly by: (1) reactivating p53-transactivity. Small molecules modulate the conformation of Mut-p53 protein to increase transcription of p53-responsive genes. (2) degrading Mut-p53. Small molecules modulate signaling pathways to increase the ubiquitination of Mut-p53 proteins. (3) restoring wt-p53 expression. m^6A, N^6-methyladenosine; wt, wild-type; Mut, mutant; GOF, gain-of-function.

effects of APR-246 have been demonstrated in a range of *in vitro* and *in vivo* preclinical cancer systems [124, 125]. In cancer patients, APR-246 monotherapy has been shown to induce p53-dependent biologic effects against malignancy. In clinical trials enrolling patients with cancers, APR-246 was found to be safe and to have therapeutic activity when combined with particular medications, like azacitidine or pembrolizumab (targeting PD-1) [22]. The FDA granted breakthrough designation to APR-246 treatment for myelodysplastic syndrome (MDS), and a phase III randomized trial for the combined treatment was initiated in multicenter (NCT03745716). Recently, a phase II trial announced encouraging results, for evaluating APR-246 plus azacitidine as a post-transplant management therapy in patients with MDS and AML with mut-p53. Combined treatment with APR-246 and azacitidine achieved significant increased relapse-free survival (RFS, 58 *vs.* 30%) with median overall survival (OS, 19.3 *vs.* 5–8 months) after transplantation, compared to previous trials [126].

Decreasing mut-p53 Aggregation: Tripyridyl amide ADH-6, which inhibits amyloid formation with Alzheimer's disease, was identified as an inhibitor of mut-p53 aggregation. ADH-6 enhances cell death and inhibits tumor growth, with high selectivity for cancer cells expressing mut-p53 (R175H, R248W/Q, R273C/H), no toxicity to healthy tissues, p53-null cells or cells with wt-p53. ADH-6 has a greater efficacy than ReACp53, which is a cell-penetrating peptide for inhibiting mut-p53 (R282W) amyloid formation [127, 128]. In this group, none of the agents have been applied in clinical trial. Whereas, above compounds are relatively broad spectrum, further studies aimed at targeting specific single mutant or a distinct group of similar mutants effectively should be pursued.

Specific Codon Revealing: The small molecule PhiKan083 as well as PK7088 was found to bind the crevice near the mutant site and thermodynamically stabilize mut-p53 (Y220C), shifting it toward a wt-p53-like state [129, 130]. Compound PK7088, which is cooperated with nutlin-3 (wt-p53 activator) to transactivate p53-target genes, induced apoptosis and decreased the viability of gastric cancer and hepatoblastoma cells that express mut-p53 (Y220C) [130]. The p53 (Y220C)-specific small molecule, PC14586, which is bioavailable orally and is now in phase I/II clinical trial (NCT04585750), has presented highly promising results [131, 132]. The discovery of p53 (Y220C)-specific drugs is encouraging, however, the p53 Y220C is not a very common mutant (~0.64% of cancer cases) and has a unique structure not shared with other mut-p53 proteins.

Stabilizing Conformation of DNA binding: The mut-p53 (R175H) results in impaired zinc binding, causing misfolding and inactivation of the p53 protein. NSC319726 (also known as ZMC1), a metal ion chelator with high affinity for zinc, has been identified as a mut-p53 (R175H)-targeting drug [133]. NSC319726 promoted p53-dependent apoptosis and tumor regression *in vivo*, in a manner highly specific to cancer cells carrying p53 R175H [133, 134]. It has been found that ZMC2 and ZMC3, which belong to the same family of thiosemicarbazones to rescue conformation via zinc, promote a wt-like conformation into mut-p53 (R175H) *in vitro* [134]. COTI-2, a third-generation thiosemicarbazone now in clinical trial phase I, showed preferential selectivity for cancer cell lines expressing p53-mut (R175H), but also had some activity in wt-p53 cells [135]. Interestingly, it was proposed that COTI-2 triggers cell death by p63 (a p53 family member), which activates p53-target genes under DNA damage and replication stress [136]. Arsenic binding can stabilize the DNA-binding loop-sheet-helix motif alongside the overall β-sandwich fold, endowing mut-p53 with transcriptional activity [137]. Arsenic trioxide (ATO; Trisenox) is an FDA-approved drug for the treatment of acute promyelocytic leukemia. Through *in silico* analysis, it was found that ATO can rescue the functionality of mut-p53 with only a limited effect on DNA contact mutants [137]. ATO can restore the proper folding of several mut-p53 (R175, G245, R249, R282), however, only a subset of those regain wt-p53 transcriptional activity [137]. ATO is involved in several trials, treating patients with *TP53*-mutated AML, multiple tumors, and MDS alone or with decitabine (**Table 2**).

Peptides Competitive Binding: Both *N*- and *C*-terminal peptides have been produced to improve or restore p53 function in mut-p53 status. To disrupt the *C*-terminal negative transcriptional regulatory element of p53, a series of carboxy-terminal peptides were employed [138–140]. Among them, in some mut-p53 containing cell lines, a peptide (from p53 protein-seq 361–382) showed a strong potential for restoring DNA binding and transcriptional activity to altered p53. The effect was dependent on mutant p53 expression, and the peptide had no toxic effect on wt-p53 or p53-null cells. Further study revealed that the peptide not only binds to the *C*-terminus but also to the central domain, thus inducing Fas/APO-1-mediated apoptosis [140]. A peptide that binds to and stabilizes the p53 core domain can function as a chaperone, restoring a wt-like conformation [141].

p53 *N*-terminal peptides have also been generated to prevent MDM2 binding to p53, and so liberate p53 from MDM2-mediated proteasomal degradation. Two peptides that resemble the *N*-terminus of p53 can attach to MDM2 with an affinity that is 100 times greater than p53, thus preventing MDM2-mediated p53 degradation. Cells that have wt-p53 experience apoptosis after being treated with the peptides [138].

A panel of mut-p53 reactivating small peptides (pCAPs) that were developed using phage display selection showed p53-dependent effects *in vitro* and *in vivo* when applied to cancer cells expressing mut-53. Mechanistic studies suggested that pCAPs bind preferentially to the wt-p53 conformation; when a mut-p53 molecule assumes transiently a wild-type-like conformation, the peptide binds and stabilizes it, gradually shifting the dynamic equilibrium of the p53 population in that direction [142].

5.2 Degradation of Mut-p53

TP53-mutated cancer cells are addicted to mut-p53 proteins that execute oncogenic GOF [143]. Decrease of mut-p53 proteins in cancer cells by promoting degradation exhibits antitumor effects (**Figure 4**) [144, 145]. Some drugs such as gambogic acid [146], capsaicin [147], MCB-613 [144], and NSC59984 [148] can induce the degradation of mut-p53 in several different types of cancer cells. Among these agents, compound MCB-613 that inhibits deubiquitinase USP15 causes rapid ubiquitination, nuclear export, and degradation of mut-p53 (R175, less effects to others) in ovarian cancer cells [144].

Inhibition of HDAC6/HSP90 chaperone axis. Recent studies found that the accumulation of mmt-p53 (R175H, R273H) depends on the histone deacetylase 6 (HDAC6)/HSP90 chaperone axis that is sustained by RhoA geranylgeranylation downstream of the mevalonate pathways [145, 149]. Ganetespib (formerly known as STA-90909), a potent HSP90 inhibitor synergizes with cyclophosphamide to improve survival of mice with autochthonous tumors in a mutant p53-dependent manner [150]. Treatment of mut-p53 mice (R172H, R248Q$^{/-}$) with ganetespib inhibits tumor growth and prolongs survival in a mut-p53 dependent manner. Currently, the suberoylanilide hydroxamic acid (SAHA, a HDAC inhibitor) and ganetespib are in clinical trials (**Table 2**). Vorinostat (a HDAC inhibitor) with pazopanib is used as a therapeutic approach for inhibiting p53-mediated angiogenesis and facilitating mutant p53 (R175H, R273H) degradation in a phase I study. This evidence supports further evaluation of the combined treatment in patients with mut-p53 cancers, especially metastatic sarcoma or metastatic colorectal cancer [151].

5.3 Restoration wt-p53 protein expression

TP53 mutation is usually heterozygous in either germline or somatic cells, including cancer cells [8, 25, 30]. This may provide opportunities to modulate the transcriptional and post-transcriptional processes to restore wt-p53 expression in mut-p53 cancer cells. Restoration of wt-p53 expression with depletion of mut-p53, which avoids the adverse effects of heterotetramer in cancer cells, would be more effective than other strategies for targeting mut-p53 (**Figure 4**) [121]. It is an intriguing finding that suppression of glucosylceramide synthase (GCS) restores p53-dependent apoptosis in ovarian cancer cells expressing deletion-mutant p53 (6 amino acids in exon-5) [30]. Inhibition of GCS eliminates the oncogenic function of mut-p53 (R273H) in the epithelial-mesenchymal transition and induced pluripotency of colon cancer cells [29]. GCS converts ceramide into glucosylceramide and regulates the synthesis of glycosphingolipids, including Gb3 [152]. Suppression of GCS, by either silencing its expression or inhibiting its activity with PDMP and Genz667161, restores p53-dependent tumor suppression [29, 30, 80, 153]. It is ceramide that can restore the expression of wt-p53 via SRSF1-mediated RNA splicing in these deletion-mutant cancer cells [154]. Our further works indicate that N^6-methyladenosine (m^{6}A) catalyzed by methyltransferase like-3 (METTL3) at the mutant codon promotes the expression of mut-p53 (R273H) and its GOF by enhanced m^{6}A-mRNA splicing [155]. Decreased METTL3 expression by treatments with small interfering RNA (siRNA) or with neplanocin A (NPC) restored wt-p53 expression and function in suppressing tumor growth (**Table 2**) [155]. These clearly indicate that m^{6}A at the mutant codon of pre-mRNA determines the protein expression of mut-p53 (R273H). Interestingly, either the suppression of ceramide glycosylation with GCS inhibitors (PDMP, Genz667161) or the provision of cell-permeable ceramide (C6-ceramide, Cer-RUB nanomicelles) can restore p53-dependent functions in eliminating CSCs, reverse of drug resistance, and decrease of tumor growth of ovarian cancer and colon cancer cells carrying mut-p53 (R273H, R248Q) (**Table 2**) [29, 58, 80]. These are proof of concept for restoring wt-p53 expression and its tumor suppression to target cancers expressing mut-p53.

6. Conclusion

Recent progression in p53 and cancer studies has characterized the critical role played by GOF mut-p53 in cancer stemness and immune evasion. GOF mut-p53 can reprogram and dedifferentiate cancer cells or normal epithelial progenitors by overexpression of pluripotent factors and forward activate the downstream signaling pathways, thus promoting cancer stemness. Cancer cells expressing mut-p53 can remarkably deactivate NK cells or CD8+ T-cells so as sheltering tumors against immunosurveillance and immune attack. These situations could be clearly observed in tumors or cancer cells under cell stress, such as chemotherapy or radiation therapy, within mut-p53 is overexpressed. Altogether, targeting mut-p53 would be more effective means than others to eliminate cancer progression and recurrence. Discovery of small molecule drug restoring p53 function is showing increasing promise, even major challenges still remain and multiple clinical trials are attempted to bring such molecules into the clinic. It is realized that the cellular processes and underlying regulatory mechanisms for the expression and degradation of mut-p53 proteins are distinguished from those for wt-p53. Enhancing ubiquitination to degrade mut-p53 and modulating m6A methylation-RNA splicing to restore wt-p53 expression are emerged as feasible approaches for targeting cancers expressing mut-p53.

Specifically, targeting mut-p53 proteins and the oncogenic GOF is critically important for improving the outcomes of cancer treatments. Further understanding in how mut-p53 executes oncogenic GOF in cancer stemness and how mut-p53 regulates particular ligands of CSCs to modulate host immunosurveillance and immune response, would help us to discover combined approaches against CSCs of tumors expressing mut-p53. Understanding how ubiquitination and underlying signaling pathways to degrade mut-p53 proteins, rather than wt-p53 protein in cancer cells, would help to develop new compounds or FDA-approved drugs to more effectively restore p53-dependent tumor suppression. More importantly, understanding m6A methylation at mutant codon of p53 pre-mRNA and further alternative RNA splicing process and the underlying mechanisms would help us to selectively target mut-p53 and more effectively combat most cancers.

Conflicts of interest

YY Liu is a member of Scientific Advisory Board for Sanofi-Genzyme and Board of Director of Mycobacterium DX Research Lab, and no other authors have competing interests.

Funding

The present study was supported by an Institutional Development Award (IDeA) from the National Institute of General Medicine Sciences of the National Institutes of Health under grant number P20 GM103424–21 (to Y.Y.L.).

Author details

Mohammad Nurul Amin and Yong-Yu Liu*
School of Basic Pharmaceutical and Toxicological Sciences, University of Louisiana at Monroe, Monroe, Louisiana, United States of America

*Address all correspondence to: yliu@ulm.edu

References

[1] Chen J. The cell-cycle arrest and apoptotic functions of p53 in tumor initiation and progression. Cold Spring Harbor Perspectives in Medicine. 2016;**6**(3):a026104

[2] Koifman G, Shetzer Y, Eizenberger S, Solomon H, Rotkopf R, Molchadsky A, et al. A mutant p53-dependent embryonic stem cell gene signature is associated with augmented tumorigenesis of stem cells. Cancer Research. 2018;**78**(20):5833-5847

[3] Blagih J, Buck MD, Vousden KH. p53, cancer and the immune response. Journal of Cell Science. 2020;**133**(5):jcs237453

[4] Olivier M, Hollstein M, Hainaut P. TP53 mutations in human cancers: Origins, consequences, and clinical use. Cold Spring Harbor Perspectives in Biology. 2010;**2**(1):a001008

[5] Joerger AC, Fersht AR. The tumor suppressor p53: From structures to drug discovery. Cold Spring Harbor Perspectives in Biology. 2010;**2**(6):a000919

[6] Freed-Pastor WA, Prives C. Mutant p53: One name, many proteins. Genes & Development. 2012;**26**(12):1268-1286

[7] Sabapathy K, Lane DP. Therapeutic targeting of p53: All mutants are equal, but some mutants are more equal than others. Nature Reviews. Clinical Oncology. 2018;**15**(1):13-30

[8] Brosh R, Rotter V. When mutants gain new powers: News from the mutant p53 field. Nature Reviews Cancer. 2009;**9**(10):701-713

[9] Oren M, Rotter V. Mutant p53 gain-of-function in cancer. Cold Spring Harbor Perspectives in Biology. 2010;**2**(2):a001107

[10] Aschauer L, Muller PA. Novel targets and interaction partners of mutant p53 gain-of-function. Biochemical Society Transactions. 2016;**44**(2):460-466

[11] Donghi R, Longoni A, Pilotti S, Michieli P, Della Porta G, Pierotti MA. Gene p53 mutations are restricted to poorly differentiated and undifferentiated carcinomas of the thyroid gland. The Journal of Clinical Investigation. 1993;**91**(4):1753-1760

[12] Robles AI, Harris CC. Clinical outcomes and correlates of TP53 mutations and cancer. Cold Spring Harbor Perspectives in Biology. 2010;**2**(3):a001016

[13] Sarig R, Rivlin N, Brosh R, Bornstein C, Kamer I, Ezra O, et al. Mutant p53 facilitates somatic cell reprogramming and augments the malignant potential of reprogrammed cells. The Journal of Experimental Medicine. 2010;**207**(10):2127-2140

[14] Uddin MB, Roy KR, Hill RA, Roy SC, Gu X, Li L, et al. p53 missense mutant G242A subverts natural killer cells in sheltering mouse breast cancer cells against immune rejection. Experimental Cell Research. 2022;**417**(1):113210

[15] Vousden KH, Prives C. Blinded by the light: The growing complexity of p53. Cell. 2009;**137**(3):413-431

[16] Sakamoto H, Lewis MS, Kodama H, Appella E, Sakaguchi K. Specific sequences from the carboxyl terminus of human p53 gene product form anti-parallel tetramers in solution. Proceedings of the National Academy of

Sciences of the United States of America. 1994;**91**(19):8974-8978

[17] Fischer M. Census and evaluation of p53 target genes. Oncogene. 2017;**36**(28):3943-3956

[18] Cho Y, Gorina S, Jeffrey PD, Pavletich NP. Crystal structure of a p53 tumor suppressor-DNA complex: Understanding tumorigenic mutations. Science. 1994;**265**(5170):346-355

[19] Wang Y, Rosengarth A, Luecke H. Structure of the human p53 core domain in the absence of DNA. Acta Crystallographica. Section D, Biological Crystallography. 2007;**63**(Pt 3):276-281

[20] Ang HC, Joerger AC, Mayer S, Fersht AR. Effects of common cancer mutations on stability and DNA binding of full-length p53 compared with isolated core domains. The Journal of Biological Chemistry. 2006;**281**(31):21934-21941

[21] Joerger AC, Ang HC, Fersht AR. Structural basis for understanding oncogenic p53 mutations and designing rescue drugs. Proceedings of the National Academy of Sciences of the United States of America. 2006;**103**(41):15056-15061

[22] Hassin O, Oren M. Drugging p53 in cancer: One protein, many targets. Nature Reviews. Drug Discovery. 2023;**22**(2):127-144

[23] Lee MK, Teoh WW, Phang BH, Tong WM, Wang ZQ, Sabapathy K. Cell-type, dose, and mutation-type specificity dictate mutant p53 functions *in vivo*. Cancer Cell. 2012;**22**(6):751-764

[24] Phang BH, Othman R, Bougeard G, Chia RH, Frebourg T, Tang CL, et al. Amino-terminal p53 mutations lead to expression of apoptosis proficient p47 and prognosticate better survival, but predispose to tumorigenesis. Proceedings of the National Academy of Sciences of the United States of America. 2015;**112**(46):E6349-E6358

[25] Hollstein M, Sidransky D, Vogelstein B, Harris CC. p53 mutations in human cancers. Science. 1991;**253**(5015):49-53

[26] Leroy B, Anderson M, Soussi T. TP53 mutations in human cancer: Database reassessment and prospects for the next decade. Human Mutation. 2014;**35**(6):672-688

[27] Muller PA, Vousden KH. Mutant p53 in cancer: New functions and therapeutic opportunities. Cancer Cell. 2014;**25**(3):304-317

[28] Muller PA, Caswell PT, Doyle B, Iwanicki MP, Tan EH, Karim S, et al. Mutant p53 drives invasion by promoting integrin recycling. Cell. 2009;**139**(7):1327-1341

[29] Hosain SB, Khiste SK, Uddin MB, Vorubindi V, Ingram C, Zhang S, et al. Inhibition of glucosylceramide synthase eliminates the oncogenic function of p53 R273H mutant in the epithelial-mesenchymal transition and induced pluripotency of colon cancer cells. Oncotarget. 2016;**7**(37):60575-60592

[30] Liu YY, Patwardhan GA, Bhinge K, Gupta V, Gu X, Jazwinski SM. Suppression of glucosylceramide synthase restores p53-dependent apoptosis in mutant p53 cancer cells. Cancer Research. 2011;**71**(6):2276-2285

[31] Chen X, Zhang T, Su W, Dou Z, Zhao D, Jin X, et al. Mutant p53 in cancer: From molecular mechanism to therapeutic modulation. Cell Death & Disease. 2022;**13**(11):974

[32] Chasov V, Mirgayazova R, Zmievskaya E, Khadiullina R,

Valiullina A, Stephenson Clarke J, et al. Key players in the mutant p53 team: Small molecules, gene editing, immunotherapy. Frontiers in Oncology. 2020;**10**:1460

[33] Pfister NT, Prives C. Transcriptional regulation by wild-type and cancer-related mutant forms of p53. Cold Spring Harbor Perspectives in Medicine. 2017;**7**(2):a026054

[34] Di Agostino S, Strano S, Emiliozzi V, Zerbini V, Mottolese M, Sacchi A, et al. Gain of function of mutant p53: The mutant p53/NF-Y protein complex reveals an aberrant transcriptional mechanism of cell cycle regulation. Cancer Cell. 2006;**10**(3):191-202

[35] Deppert W, Gohler T, Koga H, Kim E. Mutant p53: "gain of function" through perturbation of nuclear structure and function? Journal of Cellular Biochemistry. Supplement. 2000; **Suppl 35**:115-122

[36] Zhang J, Sun W, Kong X, Zhang Y, Yang HJ, Ren C, et al. Mutant p53 antagonizes p63/p73-mediated tumor suppression via Notch1. Proceedings of the National Academy of Sciences of the United States of America. 2019;**116**(48):24259-24267

[37] Morselli E, Tasdemir E, Maiuri MC, Galluzzi L, Kepp O, Criollo A, et al. Mutant p53 protein localized in the cytoplasm inhibits autophagy. Cell Cycle. 2008;**7**(19):3056-3061

[38] Duffy MJ, Synnott NC, Crown J. Mutant p53 in breast cancer: Potential as a therapeutic target and biomarker. Breast Cancer Research and Treatment. 2018;**170**(2):213-219

[39] Ghatak D, Das Ghosh D, Roychoudhury S. Cancer stemness: p53 at the wheel. Frontiers in Oncology. 2020;**10**:604124

[40] Takahashi K, Tanabe K, Ohnuki M, Narita M, Ichisaka T, Tomoda K, et al. Induction of pluripotent stem cells from adult human fibroblasts by defined factors. Cell. 2007;**131**(5):861-872

[41] Zhao Y, Yin X, Qin H, Zhu F, Liu H, Yang W, et al. Two supporting factors greatly improve the efficiency of human iPSC generation. Cell Stem Cell. 2008;**3**(5):475-479

[42] Kawamura T, Suzuki J, Wang YV, Menendez S, Morera LB, Raya A, et al. Linking the p53 tumour suppressor pathway to somatic cell reprogramming. Nature. 2009;**460**(7259):1140-1144

[43] Wang J, He Q, Han C, Gu H, Jin L, Li Q, et al. p53-facilitated miR-199a-3p regulates somatic cell reprogramming. Stem Cells. 2012;**30**(7):1405-1413

[44] Escoll M, Gargini R, Cuadrado A, Anton IM, Wandosell F. Mutant p53 oncogenic functions in cancer stem cells are regulated by WIP through YAP/TAZ. Oncogene. 2017;**36**(25):3515-3527

[45] Solomon H, Dinowitz N, Pateras IS, Cooks T, Shetzer Y, Molchadsky A, et al. Mutant p53 gain of function underlies high expression levels of colorectal cancer stem cells markers. Oncogene. 2018;**37**(12):1669-1684

[46] Alcantara Llaguno S, Chen J, Kwon CH, Jackson EL, Li Y, Burns DK, et al. Malignant astrocytomas originate from neural stem/progenitor cells in a somatic tumor suppressor mouse model. Cancer Cell. 2009;**15**(1):45-56

[47] Shetzer Y, Molchadsky A, Rotter V. Oncogenic mutant p53 gain of function nourishes the vicious cycle of tumor development and cancer stem-cell formation. Cold Spring Harbor Perspectives in Medicine. 2016;**6**(10):a026203

[48] Zhao Y, Li Y, Sheng J, Wu F, Li K, Huang R, et al. P53-R273H mutation enhances colorectal cancer stemness through regulating specific lncRNAs. Journal of Experimental & Clinical Cancer Research. 2019;**38**(1):379

[49] Ben-Porath I, Thomson MW, Carey VJ, Ge R, Bell GW, Regev A, et al. An embryonic stem cell-like gene expression signature in poorly differentiated aggressive human tumors. Nature Genetics. 2008;**40**(5):499-507

[50] Grespi F, Landre V, Molchadsky A, Di Daniele N, Marsella LT, Melino G, et al. Differential regulated microRNA by wild type and mutant p53 in induced pluripotent stem cells. Cell Death & Disease. 2016;**7**(12):e2567

[51] Sorrentino G, Ruggeri N, Specchia V, Cordenonsi M, Mano M, Dupont S, et al. Metabolic control of YAP and TAZ by the mevalonate pathway. Nature Cell Biology. 2014;**16**(4):357-366

[52] Chaffer CL, Weinberg RA. A perspective on cancer cell metastasis. Science. 2011;**331**(6024):1559-1564

[53] Nieto MA. Epithelial plasticity: A common theme in embryonic and cancer cells. Science. 2013;**342**(6159):1234850

[54] Thiery JP, Acloque H, Huang RY, Nieto MA. Epithelial-mesenchymal transitions in development and disease. Cell. 2009;**139**(5):871-890

[55] Peinado H, Olmeda D, Cano A. Snail, Zeb and bHLH factors in tumour progression: An alliance against the epithelial phenotype? Nature Reviews Cancer. 2007;**7**(6):415-428

[56] Ocana OH, Corcoles R, Fabra A, Moreno-Bueno G, Acloque H, Vega S, et al. Metastatic colonization requires the repression of the epithelial-mesenchymal transition inducer Prrx1. Cancer Cell. 2012;**22**(6):709-724

[57] Brabletz T, Jung A, Spaderna S, Hlubek F, Kirchner T. Opinion: Migrating cancer stem cells—An integrated concept of malignant tumour progression. Nature Reviews Cancer. 2005;**5**(9):744-749

[58] Khiste SK, Liu Z, Roy KR, Uddin MB, Hosain SB, Gu X, et al. Ceramide-rubusoside nanomicelles, a potential therapeutic approach to target cancers carrying p53 missense mutations. Molecular Cancer Therapeutics. 2020;**19**(2):564-574

[59] Chang CJ, Chao CH, Xia W, Yang JY, Xiong Y, Li CW, et al. p53 regulates epithelial-mesenchymal transition and stem cell properties through modulating miRNAs. Nature Cell Biology. 2011;**13**(3):317-323

[60] Brabletz S, Bajdak K, Meidhof S, Burk U, Niedermann G, Firat E, et al. The ZEB1/miR-200 feedback loop controls Notch signalling in cancer cells. The EMBO Journal. 2011;**30**(4):770-782

[61] Shimono Y, Zabala M, Cho RW, Lobo N, Dalerba P, Qian D, et al. Downregulation of miRNA-200c links breast cancer stem cells with normal stem cells. Cell. 2009;**138**(3):592-603

[62] Pinho AV, Rooman I, Real FX. p53-dependent regulation of growth, epithelial-mesenchymal transition and stemness in normal pancreatic epithelial cells. Cell Cycle. 2011;**10**(8):1312-1321

[63] Singh SK, Chen NM, Hessmann E, Siveke J, Lahmann M, Singh G, et al. Antithetical NFATc1-Sox2 and p53-miR200 signaling networks govern pancreatic cancer cell plasticity. The EMBO Journal. 2015;**34**(4):517-530

[64] Ren D, Wang M, Guo W, Zhao X, Tu X, Huang S, et al. Wild-type p53

suppresses the epithelial-mesenchymal transition and stemness in PC-3 prostate cancer cells by modulating miR-145. International Journal of Oncology. 2013;**42**(4):1473-1481

[65] Dong P, Karaayvaz M, Jia N, Kaneuchi M, Hamada J, Watari H, et al. Mutant p53 gain-of-function induces epithelial-mesenchymal transition through modulation of the miR-130b-ZEB1 axis. Oncogene. 2013;**32**(27):3286-3295

[66] Begicevic RR, Falasca M. ABC transporters in cancer stem cells: Beyond chemoresistance. International Journal of Molecular Sciences. 2017;**18**(11):2362

[67] Wang X, Wu X, Wang C, Zhang W, Ouyang Y, Yu Y, et al. Transcriptional suppression of breast cancer resistance protein (BCRP) by wild-type p53 through the NF-kappaB pathway in MCF-7 cells. FEBS Letters. 2010;**584**(15):3392-3397

[68] Chin KV, Ueda K, Pastan I, Gottesman MM. Modulation of activity of the promoter of the human MDR1 gene by Ras and p53. Science. 1992;**255**(5043):459-462

[69] Linn SC, Honkoop AH, Hoekman K, van der Valk P, Pinedo HM, Giaccone G. p53 and P-glycoprotein are often co-expressed and are associated with poor prognosis in breast cancer. British Journal of Cancer. 1996;**74**(1):63-68

[70] Ralhan R, Swain RK, Agarwal S, Kaur J, Nath N, Sarkar G, et al. P-glycoprotein is positively correlated with p53 in human oral pre-malignant and malignant lesions and is associated with poor prognosis. International Journal of Cancer. 1999;**84**(1):80-85

[71] Zhou S, Schuetz JD, Bunting KD, Colapietro AM, Sampath J, Morris JJ, et al. The ABC transporter Bcrp1/ABCG2 is expressed in a wide variety of stem cells and is a molecular determinant of the side-population phenotype. Nature Medicine. 2001;**7**(9):1028-1034

[72] Alam SK, Yadav VK, Bajaj S, Datta A, Dutta SK, Bhattacharyya M, et al. DNA damage-induced ephrin-B2 reverse signaling promotes chemoresistance and drives EMT in colorectal carcinoma harboring mutant p53. Cell Death and Differentiation. 2016;**23**(4):707-722

[73] Zhou X, Hao Q, Lu H. Mutant p53 in cancer therapy-the barrier or the path. Journal of Molecular Cell Biology. 2019;**11**(4):293-305

[74] Wang YH, Scadden DT. Harnessing the apoptotic programs in cancer stem-like cells. EMBO Reports. 2015;**16**(9):1084-1098

[75] Schulz A, Meyer F, Dubrovska A, Borgmann K. Cancer stem cells and radioresistance: DNA repair and beyond. Cancers (Basel). 2019;**11**(6):862

[76] Shetzer Y, Kagan S, Koifman G, Sarig R, Kogan-Sakin I, Charni M, et al. The onset of p53 loss of heterozygosity is differentially induced in various stem cell types and may involve the loss of either allele. Cell Death and Differentiation. 2014;**21**(9):1419-1431

[77] Januchowski R, Wojtowicz K, Zabel M. The role of aldehyde dehydrogenase (ALDH) in cancer drug resistance. Biomedicine & Pharmacotherapy. 2013;**67**(7):669-680

[78] Datta A, Das P, Dey S, Ghuwalewala S, Ghatak D, Alam SK, et al. Genome-wide small RNA sequencing identifies microRNAs deregulated in non-small cell lung carcinoma harboring gain-of-function mutant p53. Genes (Basel). 2019;**10**(11):852

[79] Gupta V, Bhinge KN, Hosain SB, Xiong K, Gu X, Shi R, et al. Ceramide glycosylation by glucosylceramide synthase selectively maintains the properties of breast cancer stem cells. The Journal of Biological Chemistry. 2012;**287**(44):37195-37205

[80] Roy KR, Uddin MB, Roy SC, Hill RA, Marshall J, Li YT, et al. Gb3-cSrc complex in glycosphingolipid-enriched microdomains contributes to the expression of p53 mutant protein and cancer drug resistance via beta-catenin-activated RNA methylation. FASEB Bioadvances. 2020;**2**(11):653-667

[81] Liu YY, Gupta V, Patwardhan GA, Bhinge K, Zhao Y, Bao J, et al. Glucosylceramide synthase upregulates MDR1 expression in the regulation of cancer drug resistance through cSrc and beta-catenin signaling. Molecular Cancer. 2010;**9**:145

[82] Carlsen L, Zhang S, Tian X, De La Cruz A, George A, Arnoff TE, et al. The role of p53 in anti-tumor immunity and response to immunotherapy. Frontiers in Molecular Biosciences. 2023;**10**:1148389

[83] Zhang C, Ni J, Fan W, Hou J. Nutlin-3 promotes TRAIL-induced liver cancer cells apoptosis by activating p53 to inhibit bcl-2 and surviving expression. Annals of Clinical and Laboratory Science. 2022;**52**(4):601-610

[84] Soussi T. p53 alterations in human cancer: More questions than answers. Oncogene. 2007;**26**(15):2145-2156

[85] Taura M, Eguma A, Suico MA, Shuto T, Koga T, Komatsu K, et al. p53 regulates toll-like receptor 3 expression and function in human epithelial cell lines. Molecular and Cellular Biology. 2008;**28**(21):6557-6567

[86] Mori T, Anazawa Y, Iiizumi M, Fukuda S, Nakamura Y, Arakawa H. Identification of the interferon regulatory factor 5 gene (IRF-5) as a direct target for p53. Oncogene. 2002;**21**(18):2914-2918

[87] Takahashi T, Tanaka M, Brannan CI, Jenkins NA, Copeland NG, Suda T, et al. Generalized lymphoproliferative disease in mice, caused by a point mutation in the Fas ligand. Cell. 1994;**76**(6):969-976

[88] Hingorani R, Bi B, Dao T, Bae Y, Matsuzawa A, Crispe IN. CD95/Fas signaling in T lymphocytes induces the cell cycle control protein p21cip-1/WAF-1, which promotes apoptosis. Journal of Immunology. 2000;**164**(8):4032-4036

[89] Lu B, Nakamura T, Inouye K, Li J, Tang Y, Lundback P, et al. Novel role of PKR in inflammasome activation and HMGB1 release. Nature. 2012;**488**(7413):670-674

[90] Yoon CH, Lee ES, Lim DS, Bae YS. PKR, a p53 target gene, plays a crucial role in the tumor-suppressor function of p53. Proceedings of the National Academy of Sciences of the United States of America. 2009;**106**(19):7852-7857

[91] Textor S, Fiegler N, Arnold A, Porgador A, Hofmann TG, Cerwenka A. Human NK cells are alerted to induction of p53 in cancer cells by upregulation of the NKG2D ligands ULBP1 and ULBP2. Cancer Research. 2011;**71**(18):5998-6009

[92] Fei L, Ren X, Yu H, Zhan Y. Targeting the CCL2/CCR2 Axis in cancer immunotherapy: One stone, three birds? Frontiers in Immunology. 2021;**12**:771210

[93] Ham SW, Jeon HY, Jin X, Kim EJ, Kim JK, Shin YJ, et al. TP53 gain-of-function mutation promotes inflammation in glioblastoma. Cell Death and Differentiation. 2019;**26**(3):409-425

[94] Thomas L. On immunosurveillance in human cancer. The Yale

Journal of Biology and Medicine. 1982;**55**(3-4):329-333

[95] Baudot AD, Ryan KM. p53 and tumor surveillance: Killer finds way to recruit assassins. Cell Cycle. 2011;**10**(22):3818

[96] Smyth MJ, Godfrey DI, Trapani JA. A fresh look at tumor immunosurveillance and immunotherapy. Nature Immunology. 2001;**2**(4):293-299

[97] Diefenbach A, Raulet DH. The innate immune response to tumors and its role in the induction of T-cell immunity. Immunological Reviews. 2002;**188**:9-21

[98] Vogler M, Shanmugalingam S, Sarchen V, Reindl LM, Greze V, Buchinger L, et al. Unleashing the power of NK cells in anticancer immunotherapy. Journal of Molecular Medicine (Berlin, Germany). 2022;**100**(3):337-349

[99] Lopez-Soto A, Huergo-Zapico L, Acebes-Huerta A, Villa-Alvarez M, Gonzalez S. NKG2D signaling in cancer immunosurveillance. International Journal of Cancer. 2015;**136**(8):1741-1750

[100] Belkahla S, Brualla JM, Fayd'herbe de Maudave A, Falvo P, Allende-Vega N, Constantinides M, et al. The metabolism of cells regulates their sensitivity to NK cells depending on p53 status. Scientific Reports. 2022;**12**(1):3234

[101] Chollat-Namy M, Ben Safta-Saadoun T, Haferssas D, Meurice G, Chouaib S, Thiery J. The pharmalogical reactivation of p53 function improves breast tumor cell lysis by granzyme B and NK cells through induction of autophagy. Cell Death & Disease. 2019;**10**(10):695

[102] McCarty TM, Liu X, Sun JY, Peralta EA, Diamond DJ, Ellenhorn JD. Targeting p53 for adoptive T-cell immunotherapy. Cancer Research. 1998;**58**(12):2601-2605

[103] Coronella JA, Telleman P, Kingsbury GA, Truong TD, Hays S, Junghans RP. Evidence for an antigen-driven humoral immune response in medullary ductal breast cancer. Cancer Research. 2001;**61**(21):7889-7899

[104] Deniger DC, Pasetto A, Robbins PF, Gartner JJ, Prickett TD, Paria BC, et al. T-cell responses to TP53 "hotspot" mutations and unique neoantigens expressed by human ovarian cancers. Clinical Cancer Research. 2018;**24**(22):5562-5573

[105] Dong ZY, Zhong WZ, Zhang XC, Su J, Xie Z, Liu SY, et al. Potential predictive value of TP53 and KRAS mutation status for response to PD-1 blockade immunotherapy in lung adenocarcinoma. Clinical Cancer Research. 2017;**23**(12):3012-3024

[106] Sharpe AH, Pauken KE. The diverse functions of the PD1 inhibitory pathway. Nature Reviews. Immunology. 2018;**18**(3):153-167

[107] Freeman GJ, Long AJ, Iwai Y, Bourque K, Chernova T, Nishimura H, et al. Engagement of the PD-1 immunoinhibitory receptor by a novel B7 family member leads to negative regulation of lymphocyte activation. The Journal of Experimental Medicine. 2000;**192**(7):1027-1034

[108] Ai L, Xu A, Xu J. Roles of PD-1/PD-L1 pathway: Signaling, cancer, and beyond. Advances in Experimental Medicine and Biology. 2020;**1248**:33-59

[109] Cortez MA, Ivan C, Valdecanas D, Wang X, Peltier HJ, Ye Y, et al. PDL1 regulation by p53 via miR-34. Journal of the National Cancer Institute. 2016;**108**(1):djv303

[110] Hao F, Gu L, Zhong D. TP53 mutation mapping in advanced non-small cell lung cancer: A Real-world retrospective cohort study. Current Oncology. 2022;**29**(10):7411-7419

[111] Chamoto K, Hatae R, Honjo T. Current issues and perspectives in PD-1 blockade cancer immunotherapy. International Journal of Clinical Oncology. 2020;**25**(5):790-800

[112] Kerkar SP, Restifo NP. Cellular constituents of immune escape within the tumor microenvironment. Cancer Research. 2012;**72**(13):3125-3130

[113] DiLillo DJ, Yanaba K, Tedder TF. B cells are required for optimal CD4+ and CD8+ T cell tumor immunity: Therapeutic B cell depletion enhances B16 melanoma growth in mice. Journal of Immunology. 2010;**184**(7):4006-4016

[114] Togashi Y, Shitara K, Nishikawa H. Regulatory T cells in cancer immunosuppression—Implications for anticancer therapy. Nature Reviews. Clinical Oncology. 2019;**16**(6):356-371

[115] Cassetta L, Pollard JW. Targeting macrophages: Therapeutic approaches in cancer. Nature Reviews. Drug Discovery. 2018;**17**(12):887-904

[116] Kitamura T, Doughty-Shenton D, Cassetta L, Fragkogianni S, Brownlie D, Kato Y, et al. Monocytes differentiate to immune suppressive precursors of metastasis-associated macrophages in mouse models of metastatic breast cancer. Frontiers in Immunology. 2017;**8**:2004

[117] Wang HQ, Mulford IJ, Sharp F, Liang J, Kurtulus S, Trabucco G, et al. Inhibition of MDM2 promotes antitumor responses in p53 wild-type cancer cells through their interaction with the immune and stromal microenvironment. Cancer Research. 2021;**81**(11):3079-3091

[118] Ji L, Xu J, Liu J, Amjad A, Zhang K, Liu Q, et al. Mutant p53 promotes tumor cell malignancy by both positive and negative regulation of the transforming growth factor beta (TGF-beta) pathway. The Journal of Biological Chemistry. 2015;**290**(18):11729-11740

[119] Zhong Y, Macgregor-Das A, SaundersT,WhittleMC,Makohon-MooreA, Kohutek ZA, et al. Mutant p53 together with TGFbeta signaling influence organ-specific hematogenous colonization patterns of pancreatic cancer. Clinical Cancer Research. 2017;**23**(6):1607-1620

[120] Guo G, Marrero L, Rodriguez P, Del Valle L, Ochoa A, Cui Y. Trp53 inactivation in the tumor microenvironment promotes tumor progression by expanding the immunosuppressive lymphoid-like stromal network. Cancer Research. 2013;**73**(6):1668-1675

[121] Liu YY. Resuscitating wild-type p53 expression by disrupting ceramide glycosylation: A novel approach to target mutant p53 tumors. Cancer Research. 2011;**71**(20):6295-6299

[122] Nishikawa S, Iwakuma T. Drugs targeting p53 mutations with FDA approval and in clinical trials. Cancers (Basel). 2023;**15**(2):429

[123] Wiman KG. Pharmacological reactivation of mutant p53: From protein structure to the cancer patient. Oncogene. 2010;**29**(30):4245-4252

[124] Bykov VJ, Zhang Q, Zhang M, Ceder S, Abrahmsen L, Wiman KG. Targeting of mutant p53 and the cellular redox balance by APR-246 as a strategy for efficient cancer therapy. Frontiers in Oncology. 2016;**6**:21

[125] Shen J, van den Bogaard EH, Kouwenhoven EN, Bykov VJ, Rinne T, Zhang Q, et al. APR-246/PRIMA-1(MET) rescues epidermal differentiation in skin keratinocytes derived from EEC syndrome patients with p63 mutations. Proceedings of the National Academy of Sciences of the United States of America. 2013;**110**(6):2157-2162

[126] Sallman DA, DeZern AE, Garcia-Manero G, Steensma DP, Roboz GJ, Sekeres MA, et al. Eprenetapopt (APR-246) and azacitidine in TP53-mutant myelodysplastic syndromes. Journal of Clinical Oncology. 2021;**39**(14):1584-1594

[127] Palanikumar L, Karpauskaite L, Al-Sayegh M, Chehade I, Alam M, Hassan S, et al. Protein mimetic amyloid inhibitor potently abrogates cancer-associated mutant p53 aggregation and restores tumor suppressor function. Nature Communications. 2021;**12**(1):3962

[128] Soragni A, Janzen DM, Johnson LM, Lindgren AG, Thai-Quynh Nguyen A, Tiourin E, et al. A designed inhibitor of p53 aggregation rescues p53 tumor suppression in ovarian carcinomas. Cancer Cell. 2016;**29**(1):90-103

[129] Boeckler FM, Joerger AC, Jaggi G, Rutherford TJ, Veprintsev DB, Fersht AR. Targeted rescue of a destabilized mutant of p53 by an in silico screened drug. Proceedings of the National Academy of Sciences of the United States of America. 2008;**105**(30):10360-10365

[130] Liu X, Wilcken R, Joerger AC, Chuckowree IS, Amin J, Spencer J, et al. Small molecule induced reactivation of mutant p53 in cancer cells. Nucleic Acids Research. 2013;**41**(12): 6034-6044

[131] Glimmers of Hope for targeting p53. Cancer Discovery. 2022;**12**(8):OF5

[132] Guiley KZ, Shokat KM. A small molecule reacts with the p53 somatic mutant Y220C to rescue wild-type thermal stability. Cancer Discovery. 2023;**13**(1):56-69

[133] Yu X, Vazquez A, Levine AJ, Carpizo DR. Allele-specific p53 mutant reactivation. Cancer Cell. 2012;**21**(5):614-625

[134] Blanden AR, Yu X, Blayney AJ, Demas C, Ha JH, Liu Y, et al. Zinc shapes the folding landscape of p53 and establishes a pathway for reactivating structurally diverse cancer mutants. eLife. 2020;**9**:e61487

[135] Salim KY, Maleki Vareki S, Danter WR, Koropatnick J. COTI-2, a novel small molecule that is active against multiple human cancer cell lines *in vitro* and *in vivo*. Oncotarget. 2016;**7**(27):41363-41379

[136] Lindemann A, Patel AA, Silver NL, Tang L, Liu Z, Wang L, et al. COTI-2, a novel thiosemicarbazone derivative, exhibits antitumor activity in HNSCC through p53-dependent and -independent mechanisms. Clinical Cancer Research. 2019;**25**(18):5650-5662

[137] Chen S, Wu JL, Liang Y, Tang YG, Song HX, Wu LL, et al. Arsenic trioxide rescues structural p53 mutations through a cryptic allosteric site. Cancer Cell. 2021;**39**(2):225-39 e8

[138] Wang W, Rastinejad F, El-Deiry WS. Restoring p53-dependent tumor suppression. Cancer Biology & Therapy. 2003;**2**(sup1):54-62

[139] Issaeva N, Friedler A, Bozko P, Wiman KG, Fersht AR, Selivanova G. Rescue of mutants of the tumor suppressor p53 in cancer cells by a designed peptide.

Proceedings of the National Academy of Sciences of the United States of America. 2003;**100**(23):13303-13307

[140] Selivanova G, Iotsova V, Okan I, Fritsche M, Strom M, Groner B, et al. Restoration of the growth suppression function of mutant p53 by a synthetic peptide derived from the p53 C-terminal domain. Nature Medicine. 1997;**3**(6):632-638

[141] Friedler AHL, Veprintsev DB, Freund SMV, Rippin TM, Nikolova PV, et al. A peptide that binds and stabilizes p53 core domain: Chaperone strategy for rescue of oncogenic mutants. National Academy of Sciences of the United States of America. 2002;**99**(2):937-942

[142] Tal P, Eizenberger S, Cohen E, Goldfinger N, Pietrokovski S, Oren M, et al. Cancer therapeutic approach based on conformational stabilization of mutant p53 protein by small peptides. Oncotarget. 2016;**7**(11):11817-11837

[143] Mantovani F, Collavin L, Del Sal G. Mutant p53 as a guardian of the cancer cell. Cell Death and Differentiation. 2019;**26**(2):199-212

[144] Padmanabhan A, Candelaria N, Wong KK, Nikolai BC, Lonard DM, O'Malley BW, et al. USP15-dependent lysosomal pathway controls p53-R175H turnover in ovarian cancer cells. Nature Communications. 2018;**9**(1):1270

[145] Ingallina E, Sorrentino G, Bertolio R, Lisek K, Zannini A, Azzolin L, et al. Mechanical cues control mutant p53 stability through a mevalonate-RhoA axis. Nature Cell Biology. 2018;**20**(1):28-35

[146] Wang J, Zhao Q, Qi Q, Gu HY, Rong JJ, Mu R, et al. Gambogic acid-induced degradation of mutant p53 is mediated by proteasome and related to CHIP. Journal of Cellular Biochemistry. 2011;**112**(2):509-519

[147] Mori A, Lehmann S, O'Kelly J, Kumagai T, Desmond JC, Pervan M, et al. Capsaicin, a component of red peppers, inhibits the growth of androgen-independent, p53 mutant prostate cancer cells. Cancer Research. 2006;**66**(6):3222-3229

[148] Zhang S, Zhou L, El-Deiry WS. Small-molecule NSC59984 induces mutant p53 degradation through a ROS-ERK2-MDM2 Axis in cancer cells. Molecular Cancer Research. 2022;**20**(4):622-636

[149] Li D, Marchenko ND, Moll UM. SAHA shows preferential cytotoxicity in mutant p53 cancer cells by destabilizing mutant p53 through inhibition of the HDAC6-Hsp90 chaperone axis. Cell Death and Differentiation. 2011;**18**(12):1904-1913

[150] Alexandrova EM, Xu S, Moll UM. Ganetespib synergizes with cyclophosphamide to improve survival of mice with autochthonous tumors in a mutant p53-dependent manner. Cell Death & Disease. 2017;**8**(3):e2683

[151] Fu S, Hou MM, Naing A, Janku F, Hess K, Zinner R, et al. Phase I study of pazopanib and vorinostat: A therapeutic approach for inhibiting mutant p53-mediated angiogenesis and facilitating mutant p53 degradation. Annals of Oncology. 2015;**26**(5):1012-1018

[152] Liu YY, Hill RA, Li YT. Ceramide glycosylation catalyzed by glucosylceramide synthase and cancer drug resistance. Advances in Cancer Research. 2013;**117**:59-89

[153] Khiste SK, Hosain SB, Dong Y, Uddin MB, Roy KR, Hill RA, et al.

Incorporation of fluorescence ceramide-based HPLC assay for rapidly and efficiently assessing glucosylceramide synthase *in vivo*. Scientific Reports. 2017;7(1):2976

[154] Patwardhan GA, Hosain SB, Liu DX, Khiste SK, Zhao Y, Bielawski J, et al. Ceramide modulates pre-mRNA splicing to restore the expression of wild-type tumor suppressor p53 in deletion-mutant cancer cells. Biochimica et Biophysica Acta. 2014;**1841**(11):1571-1580

[155] Uddin MB, Roy KR, Hosain SB, Khiste SK, Hill RA, Jois SD, et al. An N(6)-methyladenosine at the transited codon 273 of p53 pre-mRNA promotes the expression of R273H mutant protein and drug resistance of cancer cells. Biochemical Pharmacology. 2019;**160**:134-145

Section 3

Molecular Diagnostics in Hematopathology

Chapter 5

Clonality Testing in the Diagnosis of Cutaneous T-Cell Lymphoma

Fernando Roncolato, Anna Gazzola, Claudia Mannu, Riccardo Donelli, Maryam Etebari, Mohsen Navari and Pier Paolo Piccaluga

Abstract

Cutaneous T-cell lymphomas (CTCL) are heterogeneous disorders including several different entities with variable morphology, phenotype, and clinical features. The diagnosis of CTCL is often challenging; the distinction between tumors and reactive, non-neoplastic conditions is sometimes elusive. Therefore, molecular testing for T-cell receptor gamma (TRG) clonality is often performed. In this study, we evaluated the accuracy of TRG testing protocol in 110 routinary cases and discussed the subject of clonality testing in light of novel technologies (namely next-generations sequencing advent). For TRG analysis, the BIOMED-2 protocol was adopted. Sensitivity, specificity, positive and negative predictive values were calculated using the Oxford CatMaker software following the Standards for Reporting of Diagnostic Accuracy Studies (STARD) requirements for diagnostic accuracy. We found that this approach was feasible in most cases (87%) despite the small sample dimensions and the fixation issues. In addition, we found that sensitivity and specificity were 90 and 84%, respectively; accordingly, positive predictive value (PPV) and negative predictive value (NPV) were 84 and 90%, respectively. Of note, the molecular test was somehow influential in 83% of cases, when histology and phenotyping were not conclusive. In conclusion, TRG analysis by BIOMED-2 protocols is feasible and effective in the routine diagnostics of CTCL. The integration of histological, phenotypical, molecular, and clinical data is mandatory for a correct diagnosis.

Keywords: T-cell receptor gamma, T-cell lymphoma, cutaneous T-cell lymphoma, BIOMED-2, clonality, diagnostic accuracy, evidence-based medicine, next-generation sequencing, molecular diagnostic, PCR

1. Introduction

Peripheral T-cell lymphomas (PTCLs) are clonal neoplasms deriving from mature T-lymphocytes at different stages of differentiation [1]. Clinical presentations are protean, and diagnosis involves a synthesis of clinical history and pathological data from morphological, immunophenotypic, cytogenetic, and molecular investigations. Based on such criteria, the recent WHO Classification of Tumors of Hematopoietic and Lymphoid Tissues codified many disease entities, identifying specified and not otherwise specified (NOS) forms, nodal and extranodal tumors [1]. Among the latter, cutaneous T-cell lymphomas (CTCL) are relatively common, including several distinct diseases [2]. The diagnosis of CTCL, as for other PTCLs, is challenging owing to the heterogeneous pathophysiology, complex taxonomy, and, especially, the lack of tumor-associated immunophenotypic or molecular markers. Furthermore, the clinical scenario becomes yet more complicated when the disease presents in the early phase or with the contemporaneous occurrence of a prominent reactive component overwhelming the malignant elements [2].

Nonetheless, importantly, the diagnosis of lymphoproliferative disease can benefit from the demonstration of clonality at a molecular level. Specifically, in the field of T-cell lymphomas/leukemias, the study of T-cell receptor gene (TCR) rearrangements has been used to assist in the determination of clonality for over two decades [3, 4]. The somatic assembly of TCR genes is an early event during T-cell development, occurring through a V(D)J recombination directed by site-specific recombinase (RAG1 and RAG2), which eventually leads to a diverse T-cell population [3, 5]. In 2003, the BIOMED-2 consortium established standardized protocols for multiplex PCR analysis, which improved the efficiency and reproducibility of clonality detection [6]. This protocol was validated by the BIOMED-2 group in 2007 in 188 cases of T-cell malignancy [7, 8]. Specifically, the combined analysis of TCR-gamma (TRG) and TCR-beta (TRB) led to sensitivity and specificity values above 90% [6–8].

Although the efficiency of BIOMED-2 protocols was defined, in both studies, the BIOMED-2 protocol was tested in a series of tissues with well-established histological diagnoses of T-cell malignancy, principally represented by fresh or frozen specimens [6–8]. By contrast, routine clinical diagnosis is predominantly based on formalin-fixed paraffin-embedded (FFPE) tissue blocks. FFPE blocks are convenient as they are small, easy to transport, and allow for retrospective analysis by immunohistochemistry and in situ hybridization (ISH/FISH). However, by comparison to fresh specimens, molecular analyses on FFPE blocks are more challenging owing principally to the more involved method required for extracting high-quality DNA. The interference of formalin fixation with DNA architecture and nucleoside fragmentation can lead to lower amplification yield and potentially a lower diagnostic utility [9, 10]. In this regard, small specimens, particularly those such as skin biopsies, represent a significant challenge in molecular testing. Practically, the two steps (TRG and TRB) can be performed simultaneously to save time, or consecutively, to save resources. In fact, the latter solution may allow the analysis to be limited to TRG in most instances. Noteworthy is that a formal, evidence-based diagnostic accuracy study has never been performed in this setting.

In order to properly quantify this possibility, in this study we performed a diagnostic accuracy study based on a retrospective analysis of our experience with the BIOMED-2 TRG protocol in 110 skin specimens aiming to: [1] assess the feasibility of the protocol in non-selected consecutive FFPE cases included in the routine practice; [2] assess sensitivity, specificity, PPV and NPV of the test in detecting T-cell malignancies in FFPE tissues; and [3] determine the rate and clinical significance of clonal rearrangements in cases deemed to be reactive or non-diagnosable by histopathological and morphological assessment ("TRG monoclonality of uncertain significance").

Furthermore, we discuss the issue of clonality testing in light of the new available technologies, namely next-generation sequencing (NGS).

2. Materials and methods

2.1 Case selection

We included in this study 110 consecutive cases received over 3 years at the Molecular Pathology Laboratory, Hematopathology Unit, Institute of Hematology and Medical Oncology "L. & A. Seràgnoli." Histological samples were classified by at least two experienced hematopathologists who were blinded to the TRG result using the morphological, immunohistochemical, and cytogenetic criteria of the most updated WHO classification [2]. The diagnoses were as follows: PTCL/CTCL (N = 48; 49%), B-cell lymphomas (N = 8; 8%), and inflammatory disorders (N = 42, 43%). We also studied a further 12 cases for which a definitive diagnosis was not reached based on morphology, phenotype, or clinical presentation, and where the differential between tumor and inflammatory disorders was not resolved. For all cases, a minimum of 12 months of clinical follow-up from the last PCR study was available. Patients' characteristics are reported in **Table A1**.

All specimens were formalin-fixed and paraffin-embedded (FFPE) prior to PCR analysis.

Calculations of sensitivity (ST), specificity (SP), positive predictive value (PPV), and negative predictive value (NPV) were made by CATmaker software (Centre for Evidence-Based Medicine, Oxford University, http://www.cebm.net) using the blinded histopathological review as the reference test in our case series.

For the purposes of this analysis, a distinction was not drawn between primary cutaneous T-cell lymphomas and systemic lymphomas manifesting in the skin, as the analysis was designed to assess the capacity of the molecular investigation to detect any T-cell lymphoma in the skin. The STARD Statement for diagnostic accuracy studies was fulfilled (**Table A2**) [11].

The study design is summarized in **Figure 1**.

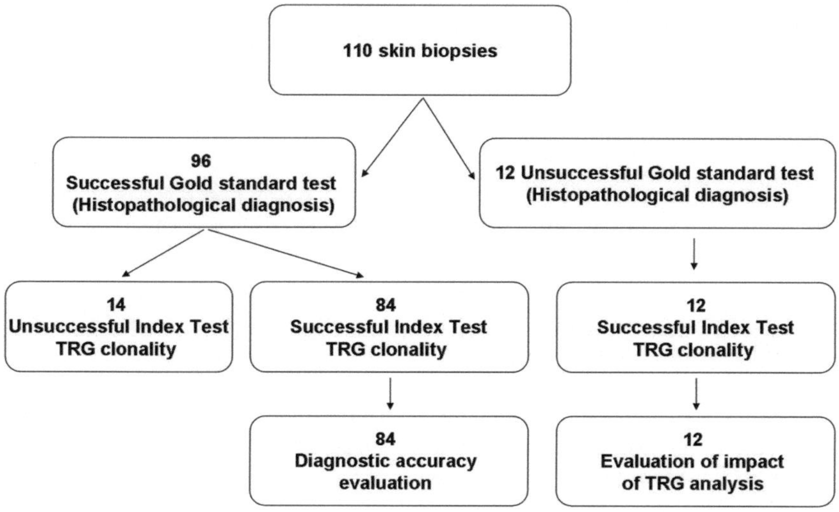

Figure 1.
Schematic representation of the diagnostic accuracy study design.

2.2 Molecular analysis

Molecular tests were performed and analyzed by at least two experienced molecular pathologists. Molecular testing was performed within 1 week of the histological evaluation. Histopathological evaluation and molecular tests were performed in a blinded manner.

Genomic DNA was extracted from paraffin-embedded tissue by using a Qiagen DNA mini kit according to the manufacturer's instructions. PLZF was studied as a control gene in order to verify the DNA integrity. PCR analysis of TRG rearrangement was executed using multiplex PCR tubes (BIOMED-2 Concerted Action) [6]. Amplification reactions were performed in an automated thermocycler (mastercycler Eppendorf) according to the BIOMED-2 multiplex PCR protocol [6]. Each 50-microliter PCR reaction included 100 ng of DNA, 10 pm of each primer, 0,2 mmol/L dNTP, 5 microliter of 10X Gold buffer, 1.5 mmol/L of MgCl2 and 1 U of Ampli-Taq Gold polymerase (Applied Biosystems). The cycling parameters were as follows: pre-activation for 7 minutes at 95°C, 35 cycles of denaturation (95°C for 30 sec), an annealing step (60°C for 30 sec), an extension step (72°C for 60 sec), finally 10 minutes of extension at 72°C. Each sample was evaluated using heteroduplex analysis and GeneScanning to determine polyclonal or monoclonal character.

2.2.1 Heteroduplex analysis

In order to allow the spontaneous formation of homoduplex or heteroduplex from DNA fragments, amplicons were denatured by heating (94°C for 5 min) and cooled at low temperatures (4°C for 1 hour). PCR products were then visualized by electrophoresis on polyacrylamide gels being separated according to their length and conformation. According to BIOMED-2 protocols, samples were defined as monoclonal when a single band was identified within a predictable size range and polyclonal when only a smear was detected [6]. This technique has a well-recognized detection limit of ~5% due to the frequency of polyclonal/reactive lymphocytes present in the tissue.

2.2.2 GeneScanning analysis

After amplification, 1 μ of PCR product with 0.5 μ of a standard molecular weight product (LIZ Applied Biosystems) was mixed with 12 μ of formamide to induce denaturation into single DNA strands (1 minute to 95C°). Subsequently, they were separated through a polymer capillary electrophoresis system and automatically detected by fluorescence reading with a laser system in an automatic DNA sequencer (ABI Prism 310 Applied Biosystems).

Tissue samples were considered to have a clonal T-cell population if 1 or 2 peaks of the amplified PCR product in question were obtained (monoclonal and biclonal/biallelic, respectively); detection of three to five peaks was counted as an oligoclonal result, while a Gaussian distribution of peaks was referred to as a polyclonal population [6]. The control gene minimum amplification requirement was 300 bps, and when this was not reached, or the target gene was not amplified, the sample was considered "not evaluable."

3. Results

A total of 110 case samples were interrogated using the BIOMED-2 protocol for TRG analysis. Fourteen cases did not have an evaluable molecular result (14/110, 12.7%), owing to failure to amplify either the target gene product or the control gene, and were then excluded from the final analysis. 96/110 samples (87.3%) could be evaluated and were included in the final analysis.

Of the specimens that allowed a clear and definitive histopathological diagnosis, 84/96 had an evaluable molecular result (87.5%).

Based on TRG analysis, there was evidence of clonal rearrangement in 42/84 (50%) of cases, oligoclonal in 3/84 (4%), and a polyclonal pattern was detected in 39/84 (46%) cases, respectively.

Mono/biclonality was detected in 36/47 (77%) of the CTCL cases, 2/8 (25%) of the B-NHL cases, and 4/42 (10%) of the inflammatory reactions.

The ST and SP of the molecular test in discriminating malignant T-cell lymphoproliferation vs. other conditions (including B-NHL and inflammatory reactions) were 90.0 and 84%, respectively. Accordingly, PPV and NPV were 84.0 and 90%, respectively (**Table 1**).

Target: Differential diagnosis CTCL vs. Other			
		Histopathological diagnosis	
		CTCL	**Other**
TRG	Clonal vs. Oligo-polyclonal	36	7
		4	37
	Parameter	**Value**	**95% CI**
	ST	90%	81–99
	SP	84%	73–95
	Pre-test probability	48%	37–58
	PPV	84%	73–95
	NPV	90%	81–99
	LR+	5.66	2.85 to 11.25
	LR-	0.12	0.05–0.30
ST = sensitivity			
SP = specificity			
PPV = positive predictive value			
NPV = negative predictive value			
LR + = likelyhood ratio positive			
LR- = likelyhood ratio negative			
CATmaker software (Centre for Evidence-Based Medicine, Oxford University, http://www.cebm.net).			

Table 1.
Calculation of sensitivity (ST), specificity (SP), positive predictive value (PPV) and negative predictive value (NPV), basing on the histopathological analysis taken as diagnostic gold standard.

	Number of cases	Diagnosis	
		TCL	Non-TCL
TRG			
Monoclonal	4	3 (75%)	1 (25%)
polyclonal/oligoclonal	8	1/0 (12.5%)	4/3 (87.5%)

Table 2.
Impact of the molecular result in cases with undefined diagnosis.

Lymphoma type	Number of cases	Evidence of clonality (number of cases)	Evidence of clonality (percentage of cases)
Mycosis fungoides	18	16	88.89
PTCL/NOS	15	13	86.67
CTCL/NOS	5	5	100.00
T-LGL	1	1	100.00
ALCL, ALK-	1	1	100.00
Total	**40**	**36**	**90.00**

Table 3.
TRG *clonality according to lymphoma histotype.*

Subsequently, we evaluated the 12 cases for which a conclusive diagnosis was not made by histopathological review. Specifically, we detected monoclonal rearrangement in 4/12 cases, oligoclonal rearrangement in 3/12, and 5/12 presented with a polyclonal pattern. In the monoclonal group, 3/4 ultimately received a diagnosis of CTCL after the integration of all diagnostic procedures. Among oligoclonal/polyclonal cases, 1 was eventually diagnosed as CTCL, while the remaining 8 were diagnosed as inflammatory conditions. Overall, based on such data, the molecular result was influential on the final diagnosis in 10/12 (83%) of the cases when morphology, immunophenotype, and molecular data were integrated (**Table 2**).

We then evaluated the molecular results in PTCLs according to the histological subtype in order to assess whether specific diseases are differentially associated with different degrees of clonality at TRG analysis (**Table 3**). We found that there were in fact no significant differences recorded, with TRG successful in detecting clonal rearrangements in the majority of cases (**Table 4**).

Finally, we investigated whether cases presenting evidence of clonal rearrangement but without clear evidence of PTCL had a higher risk of developing T-cell malignancies in the following months. Specifically, among cases that received a final diagnosis of inflammatory disorder, 4/42 (9.5%) demonstrated TRG clonality. These particular patients largely fulfilled the minimum requested follow-up of 12 months, the mean follow-up period being 35 months (range 33–36 months). Patients were then monitored by means of outpatient clinical follow-up and/or phone contact with the treating physician. No patient received a diagnosis of a T-cell neoplasm during the study period, to the best of our knowledge.

Matched histological and molecular analysis results are detailed in **Table A3**.

	Sample	Tissue	Efficiency (% of evaluable cases)	Probe	ST (%)	SP (%)	PPV (%)	NPV (%)
Seràgnoli	FFPE	Skin	88	γ	73	80	75	78
Zhang	FFPE	Skin	n/a	γ	64	84	var	var
				β	64	84	var	var
				γ + β	78	74	var	var
Lukowsky	FFPE	Skin	n/a	γ	81	n/a	n/a	n/a
				β	78	n/a	n/a	n/a
				γ + β	87	n/a	n/a	n/a
Goeldel	Frozen	Skin	0	γ	77	84	84	79
Ponti	Fresh/frozen	Skin	n/a	γ	84	98	95	92
Biomed-2 Group	Fresh/frozen	Not specified	n/a	γ	89	n/a	n/a	n/a
				β	91	n/a	n/a	n/a
				γ + β	94	n/a	n/a	n/a

n/a = not available.
var = variable PPV and NPV dependent on pre-test probability.

Table 4.
Comparison of sensitivity (ST), specificity (SP), positive predictive value (PPV), and negative predictive value (NPV) in different studies adopting the BIOMED-2 protocols.

4. Discussion

In this study, we examined the sensitivity and specificity and, accordingly, PPV and NPV, of the BIOMED-2 protocol in detecting TRG clonal rearrangements in cutaneous T-cell lymphoproliferative disorders. We included 110 consecutive cases of histologically complex FFPE skin biopsies referred to our institution over a 3-year period.

In our hands, the BIOMED-2 TRG protocol was technically successful in 87% of cases, based on a control gene minimum amplification requirement of 300 bps. In particular, it demonstrated a sensitivity of 90.0% and a specificity of 84%. The sensitivity and specificity data using this same approach have been published in previous papers (**Table 4**), and the figures obtained in our institution are comparable to previously published data in FFPE specimens. This suggests that sensitivity in FFPE specimens can approach that of fresh frozen specimens. With regard to FFPE samples, Zhang et al. reported a sensitivity and specificity of 64 and 84%, respectively, in a case series looking exclusively at MF, while Lukowsky et al. reported a sensitivity of 81% [12, 13]. In fresh/frozen tissues, Goeldel et al. reported a sensitivity and specificity of 77 and 84%, respectively [9, 14], while Ponti et al. described slightly higher figures of 83.5 and 97.7%, respectively [15]. A direct comparison with the original data from the BIOMED-2 consortium does, however, pose some problems as that group only analyzed fresh and frozen specimens and included non-skin specimens as well (**Table 4**).

Our study differs from the previous one, being the first phase 3 diagnostic accuracy study specifically designed and conducted according to the STRAD requirements for evidence-based medicine [11]. In doing so, we evaluated, for the first time in the specific setting of FFPE samples, the PPV and NPV of the BIOMED-2 TRG protocol. Importantly, such variables are strictly dependent on the incidence of the disease in the population tested (pre-test probability). In our laboratory, the use of TRG rearrangement testing is typically reserved for those cases where diagnostic uncertainty persists after morphological assessment with immunohistochemical staining, in which the pre-test probability is moderate/high and in which a positive or negative result may influence the final diagnosis [16]. In this context, the addition of a molecular tool as a diagnostic aid becomes significant. In this series, the pre-test probability was quite balanced, being 48%. We calculated a PPV of 84% with an NPV of 90% and found that most histologically "uncertain" cases could be satisfactorily resolved with the addition of the PCR information. Recently, Zhang et al. created a model that demonstrated the effect of pre-test probability on the PPV and NPV and suggested that the molecular result should only be considered when the pre-test probability lies between 0.15 and 0.75 [12], and this is actually consistent with our practice. Zhang et al. further pointed out that at the extremes of the pre-test probability range, the molecular result should be ignored [12]. Practically, based on the same SP and ST recorded in our study, a pre-test probability of 8% would lead to a positive predictive value of as low as 34%. Indeed, this underlines the importance of patient selection based on morphology and phenotype before molecular testing, which cannot represent a reliable screening test.

Regarding fresh/frozen samples, Ponti et al. described a remarkable PPV and NPV of 95 and 92%, respectively. It should be noted, however, that PPV and PNV may vary in the different studies due to differences in the considered series (i.e., research vs. routine diagnostic). In fact, at times, the clinical imperative urges contemporaneous initiation of multiple investigative strategies, including PCR, not respecting the ideal logical order (histology, immunohistochemistry, and genetics), thus affecting the pre-test probability. This real-world environment may alter the PPV and the NPV of the analysis. Further, the addition of TRB and TRD analysis, not available in this series, would potentially certainly improve the efficiency of the BIOMED-2 protocol. In this regard, it should be noted that this study did not aim to assess the accuracy of the entire protocol but rather of the TRG step, which is adopted as the first and often only one in many laboratories. For sure, the addition of the subsequent steps would increase the overall sensitivity, though negatively affecting, on the other hand, the specificity.

As mentioned, in spite of these remarkable figures for PPV and NPV, the importance of clinicopathologic integration in making a diagnosis in such a complex clinical setting must be remembered. It should be kept in mind that clonality, per sè, does not always indicate malignancy, and it is well-recognized that clonality can also be seen in reactive processes and thus cannot be considered a "sine qua non" of cancer [14, 17–20]. However, when clonality is detected without a definitive diagnosis of malignancy, a close clinical follow-up is mandatory, in order to ensure occult T-cell lymphoma is not missed [17, 21, 22]. In fact, progression to frank T-cell malignancy has been reported with variable frequency [23, 24]. Indeed, several studies have examined the fate of patients with an indeterminate diagnosis, with a variable percentage of patients who later on presented with a clear CTCL, ranging from 0 to 85% [15, 25–27]. With this in mind, we followed up on cases that demonstrated clonality, but the global picture was not indicative of lymphoma. However, in our experience, no one developed a lymphoma within the follow-up period. We cannot exclude that a later onset might occur.

Diagnostic algorithms for MF incorporating molecular testing with integrated clinicopathologic findings have been examined by a number of groups including most notably the ISCL [28–31]. Our findings suggested that TRG performed in FFPE in this subgroup remains a valid method of supporting a diagnosis in histologically challenging cases. Particularly, we had evidence that TRG clonal rearrangements were clinically useful also when a clear diagnosis of lymphoma could not be established. The role of molecular clonality testing in influencing the diagnosis of cutaneous lymphoid pathology in cases that are histologically uncertain needs further investigation. Nevertheless, it is now considered part of the diagnostic repertoire available to the pathologist and, indeed, has formed part of the ISCL and EORTC guidelines for diagnosis of MF since 2007 [29]. In our study, the most common malignancy identified was MF, in which 16/18 cases (88.9%) demonstrated TRG clonality. This compares to 68.2–88% as reported in the literature [12, 30], possibly reflecting the remarkable selection of cases based on immunomorphology in dedicated and ultra-specialistic Hematopathology Units. It is conceivable that the addiction of miRNA analysis [32] as well as comprehensive genetic testing [33–35], will further increase the importance of molecular pathology in CTCL analysis.

Finally, recent studies showed the potential efficacy of a next-generation sequencing (NGS) approach to resolve clonality testing [36]. These methods are based on the preparation of a DNA samples library amplified by PCR, using appropriate forward and reverse primers (tagged with unique barcodes) which usually target, respectively, different portions of V and J regions of the TRG gene; the amplified library is subsequently sequenced through a reversible dye-terminators technique and analyzed with bioinformatics approaches that return the proportion of the given sequences and assign them a rearrangement identity based on an alignment score [37–39]. These technologies are complex and parallelized processes that permit the simultaneous analysis of several samples returning high-throughput data. The introduction of NGS approach for the clonality assessment in CTCL can lead to useful advantages with respect to the gold standard PCR-based ones, overcoming its main limits [40, 41]: first, the possibility of distinguishing between same-sized amplified sequences, given that sequencing separates them also based on their nucleotides composition and not only on their length; further, also the possibility to better interpreting ambiguous results, as non-uniform Gaussian distributions, and better resolving a polyclonal background. In addition, this approach necessitates a minor amount of DNA (10–20 ng vs. 100–500 ng) and has the ability to detect and quantify also recurrent minor clones with small numbers of circulating tumor cells: as a result, NGS can improve the monitoring of the disease progression and treatments response, especially regarding minimal residual disease (MRD) context [42]. Hence, these new techniques could lead to a better and more objective classification, stratification, and monitoring of lymphoid malignancies, such as CTCL, which are essential proprieties in molecular diagnostics.

5. Conclusions

In conclusion, the TRG BIOMED-2 protocol appeared to be a feasible and remarkably effective method for analyzing clonality from FFPE specimens in histologically challenging cases. However, as a slight overestimation of clonal restrictions is possible, analysis repetition and careful patient follow-up are prudent. Proper clinical comparison with NGS technologies [36] is now certainly warranted.

Acknowledgements

The authors are grateful to Dr. Francesco Bacci, Dr. Elena Sabattini, and Dr. Carlo Sagramoso-Sacchetti for their contribution to diagnostic assessments as well as to Prof. Stefano A. Pileri for the precious advice.

The work reported in this publication was funded by the Italian Ministry of Health, RC-2023-2778976 (Prof. Piccaluga) and FIRB Futura 2011 RBFR12D1CB.

Conflict of interest

"The authors declare no conflict of interest."

Note

Prof. Pier Paolo Piccaluga is currently affiliated with the Jomo Kenyatta University of Agriculture and Technology (Nairobi, Kenya), The University of Nairobi (Nairobi, Kenya), and the University of Botswana (Gaborone, Botswana).

Appendix

Case number	Gender	Site of biopsy	Clinical History
1	M	skin	Skin lesion NOS
2	M	skin	Skin lesion NOS
3	F	skin	Skin lesion NOS
4	F	skin	Skin lesion in pregressed NHL
5	M	skin	Skin lesion NOS
6	M	skin	Skin lesion NOS
7	M	skin	Erythema
8	F	skin	Dermatosis
9	M	skin	Psoriasis + adenopathies
10	M	skin	Skin lesion NOS
11	F	skin	Tumoral skin lesion
12	F	skin	Hashimoto thyroiditis
13	M	skin	Abdominal erythema
14	M	skin	Skin lesion NOS
15	M	skin	Skin nodules at lower limbs
16	F	skin	Skin lesion NOS
17	M	skin	Skin lesion NOS
18	M	skin	Skin lesion NOS
19	M	skin	Suspected Lymphomatoid Papulosis

Case number	Gender	Site of biopsy	Clinical History
20	M	skin	Skin lesion NOS
21	F	skin	Scalp erythema
22	M	skin	Skin lesion in pregressed NHL
23	F	skin	Skin lesion NOS
24	F	skin	Skin lesion NOS
25	F	skin	Skin lesion NOS
26	F	skin	Skin lesion NOS
27	M	skin	Skin lesion NOS
28	M	skin	Skin lesion NOS
29	F	skin	Erythema
30	M	skin	Erythema
31	M	skin	Papulo-nodular skin lesions
32	M	skin	Suspected lymphoma
33	F	skin	Cutaneous pseudolymphoma
34	F	skin	Plaque
35	F	skin	Skin lesion NOS
36	M	skin	Mycosis fungoides
37	F	skin	Erythrodermic lesion
38	M	skin	Skin lesion NOS
39	M	skin	Skin lesion NOS
40	F	skin	Skin lesion NOS
41	M	skin	Skin lesion NOS
42	F	skin	Skin lesion NOS
43	M	skin	Skin lesion NOS
44	F	skin	Skin lesion NOS
45	M	skin	Erythema
46	M	skin	Lower limb ulcer
47	F	skin	Skin lesion NOS
48	F	skin	Suspected insect bite
49	M	skin	Skin lesion NOS
50	F	skin	Skin lesion NOS
51	M	skin	Skin lesion NOS
52	M	skin	Plaque
53	M	skin	Skin lesion + adenopathy
54	M	skin	Plaque
55	M	skin	Skin lesion NOS
56	F	skin	Skin lesion NOS
57	F	skin	Skin lesion NOS

Case number	Gender	Site of biopsy	Clinical History
58	F	skin	Tumoral skin lesion
59	F	skin	Skin lesion NOS
60	F	skin	Mycosis fungoides
61	M	skin	Skin lesions
62	M	skin	Tumoral skin lesion
63	M	skin	Mycosis fungoides
64	M	skin	Skin lesion NOS
65	M	skin	Skin lesion NOS
66	F	skin	HIV+ + skin lesions
67	M	skin	Skin lesion NOS
68	F	skin	Skin lesion NOS
69	M	skin	Skin lesion NOS
70	F	skin	Tumoral skin lesion
71	M	skin	Skin lesion NOS
72	M	skin	Skin lesion NOS
73	M	skin	Skin lesion NOS
74	M	skin	Skin lesion NOS
75	M	skin	Skin lesion NOS
76	M	skin	Skin lesion NOS
77	F	skin	Skin lesion NOS
78	F	skin	Skin lesion NOS
79	M	skin	Skin lesion NOS
80	F	skin	Tumoral skin lesion
81	F	skin	Skin lesion NOS
82	M	skin	Pregressed Cutaneous PTCL
83	F	skin	Mycosis fungoides
84	M	skin	Skin lesion NOS
85	F	skin	Plaque
86	M	skin	Skin lesion NOS
87	F	skin	Diffuse pruritis
88	F	skin	Skin lesion NOS
89	M	skin	Erythema + axillary adenopathy
90	M	skin	Skin lesion NOS
91	M	skin	Skin lesion NOS
92	F	skin	Skin nodules
93	M	skin	Skin lesion NOS
94	M	skin	Plaque
95	F	skin	Skin lesion NOS

Case number	Gender	Site of biopsy	Clinical History
96	M	skin	Papular skin lesions
97	F	skin	Skin lesion NOS
98	M	skin	Skin nodules
99	F	skin	Skin lesion NOS
100	M	skin	Skin lesion NOS
101	M	skin	HIV+, skin lesions, adenopathies
102	M	skin	Suspected follicular mucinosis
103	M	skin	Skin lesion NOS
104	M	skin	Erythema and pruritis
105	M	skin	Plaque
106	F	skin	Dermatosis
107	F	skin	Skin lesion NOS
108	M	skin	Skin lesion NOS
109	F	skin	Skin lesion NOS
110	M	skin	Plaque

NOS = not otherwise specified.

Table A1.
Patients' characteristics.

Section and Topic	Item #		On page #
TITLE/ ABSTRACT/ KEYWORDS	1	Identify the article as a study of diagnostic accuracy	2
INTRODUCTION	2	State the research questions or study aims, such as estimating diagnostic accuracy or comparing accuracy between tests or across participant groups.	4
METHODS			
Participants	3	Describe the study population: The inclusion and exclusion criteria, setting and locations where the data were collected.	5
	4	Describe participant recruitment: Was recruitment based on presenting symptoms, results from previous tests, or the fact that the participants had received the index tests or the reference standard?	Consecutive patients who received the index test (Figure 1)
	5	Describe participant sampling: Was the study population a consecutive series of participants defined by the selection criteria in items 3 and 4? If not, specify how participants were further selected.	Consecutive cases
	6	Describe data collection: Was data collection planned before the index test and reference standard were performed (prospective study) or after (retrospective study)?	Restrospective study

Section and Topic	Item #		On page #
Test methods	7	Describe the reference standard and its rationale.	5
	8	Describe technical specifications of material and methods involved including how and when measurements were taken, and/or cite references for index tests and reference standard.	5-7
	9	Describe definition of and rationale for the units, cutoffs and/or categories of the results of the index tests and the reference standard.	5-7
	10	Describe the number, training and expertise of the persons executing and reading the index tests and the reference standard.	5-6
	11	Describe whether or not the readers of the index tests and reference standard were blind (masked) to the results of the other test and describe any other clinical information available to the readers.	5-7
Statistical methods	12	Describe methods for calculating or comparing measures of diagnostic accuracy, and the statistical methods used to quantify uncertainty (e.g. 95% confidence intervals).	5-6
	13	Describe methods for calculating test reproducibility, if done.	6-7
RESULTS			
Participants	14	Report when study was done, including beginning and ending dates of recruitment.	5
	15	Report clinical and demographic characteristics of the study population (e.g. age, sex, spectrum of presenting symptoms, comorbidity, current treatments, recruitment centers).	**Table A1**
	16	Report the number of participants satisfying the criteria for inclusion that did or did not undergo the index tests and/or the reference standard; describe why participants failed to receive either test (a flow diagram is strongly recommended).	8
Test results	17	Report time interval from the index tests to the reference standard, and any treatment administered between.	6
	18	Report distribution of severity of disease (define criteria) in those with the target condition; other diagnoses in participants without the target condition.	8
	19	Report a cross tabulation of the results of the index tests (including indeterminate and missing results) by the results of the reference standard; for continuous results, the distribution of the test results by the results of the reference standard.	**Table A3**
	20	Report any adverse events from performing the index tests or the reference standard.	/
Estimates	21	Report estimates of diagnostic accuracy and measures of statistical uncertainty (e.g. 95% confidence intervals).	**Tables 1** and **2**

Section and Topic	Item #		On page #
	22	Report how indeterminate results, missing responses and outliers of the index tests were handled.	6
	23	Report estimates of variability of diagnostic accuracy between subgroups of participants, readers or centers, if done.	/
	24	Report estimates of test reproducibility, if done.	/
DISCUSSION	25	Discuss the clinical applicability of the study findings.	8-13

Table A2.
STARD requirements for evidence based medicine diagnostic accuracy studies.

Case number	Gold standard	Index test: TCRG analysis
1	Inflammatory disorder	Polyclonal
2	MF/SS	Clonal
3	Inflammatory disorder	Clonal
4	Inflammatory disorder	Polyclonal
5	MF/SS	Clonal
6	Inflammatory disorder	Clonal
7	Inflammatory disorder	Polyclonal
8	MF/SS	Clonal
9	Inflammatory disorder	Oligoclonal
11	Inflammatory disorder	Polyclonal
12	non-diagnostic	Polyclonal
13	Inflammatory disorder	Polyclonal
14	PTCL/NOS	Clonal
16	B-NHL	Polyclonal
17	B-NHL	Clonal
18	MF/SS	Clonal
19	non-diagnostic	Clonal
20	PTCL/NOS	Clonal
21	Inflammatory disorder	Polyclonal
22	non-diagnostic	Polyclonal
24	Inflammatory disorder	Clonal
25	non-diagnostic	Clonal
26	Inflammatory disorder	Clonal
27	MF/SS	Clonal
28	non-diagnostic	Clonal
30	MF/SS	Clonal
32	B-NHL	Clonal

Case number	Gold standard	Index test: TCRG analysis
33	Inflammatory disorder	Polyclonal
34	Inflammatory disorder	Polyclonal
35	PTCL/NOS	Clonal
37	MF/SS	Clonal
38	Inflammatory disorder	Polyclonal
39	MF/SS	Clonal
40	PTCL/NOS	Clonal
41	B-NHL	Oligoclonal
42	PTCL/NOS	Clonal
43	Inflammatory disorder	Polyclonal
44	Inflammatory disorder	Polyclonal
45	PTCL/NOS	Clonal
46	T-LGL	Clonal
47	Inflammatory disorder	Polyclonal
48	Inflammatory disorder	Polyclonal
50	CTCL/NOS	Clonal
51	Inflammatory disorder	Polyclonal
52	MF/SS	Polyclonal
53	PTCL/NOS	Clonal
54	MF/SS	Clonal
55	non-diagnostic	Polyclonal
56	MF/SS	Clonal
57	Inflammatory disorder	Polyclonal
58	CTCL/NOS	Clonal
59	non-diagnostic	Oligoclonal
60	PTCL/NOS	Clonal
61	MF/SS	Polyclonal
62	Inflammatory disorder	Polyclonal
64	MF/SS	Clonal
65	non-diagnostic	Polyclonal
67	non-diagnostic	Polyclonal
68	non-diagnostic	Oligoclonal
69	ALK neg ALCL	Clonal
70	CTCL/NOS	Clonal
71	PTCL/NOS	Clonal
72	non-diagnostic	Clonal
73	Inflammatory disorder	Polyclonal
74	Inflammatory disorder	Polyclonal

Case number	Gold standard	Index test: TCRG analysis
75	Inflammatory disorder	Polyclonal
76	MF/SS	Clonal
77	Inflammatory disorder	Polyclonal
78	Inflammatory disorder	Polyclonal
79	B-NHL	Polyclonal
80	CTCL/NOS	Clonal
81	PTCL/NOS	Polyclonal
82	MF/SS	Clonal
83	Inflammatory disorder	Polyclonal
85	Inflammatory disorder	Polyclonal
86	PTCL/NOS	Polyclonal
87	Inflammatory disorder	Polyclonal
88	Inflammatory disorder	Polyclonal
91	Inflammatory disorder	Polyclonal
92	PTCL/NOS	Clonal
93	B-NHL	Oligoclonal
94	MF/SS	Clonal
95	non-diagnostic	Oligoclonal
96	Inflammatory disorder	Polyclonal
98	MF/SS	Clonal
99	PTCL/NOS	Clonal
101	PTCL/NOS	Clonal
102	MF/SS	Clonal
103	PTCL/NOS	Clonal
104	Inflammatory disorder	Polyclonal
105	B-NHL	Polyclonal
106	Inflammatory disorder	Polyclonal
107	CTCL/NOS	Clonal
108	Inflammatory disorder	Polyclonal
109	Inflammatory disorder	Polyclonal
110	B-NHL	Polyclonal

B-NHL = B-non Hodgkin lymphoma; CTCL = cutaneus T-ceel lymphoma; DLBCL = diffuse large B-cell lymphoma; FL = follicular lymphoma; LGL = large granular lymphocyte leukemia; MF = mycosiss fungoides; MZL = marginal zone lymphoma; NOS = not otherwise specified; PTCL = peripheral T-cell lymphoma; SS = Sezary syndrome.

Table A3.
Comparison of Gold standard (histopathological diagnosis) and Index Test (TRG clonality testing).

Author details

Fernando Roncolato[1,2], Anna Gazzola[3], Claudia Mannu[3], Riccardo Donelli[2,4], Maryam Etebari[5,6], Mohsen Navari[5,6,7] and Pier Paolo Piccaluga[2,4]*

1 Department of Haematology, St. George Hospital, Sydney, Australia

2 Department of Medical and Surgical Sciences, Bologna University School of Medicine, Bologna, Italy

3 Hematopathology Unit, IRCCS Azienda Opedaliera-Universitaria di Bologna, Italy

4 Biobank of Research, IRCCS Azienda Opedaliera-Universitaria di Bologna, Bologna, Italy

5 Department of Medical Biotechnology, School of Paramedical Sciences, Torbat Heydariyeh University of Medical Sciences, Torbat Heydariyeh, Iran

6 Research Center of Advanced Technologies in Medicine, Torbat Heydariyeh University of Medical Sciences, Torbat Heydariyeh, Iran

7 Bioinformatics Research Center, Mashhad University of Medical Sciences, Mashhad, Iran

*Address all correspondence to: pierpaolo.piccaluga@unibo.it

References

[1] Alaggio R, Amador C, Anagnostopoulos I, et al. The 5th edition of the World Health Organization classification of Haematolymphoid Tumours: Lymphoid neoplasms. Leukemia. 2022;**36**:1720-1748

[2] Wilcox RA. Cutaneous T-cell lymphoma: 2016 update on diagnosis, risk-stratification, and management. American Journal of Hematology. 2016; **91**(1):151-165

[3] Weiss LM, Hu E, Wood GS, et al. Clonal rearrangements of T-cell receptor genes in mycosis fungoides and dermatopathic lymphadenopathy. The New England Journal of Medicine. 1985; **313**(9):539-544

[4] Bertness V, Kirsch I, Hollis G, et al. T-cell receptor gene rearrangements as clinical markers of human T-cell lymphomas. The New England Journal of Medicine. 1985; **313**(9):534-538

[5] Krangel MS. Mechanics of T cell receptor gene rearrangement. Current Opinion in Immunology. 2009;**21**(2): 133-139

[6] van Dongen JJ, Langerak AW, Bruggemann M, et al. Design and standardization of PCR primers and protocols for detection of clonal immunoglobulin and T-cell receptor gene recombinations in suspect lymphoproliferations: Report of the BIOMED-2 concerted action BMH4-CT98-3936. Leukemia. 2003;**17**(12): 2257-2317

[7] Bruggemann M, White H, Gaulard P, et al. Powerful strategy for polymerase chain reaction-based clonality assessment in T-cell malignancies report of the BIOMED-2 concerted action BHM4 CT98-3936. Leukemia. 2007; **21**(2):215-221

[8] Sandberg Y, Verhaaf B, van Gastel-Mol EJ, et al. Human T-cell lines with well-defined T-cell receptor gene rearrangements as controls for the BIOMED-2 multiplex polymerase chain reaction tubes. Leukemia. 2007;**21**(2): 230-237

[9] Bagg A, Braziel RM, Arber DA, et al. Immunoglobulin heavy chain gene analysis in lymphomas: A multi-center study demonstrating the heterogeneity of performance of polymerase chain reaction assays. The Journal of Molecular Diagnostics. 2002;**4**(2):81-89

[10] Liu H, Bench AJ, Bacon CM, et al. A practical strategy for the routine use of BIOMED-2 PCR assays for detection of B- and T-cell clonality in diagnostic haematopathology. British Journal of Haematology. 2007;**138**(1):31-43

[11] Cohen J, Korevaar D, Altman D, et al. STARD 2015 guidelines for reporting diagnostic accuracy studies: Explanation and elaboration. BMJ Open. 2016;**6**(11):e012799

[12] Zhang B, Beck AH, Taube JM, et al. Combined use of PCR-based TCRG and TCRB clonality tests on paraffin-embedded skin tissue in the differential diagnosis of mycosis fungoides and inflammatory dermatoses. The Journal of Molecular Diagnostics. 2010;**12**(3): 320-327

[13] Lukowsky A, Muche JM, Mobs M, et al. Evaluation of T-cell clonality in archival skin biopsy samples of cutaneous T-cell lymphomas using the biomed-2 PCR protocol. Diagnostic Molecular Pathology. 2010;**19**(2):70-77

[14] Goeldel AL, Cornillet-Lefebvre P, Durlach A, et al. T-cell receptor gamma gene rearrangement in cutaneous T-cell lymphoma: Comparative study of polymerase chain reaction with denaturing gradient gel electrophoresis and GeneScan analysis. The British Journal of Dermatology. 2009;**162**(4): 822-829

[15] Ponti R, Quaglino P, Novelli M, et al. T-cell receptor gamma gene rearrangement by multiplex polymerase chain reaction/heteroduplex analysis in patients with cutaneous T-cell lymphoma (mycosis fungoides/Sezary syndrome) and benign inflammatory disease: Correlation with clinical, histological and immunophenotypical findings. The British Journal of Dermatology. 2005;**153**(3):565-573

[16] Hagen MD. Test characteristics. How good is that test? Primary Care. 1995;**22**(2):213-233

[17] Langerak AW, Molina TJ, Lavender FL, et al. Polymerase chain reaction-based clonality testing in tissue samples with reactive lymphoproliferations: Usefulness and pitfalls. A report of the BIOMED-2 concerted action BMH4-CT98-3936. Leukemia. 2007;**21**(2):222-229

[18] Schiller PI, Flaig MJ, Puchta U, et al. Detection of clonal T cells in lichen planus. Archives of Dermatological Research. 2000;**292**(11):568-569

[19] Dereure O, Levi E, Kadin ME. T-cell clonality in pityriasis lichenoides et varioliformis acuta: A heteroduplex analysis of 20 cases. Archives of Dermatology. 2000;**136**(12):1483-1486

[20] Lukowsky A, Muche JM, Sterry W, et al. Detection of expanded T cell clones in skin biopsy samples of patients with lichen sclerosus et atrophicus by T cell receptor-gamma polymerase chain reaction assays. The Journal of Investigative Dermatology. 2000;**115**(2): 254-259

[21] Meyer N, Mazereeuw-Hautier J, Launay F, et al. Cutaneous T cell lymphoma complicating severe atopic dermatitis. Is making a diagnosis the main challenge? Dermatology. 2009; **218**(2):168-171

[22] Arana A, Wentworth CE, Fernandez-Vidaurre C, et al. Incidence of cancer in the general population and in patients with or without atopic dermatitis in the U.K. The British Journal of Dermatology. 2010;**163**(5):1036-1043

[23] Ponti R, Fierro MT, Quaglino P, et al. TCRgamma-chain gene rearrangement by PCR-based GeneScan: Diagnostic accuracy improvement and clonal heterogeneity analysis in multiple cutaneous T-cell lymphoma samples. The Journal of Investigative Dermatology. 2008;**128**(4):1030-1038

[24] Wood GS, Tung RM, Haeffner AC, et al. Detection of clonal T-cell receptor gamma gene rearrangements in early mycosis fungoides/Sezary syndrome by polymerase chain reaction and denaturing gradient gel electrophoresis (PCR/DGGE). The Journal of Investigative Dermatology. 1994;**103**(1): 34-41

[25] Thurber SE, Zhang B, Kim YH, et al. T-cell clonality analysis in biopsy specimens from two different skin sites shows high specificity in the diagnosis of patients with suggested mycosis fungoides. Journal of the American Academy of Dermatology. 2007;**57**(5): 782-790

[26] Eros N, Karolyi Z, Marschalko M, et al. Clinical, histopathological, immunophenotypic and molecular

analysis of 60 patients with cutaneous T-cell infiltrates with follow up of indeterminate cases to identify T-cell lymphoma. Pathology Oncology Research. 2008;**14**(1):63-67

[27] Foo CC, Tang MB, Chong TK, et al. T-cell receptor-gamma gene analysis in evolving to advancing cutaneous T-cell lymphoma. The Australasian Journal of Dermatology. 2007;**48**(3):156-160

[28] Vonderheid EC, Bernengo MG, Burg G, et al. Update on erythrodermic cutaneous T-cell lymphoma: Report of the International Society for Cutaneous Lymphomas. Journal of the American Academy of Dermatology. 2002;**46**(1): 95-106

[29] Olsen E, Vonderheid E, Pimpinelli N, et al. Revisions to the staging and classification of mycosis fungoides and Sezary syndrome: A proposal of the International Society for Cutaneous Lymphomas (ISCL) and the cutaneous lymphoma task force of the European Organization of Research and Treatment of cancer (EORTC). Blood. 2007;**110**(6):1713-1722

[30] Furmanczyk PS, Wolgamot GM, Kussick SJ, et al. Diagnosis of mycosis fungoides with different algorithmic approaches. Journal of Cutaneous Pathology. 2009;**37**(1):8-14

[31] Ferrara G, Di Blasi A, Zalaudek I, et al. Regarding the algorithm for the diagnosis of early mycosis fungoides proposed by the International Society for Cutaneous Lymphomas: Suggestions from routine histopathology practice. Journal of Cutaneous Pathology. 2008; **35**(6):549-553

[32] Ralfkiaer U, Hagedorn PH, Bangsgaard N, et al. Diagnostic microRNA profiling in cutaneous T-cell lymphoma (CTCL). Blood. 2011;**118**(22): 5891-5900

[33] Wang L, Ni X, Covington K, et al. Genomic profiling of Sézary syndrome identifies alterations of key T cell signaling and differentiation genes. Nature Genetics. 2015;**47**(12):12

[34] da Silva AA, Abate F, Khiabanian H, et al. The mutational landscape of cutaneous T cell lymphoma and Sézary syndrome. Nature Genetics. 2015; **47**(12):5

[35] Choi J, Goh G, Walradt T, et al. Genomic landscape of cutaneous T cell lymphoma. Nature Genetics. 2015; **47**(9):8

[36] Sufficool K, Lockwood C, Abel H, et al. T-cell clonality assessment by next-generation sequencing improves detection sensitivity in mycosis fungoides. Journal of the American Academy of Dermatology. 2015;**73**(2):8

[37] Gazzola A, Mannu C, Rossi M, Laginestra MA, Sapienza MR, Fuligni F, et al. The evolution of clonality testing in the diagnosis and monitoring of hematological malignancies. Therapeutic Advances in Hematology. 2014;**5**:35-47

[38] Greiner TC. Clinical use of next-generation sequencing of trg gene rearrangements has arrived. American Journal of Clinical Pathology. American Society of Clinical Pathologists. 2014; **141**:302-304

[39] Kohlmann A, Grossmann V, Nadarajah N, Haferlach T. Next-generation sequencing - feasibility and practicality in haematology. British Journal of Haematology. 2013;**160**: 736-753

[40] Walia R, Yeung CCS. An update on molecular biology of cutaneous T cell

lymphoma. Frontiers in Oncology. 2020; **9**:1558. Published 2020 Jan 22. DOI: 10.3389/fonc.2019.01558

[41] Phyo ZH, Shanbhag S, Rozati S. Update on biology of cutaneous T-cell lymphoma. Frontiers in Oncology. 2020; **10**:765. Published 2020 May 12. DOI: 10.3389/fonc.2020.00765

[42] Weng WK, Armstrong R, Arai S, Desmarais C, Hoppe R, Kim YH. Minimal residual disease monitoring with high-throughput sequencing of T cell receptors in cutaneous T cell lymphoma. Science Translational Medicine. 2013;**5**(214):214-171

Chapter 6

Integrated Histomolecular Diagnosis in Mediastinal Gray Zone Lymphomas

Alexandra Traverse-Glehen and Marie Donzel

Abstract

Mediastinal gray zone lymphoma is now recognized as a distinct entity in the newly updated classification of hematolymphoid malignancies. In recent years, several clinicopathological and molecular studies have helped to clarify the spectrum of this entity, which is intermediate between Classical Hodgkin Lymphoma and Primary Mediastinal B-cell Lymphoma. The mediastinal location remains an important feature of the disease and it needs to be cautious to do this diagnosis in extramediastinal location. In addition, cases with EBV association should be better classified in polymorphic EBV+ B-cell lymphomas until a better understanding of this entity. As in PMBCL and CHL, MGZ exhibits a high rate of immune escape with *CIITA* break and *PDL1/PDL2* abnormalities.

Keywords: mediastinal gray zone lymphoma, classical Hodgkin lymphoma, primary mediastinal large B-cell lymphoma, EBV, molecular pathology

1. Introduction

Mediastinal Gray Zone Lymphoma (MGZL) was first described in 1998 [1] and recognized as a provisional entity in the 2008 WHO classification [2, 3], referred to as "B-cell lymphoma, unclassifiable, with features intermediate between Diffuse Large B-Cell Lymphoma (DLBCL) and Classic Hodgkin Lymphoma (CHL)". It is now a definitive entity of the 2022 WHO (World Health classification of hematologic malignancies) and the ICC (International Consensus Conferences), so-called "Mediastinal gray zone lymphoma" [4].

It is indeed a B-cell lymphoma with overlapping clinical, morphological, phenotypic, and molecular features between Primary Mediastinal (thymic) B-Cell Lymphoma (PMBL) and Classical Hodgkin Lymphoma (CHL), more particularly Nodular Sclerosis CHL (NSCHL). The definition of this entity has evolved over the years, in particular thanks to the development of molecular techniques which made it possible to dismember this entity. MGZL is classified into two subtypes, CHL-like-GZL and PMBCL-like-GZL [5]. CHL-like-GZL is identified based on its morphological similarity to CHL, but with a PMBCL-like immunophenotype characterized by strong and homogeneous expression of B-cell markers on all tumor cells. The second, so-called PMBL- or LBCL-like-GZL corresponds to cases that were morphologically more closely related to LBCL, in particular PMBL, but harbored a CHL immunophenotype. The introduction of Gene Expression Profiling (GEP) [6] and Next Generation Sequencing [7] has led to the reclassification of LBCL-like GZL into two distinct categories. True PMBL-type GZL, which is related to lymphomas of thymic origin (such as CHL and PMBL), and DLBCL-like GZL, which seems to have a different cell of origin and will therefore be excluded from the spectrum of MGZ in the future. In addition, EBV-associated gray zone lesions can be more accurately classified as polymorphic-EBV-Large B-cell lymphoma. In the new 2022 WHO classification, as well as in the ICC, the term inclassable B-cell lymphoma with features intermediate between CHL and Large B-cell lymphoma has been replaced by MGZ. This new nomenclature is used to specifically identify this entity as a primary mediastinal disease.

All studies suggest a common cell of origin for lymphomas of the thymic-anatomic niche, including CHL, PMBL, and MGZL, which may be derived from the same cell of origin, a thymic B lymphocyte [6, 8], although the etiology is unknown. This may explain overlapping disease evolution of these entities [9].

2. Mediastinal gray zone lymphoma

2.1 Epidemiology and clinical presentation

The epidemiology of MGZ is not well known.

Mediastinal Gray Zone Lymphoma commonly affects people between the ages of 20 and 40, with a median age of 32 years (13–83 years) [10] and it is slightly more common in men than in women [10]. The age of onset is thus common with CHL and PMBL, but the latter is more frequent in young female [11]. Most cases have been reported from North America. Like NSCHL, the disease appears to be less common in black people and Asians.

Clinical presentation of GZL includes general symptoms of lymphomas, such as alteration of the general condition (tiredness, loss of appetite, loss of weight), B-symptoms (night sweats, fever), itchy skin or cytopenia (anemia, lymphopenia...). There are signs associated with the presence of a mediastinal mass, which is classically a large anterior prevascular mass. These symptoms include vena cava syndrome, and which sometimes causes noisy symptoms such as tracheal compression and respiratory distress in cases of bulky disease (one third of cases) [10]. Disease is more often disseminated at diagnosis, with predominance of Ann Arbor stages III–IV [8, 10]. In these cases, supraclavicular lymph nodes involvement is frequent, but other peripheral lymph node groups are less commonly involved. Pleural or pericardial effusion/extension is common, and there is a possibility of direct spread to the lung. However, involvement in subdiaphragmatic locations and/or bone marrow extension is uncommon (less than 10% of cases) [10], except in the rare cases of disseminated disease [6].

Rare cases without anterior mediastinal involvement, referred to as non-mediastinal GZL with primary extra-mediastinal presentation (PEMGZL), have been previously reported. These cases generally occur in older patients (median age 65 years), and there is no gender predisposition associated with this condition. The definition of PEMGZL is a topic of ongoing discussion. It is important to note that this diagnosis should be made with caution and restricted primarily to (clinical) research studies.

2.2 Diagnosis

2.2.1 Histology

Most cases of MGZL are composed of a diffuse proliferation of pleomorphic tumor cells in a diffusely fibrotic stroma, sometimes giving the impression of a vaguely nodular architecture in cases with fibrous band. The cells are medium or large, round or oval, and may even appear spindle-shaped due to cell crush artifacts, similar to what can be observed in PMBL. However, the proliferation is more pleomorphic than in the typical case of PMBL, due to the association with lacunar cells and/or Hodgkin cells. The neoplastic lymphocytes show indeed a broad spectrum of cytological appearances, resembling typical Hodgkin and Reed-Sternberg cells, lacunar cells, centroblasts and immunoblasts. This broad spectrum of cytological appearance, with different areas of the tumor showing variations in cytological appearance, is a characteristic feature of MGZL. The background inflammatory infiltrate may contain eosinophils, lymphocytes, plasma cells, and histiocytes, although eosinophils are less abundant than in NSCHL. Sheets of necrosis are usually present, classically without neutrophilic infiltrate.

As seen before, the morphological spectrum of MGZL is broad, extending from CHL-like-GZL to PMBCL-like-GZL. These subtypes may coexist within the same tumor specimen [6].

The majority of MGZL resemble to CHL, particularly the nodular sclerosis CHL (NSCHL) (60%) [5] and are called CHL-like-GZL. Typical cases (group 0) have a morphology closely related to NSCHL and often show confluent, sheet-like growth of pleomorphic cells within a variable abundant microenvironment (including eosinophils and plasma cells) and dense fibrotic stroma. Some cases are less typical (group 1), including some CHL features but associated with intermediate cells and/or diffuse areas, with a background less rich in eosinophils and plasma cells. In this second case, the differential diagnosis with PMBL can be difficult based on morphologic criteria alone.

A minority of MGZL mimic PMBL and are called PMBL-like-GZL. Typical cases (group 3) have a morphology closely related to large B-cell lymphomas, in particular PMBL. These cases present with a rather monomorphic appearance, with sheets of medium to large atypical cells in a variable, dense fibrotic stroma with paucicellular inflammatory infiltrate. Marked pleomorphism and some Hodgkin cells may be encountered. Some cases are also less typical (group 2), with predominance of medium to large atypical and pleomorphic tumor cells, with clear cells, Hodgkin cells, and/or Reed-Sternberg (RS) cells.

2.2.2 Immunohistochemistry

The spectrum of MGZL ranges from cases with a morphology more closely related to CHL but showing a strong B-cell phenotype to cases in which morphology is more closely related to DLBCL but with a CHL-like immunophenotype. This challenging diagnosis should not be overdone and must be considered after exclusion of CHL and PMBL.

The diagnosis of CHL-like-GZL, especially in its classical form (group 0), is based on the discrepancy between morphological appearance and immunophenotype. Indeed, the diagnosis of MGZL should be evoked in case of conservation of the B-cell program on Hodgkin cells, with expression of membranous B-cell marker (CD20,

CD19, and CD79a) and of nuclear transcription factor (PAX5, OCT2, BOB1). Both CD30 and IRF4 (MUM1) are usually diffusely positive, with variable intensity, but CD15 may be inconstant [5, 10]. CD23 expression is not classical but may be seen in about 30% of CHL-like-GZL [5]. MAL expression is seen in 49% of cases [5, 12]. Expression of BCL6 is variable. CD10 and ALK are negative, such as surface and cytoplasmic immunoglobulins [5]. The background lymphocytes are predominantly CD3+/CD4+ T-cells, as seen in CHL. MGZL is infrequently positive for EBV, and EBV positivity should prompt suspicion for EBV-positive CHL [5, 13].

PMBL-like-GZL are, at the contrary, characterized by loss of the B-cell program, including loss of CD20 expression (22% of cases) [5] or loss of another B-cell marker. Most cases show intense and diffuse expression of CD30 and CD15. In cases where CD30 intensity is medium to low, CD15 must be diffuse and intense, and vice versa. MAL expression is reported in 61% of cases, and CD23 expression in 49% of cases [5, 12]. MGZL is infrequently positive for EBV, and EBV positivity should prompt suspicion for EBV-positive DLBCL [5, 13].

Morphological and phenotypical data are resumed in **Table 1** and illustrated in **Figure 1**. As these complex histological features are often not reliably identifiable in core needle biopsies, an excisional biopsy is required to arrive at the diagnosis of MGZL. Moreover, this diagnosis rests on the mismatch between morphological and immunohistochemical findings and require therefore a large panel of antibodies.

Moreover, patients may present with an unambiguous diagnosis of CHL and PMBL at different time points during the course of the disease, in the same or different anatomic sites, with some composite or sequential/metachronous cases, suggesting a certain degree of plasticity between these entities. These cases should not be classified as MGZL, instead, it is recommended to name and classify the individual components separately. The same holds true for "composite" lymphomas diagnosed at any localization composed of DLBCL and CHL, which are generally not biologically related [2, 14, 15]. For these reasons, this diagnosis is very difficult on core needle biopsy, and an excision biopsy is recommended, and if necessary an expert pathological review and a multidisciplinary integration of clinical and pathological.

	CHL-like-GZL (group 0)	**CHL-like-GZL (group 1)**	**PMBL-type GZL (group 2)**	**PMBL-type GZL (group 3)**
Morphology	≈ CHL Pleomorphic cells with lacunar and Hodgkin/RS cells. Inflammatory background.	CHL features associated with intermediate cells and/or diffuse areas. Less inflammatory background.	Predominance of medium to large atypical and pleomorphic tumor cells, with clear cells, Hodgkin cells, or RS cells.	≈ PMBL Monomorphic appearance. Paucicellular inflammatory infiltrate.
B-cell markers	CD20 + PAX5 + and another B-cell marker + (CD19, CD79a, BOB1, OCT2).		Partial or complete loss of B-cell marker.	
CD30 CD15	+++ (variable intensity) +/−		Strong and uniform positive expression of CD30 and/or CD15.	

Table 1.
Summary of morphological and immunohistochemical features to differentiate mediastinal gray zone lymphoma (MGZL) subtypes.

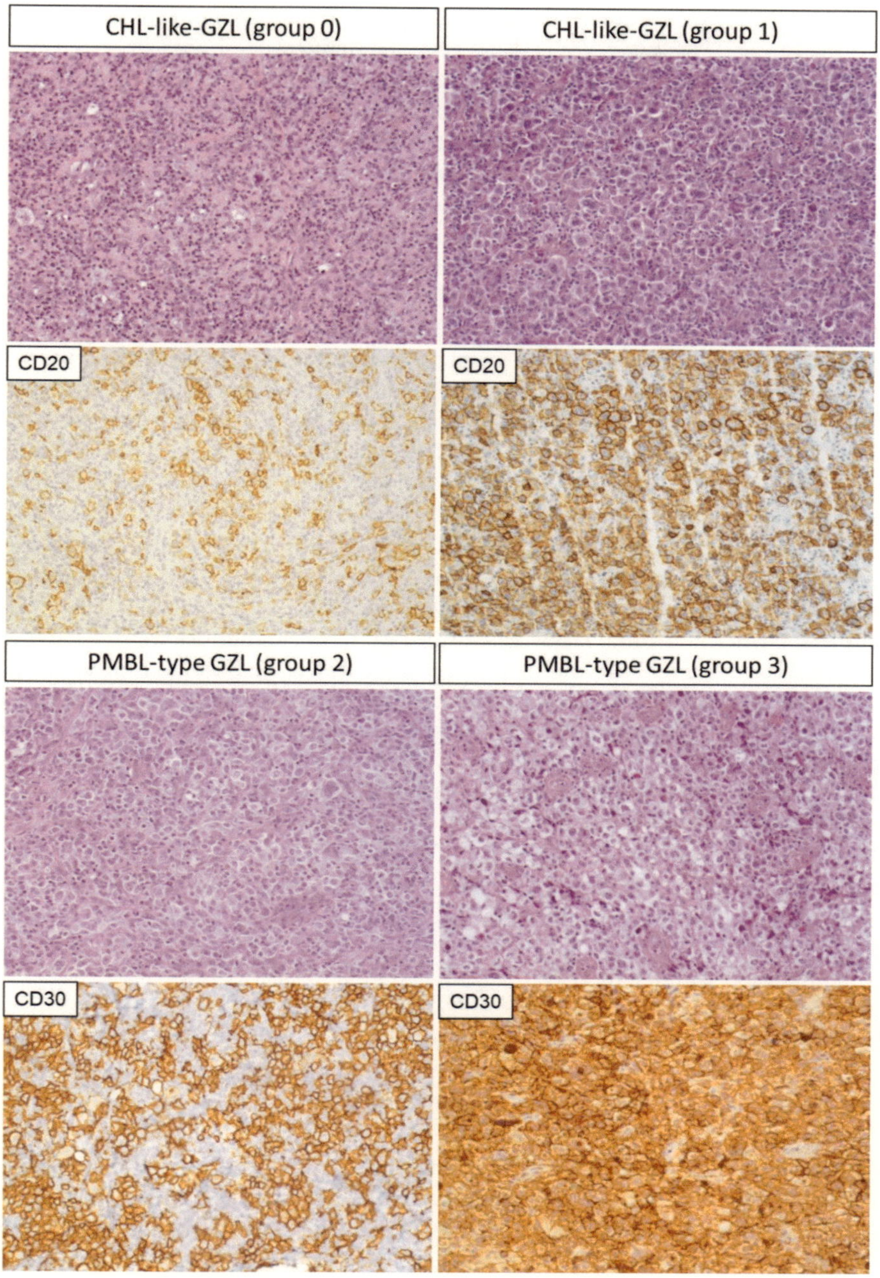

Figure 1.
Illustration of morphological and immunohistochemical features to differentiate mediastinal gray zone lymphoma (MGZL) subtypes.

2.3 Molecular pathology

Using fluorescence in situ hybridization, cases with PMBL-like morphology harbor more frequent PDL1/PDL2 or CIITA rearrangements than CHL-like-GZL (63 vs. 32% using a CIITA break-apart probe, and 32 vs. 6% using a PDL1/PDL2 break apart probe) [5]. MYC rearrangement is rare, but some studies demonstrated gains of 8q24 (MYC) in among 27% of cases [5]. BCL2 and BCL6 rearrangements are rare (respectively 6 and 0%) [7] in MGZL and their detection should lead to a re-evaluation of the diagnosis of DLBCL with secondary mediastinal location. In cytogenetics, gains at 2p16.1 (REL/BCL11A locus) and alterations at 9p24.1 (JAK2/PDL2 locus) are observed in 33 and 55% of cases respectively [14]. Cytogenetic abnormalities involving the JAK2/PDL2 may be responsible of an increased expression of PDL1 (CD274).

Studies using gene expression profiling (GEP) have further dismembered the CHL/MGZL/PMBL spectrum [6, 16]. Expression signatures revealed differences between CHL and PMBL, and confirmed the presence of different subtypes of MGZL, some clustering more with CHL, corresponding to CHL-like GZL from a morphological and immunohistochemical point of view, and others clustering with PMBL, corresponding to PMBL-like GZL. They also highlighted some characteristics of CHL, shared with the CHL-like GZL, as the lower expression of germinal center genes (GCB) and IFN regulatory factor 4 (IRF4) genes in MGZL and CHL, indicating downregulation of the B-cell program in these entities compared with PMBL and PMBL-like GZL. Conversely, infiltrating T-cells genes (IL6ST, CTLA4, CD28, and ICOS), immune regulation genes (IL1R2, IL32, IL7R, and TNIP3), and macrophage signature were higher in CHL and CHL-like GZL consistent with the presence of an inflammatory background [10, 16].

Studies on the mutational landscape of MGZL have further clarified its characteristics and have allowed distinguishing it from other large B-cell lymphomas that do not have a mediastinal origin/location. The genetical landscape of MGZL shows many similarities to PMBL and NSCHL, reinforcing the hypothesis that it can be the missing link between these two entities. MGZL cases with thymic niche involvement exhibit a pattern of mutation which was very similar to CHL and PMBL, including SOCS1 (45%), B2M (45%), TNFAIP3 (35%), GNA13 (35%), LRRN3 (32%), and NFKBIA (29%) mutations, involving the JAK/STAT and NF-κB pathways. In contrast, cases without thymic niche involvement, so-called DLBCL-like GZL, have a significantly distinct pattern, enriched in mutations related to apoptosis defects (TP53 [39%], BCL2 [28%], BIRC6 [22%]) and depleted in GNA13, XPO1, or NF-κB signaling pathway mutations [7].

2.4 Differential diagnosis

As described earlier, the diagnosis of MGZL should only be considered after careful exclusion of other entities, in particular CHL and PMBL. In daily practice, although the exact number of B-cell markers required to be expressed for MGZL diagnosis remains controversial, the diagnosis of CHL-like-GZL should be reserved for cases with intense and diffuse expression of CD20, associated with expression of PAX5 and with the expression of another B-cell marker on Hodgkin cells [10]. If additional B-cell markers are negative (solely CD20 + and PAX5 +), the diagnosis of CHL will be favored.

Concerning PMBL-like forms, the diagnosis of MGZL should not be based on CD30 expression alone but may be made only in cases of loss of the B-cell program, or, if B-markers are retained, in cases of intense and diffuse co-expression of CD30 and CD15. Phenotypes that should favor the diagnosis of PMBL-like-GZL rather than PMBL in front of a lymphocytic infiltrate made up of large, fairly pleomorphic cells are: (i) CD20 +++, CD30 + intense and diffuse, CD15 +/−; (ii) CD20 +++, CD15 + intense and diffuse, CD30 +/−; or (iii) CD20 -, CD79A +, CD30 +, and CD15 + .

EBV+ MGZL is extremely rare and alternative differential diagnoses as mentioned should be excluded in these cases. In particular, EBV positivity must argue for the diagnosis of EBV+ DLBCL or B-cell lymphoproliferative disorder in immunodeficiency settings, as well as T-cell lymphomas with EBV-positive cells, in particular angio-immunoblastic T-cell lymphoma.

A monoclonal B population is classically present and may help the pathologist to differentiate CHL-like GZL from T-cell lymphomas with Hodgkin or RS-cells, in particular follicular subtype of T-follicular helper (TFH) lymphoma.

As discussed earlier, molecular data can help in the differential diagnosis of MGZ. Thus, the demonstration of a CIITA rearrangement can lead to the diagnosis of PMBL-like-GZL, whereas in case of MYC, BCL2 or BCL6 rearrangements, the diagnosis of DLBCL should be discussed. Similarly, the demonstration of a mutational profile similar to that observed in CHL or PMBL will reinforce the diagnosis of MGZL instead of DLBCL. Finally, techniques using RNA expression such as the nCounter NanoString Assay, developed after the model of GEP studies, can also lead the diagnosis toward CHL or PMBL instead of DLBCL. The demonstration of transcriptional enrichment in genes of the tumor microenvironment, notably those involved in immune escape, may also be an argument favoring the diagnosis of MGZL. These data illustrate the importance of a comprehensive integration of clinical, histological, and molecular data in the differential diagnosis of MGZL, PMBL, CHL, or DLBCL.

2.5 Prognosis and treatment

In retrospective series, the outcome seems to be worse when compared to PMBCL or CHL with a lower response rate to regimens effective in CHL, such as ABVD. Any consensus at this time is described for a consensus treatment.

3. Conclusions

The diagnosis of MGZL should be made with caution especially because no therapeutic consensus exists at this time. A diagnosis of CHL with few B-cell markers and PMBCL with loss of B-cell markers should be considered to adapt the therapeutic options. Not mediastinal cases and EBV cases must be included with careful integration of all data.

Conflict of interest

The authors declare no conflict of interest.

Author details

Alexandra Traverse-Glehen[1,2] and Marie Donzel[1,2*]

1 Hospices Civils de Lyon, Institut de pathologie multisite, Hôpital Lyon Sud, Lyon, France

2 Centre International de Recherche en Infectiologie (CIRI), Université Claude Bernard Lyon-1, Lyon, France

*Address all correspondence to: marie.donzel@chu-lyon.fr

References

[1] Rüdiger T, Jaffe ES, Delsol G, deWolf-Peeters C, Gascoyne RD, Georgii A, et al. Workshop report on Hodgkin's disease and related diseases (gray zone lymphoma). Annals of Oncology: Official Journal of the European Society for Medical Oncology. 1998;**9**(Suppl. 5):S31-S38

[2] Traverse-Glehen A, Pittaluga S, Gaulard P, Sorbara L, Alonso MA, Raffeld M, et al. Mediastinal gray zone lymphoma: The missing link between classic Hodgkin's lymphoma and mediastinal large B-cell lymphoma. The American Journal of Surgical Pathology. 2005;**29**(11):1411-1421

[3] Campo E, Swerdlow SH, Harris NL, Pileri S, Stein H, Jaffe ES. The 2008 WHO classification of lymphoid neoplasms and beyond: Evolving concepts and practical applications. Blood. 2011;**117**(19):5019-5032

[4] Alaggio R, Amador C, Anagnostopoulos I, Attygalle AD, Araujo IB de O, Berti E, et al. The 5th edition of the World Health Organization classification of Haematolymphoid tumours: Lymphoid neoplasms. Leukemia. 2022;**36**(7):1720-1748

[5] Sarkozy C, Copie-Bergman C, Damotte D, Ben-Neriah S, Burroni B, Cornillon J, et al. Gray-zone lymphoma between cHL and large B-cell lymphoma: A histopathologic series from the LYSA. The American Journal of Surgical Pathology. 2019;**43**(3):341-351

[6] Sarkozy C, Chong L, Takata K, Chavez EA, Miyata-Takata T, Duns G, et al. Gene expression profiling of gray zone lymphoma. Blood Advances. 2020;**4**(11):2523-2535

[7] Sarkozy C, Hung SS, Chavez EA, Duns G, Takata K, Chong LC, et al. Mutational landscape of gray zone lymphoma. Blood. 2021;**137**(13):1765-1776

[8] Kritharis A, Pilichowska M, Evens AM. How I manage patients with gray zone lymphoma. British Journal of Haematology. 2016;**174**(3):345-350

[9] Dunleavy K, Wilson WH. Primary mediastinal B-cell lymphoma and mediastinal gray zone lymphoma: Do they require a unique therapeutic approach? Blood. 2015;**125**(1):33-39

[10] Sarkozy C, Molina T, Ghesquières H, Michallet AS, Dupuis J, Damotte D, et al. Mediastinal gray zone lymphoma: Clinico-pathological characteristics and outcomes of 99 patients from the lymphoma study association. Haematologica. 2017;**102**(1):150-159

[11] Ahmed Z, Afridi SS, Shahid Z, Zamani Z, Rehman S, Aiman W, et al. Primary mediastinal B-cell lymphoma: A 2021 update on genetics, diagnosis, and novel therapeutics. Clinical Lymphoma, Myeloma & Leukemia. Nov 2021;**21**(11):e865-e875

[12] Copie-Bergman C, Plonquet A, Alonso MA, Boulland ML, Marquet J, Divine M, et al. MAL expression in lymphoid cells: Further evidence for MAL as a distinct molecular marker of primary Mediastinal large B-cell lymphomas. Modern Pathology. 2002;**15**(11):1172-1180

[13] Maracaja DLV, Puthenpura V, Pels SG, O'Malley DP, Sklar JL, Finberg KE, et al. EBV-positive primary large B-cell lymphoma: The role of immunohistochemistry and XPO1 in the

diagnosis of Mediastinal lymphomas. Applied Immunohistochemistry & Molecular Morphology AIMM. 2020;**28**(10):725-730

[14] Eberle FC, Salaverria I, Steidl C, Summers TA, Pittaluga S, Neriah SB, et al. Gray zone lymphoma: Chromosomal aberrations with immunophenotypic and clinical correlations. Modern Pathology : An Official Journal of the United States and Canadian Academy of Pathology, Inc. 2011;**24**(12):1586-1597

[15] Aussedat G, Traverse-Glehen A, Stamatoullas A, Molina T, Safar V, Laurent C, et al. Composite and sequential lymphoma between classical Hodgkin lymphoma and primary mediastinal lymphoma/diffuse large B-cell lymphoma, a clinico-pathological series of 25 cases. British Journal of Haematology. 2020;**189**(2):244-256

[16] Pittaluga S, Nicolae A, Wright GW, Melani C, Roschewski M, Steinberg S, et al. Gene expression profiling of mediastinal gray zone lymphoma and its relationship to primary mediastinal B-cell lymphoma and classical Hodgkin lymphoma. Blood Cancer Discov. 2020;**1**(2):155-161

Section 4

Molecular Diagnostic in Solid Tumors

Chapter 7

Molecular Diagnosis of Breast Cancer

Vladimir Kanstantinovich Bozhenko, Rajesh Ranjit and Elena Aleksandrovna Kudinova

Abstract

Breast cancer is the most commonly diagnosed cancer in the world. Clinical manifestation and instrumental methods like mammography, ultrasound, and MRI are widely used in detecting breast cancer, however, molecular diagnosis is an indispensable aspect of breast cancer diagnosis processes. The method is a cornerstone for assessing the risk factors, screening the potential case, diagnosing the disease accurately, selecting the proper treatment procedures, prescribing the most effective drug, and monitoring the treated patients. Along with it, the chapter has also covered the different methods of molecular genetic diagnostic procedures used in clinical practice and for research, with their advantages and shortcomings. Modern technologies have allowed oncologists to dive deeper into the different types of breast cancer in order to find the most effective treatment for the patient, leading to the era of precision medicine in the field of oncology.

Keywords: breast cancer, oncomarkers, genetics, phenotype, molecular biological subtype, precision medicine

1. Introduction

Breast cancer is a form of malignant tumour in which breast tissue grows uncontrollably. It has been enlisted to be the most commonly diagnosed cancer in the world. According to the data, around 2.26 million cases of breast cancer were recorded in 2020, followed by lung cancer (2.21 million) and prostate cancer (1.41 million) [1]. In order to identify the cancer in its early stage, screening is done routinely. The screening usually consists of instrumental methods of diagnosis like mammography and ultrasound. When there is a suspicion of cancer, the patients undergo a biopsy and various molecular studies are done to diagnose the disease, identify its molecular subtype, and select the most appropriate treatment. However new genetic tools have recently been discovered that aid in screening and diagnosing breast cancer as well. Finally, after treatment has been completed, certain biomarkers are monitored to observe the progression/stabilization of the disease.

Currently, molecular biological technologies are used to solve the whole range of tasks related to diagnosis, therapy planning, monitoring, and prognosis in breast cancer.

But, first of all, we need to understand what causes breast cancer. The most widely accepted theory of its origin is related to genetics, however exact aetiology of cancer is still shrouded in mystery. Nevertheless, there are some factors that seem to enhance the growth and development of breast cancer. For studying breast cancer, we first need to understand what those risk factors are, which are illustrated in **Table 1**.

As there are many factors that need to be accounted for determining the risk of having breast cancer, there exists a number of online calculators that compute the risk of having cancer, based on the presence/absence of these factors. Some of the calculators are as follows:

Risk factor	Remarks
Sex	Women are more common victims of breast cancer than men.
Age	It is the second most important risk factor for breast cancer. The incidence of breast cancer is found to be increased with increasing age. According to an article in 2017, the risk of breast cancer is directly proportional to age [2]: From birth till age 49: 1 in 52 50–59: 1 in 44 60–69: 1 in 29 >70: 1 in 15
Family history	Nearly 25% of breast cancers have been found to be associated with family history. In one of the UK cohort researches, individuals with one-first degree relative suffering from breast cancer has an increased risk of breast cancer by a factor of 1.75. The factor increases to 2.5 if the individual has two or more first-degree relatives with breast cancer [3]. This is partially found to be related to BRCA1 and BRCA2 genes.
Reproductive factors	The number of ovulations is directly proportional to the increased risk of developing breast cancer. Hence, reproductive characteristics like early menarche, late menopause, late age of first pregnancy, and low parity increase the risk of developing breast cancer. Breast cancer risk is increased by 3% for each 1-year delay in menopause. Each additional birth or each 1-year delay in menarche reduces the risk of breast cancer by 5% or 10%, respectively [4, 5].
Estrogen	Estrogen levels are associated with the risk of breast cancer. Estrogen is endogenously produced by the ovary in premenopausal women and exogenously received in the form of oral contraceptives or hormone replacement therapy, which may trigger breast cancer [6]. Even though formulations in oral contraceptives have been upgraded to reduce side effects, the risk was still found to be higher than 1.5 for African-American women and Iranian populations [7, 8].
Lifestyle	Breast cancer risk can be increased by contemporary lifestyle factors such as excessive alcohol use and dietary fat consumption. Alcohol drinking can stimulate the estrogen receptor pathways and raise blood levels of hormones associated with estrogen. Consumption of 35 to 44 grams of alcohol per day can raise the risk of breast cancer by 32% [9, 10]. Mutagens from cigarette smoke have been found in the breast fluid of non-lactating women, despite the fact that the link between smoking and the risk of breast cancer is still debatable. Women who smoke and drink also have a higher chance of developing breast cancer [11]. As of today, mounting data show that smoking, especially when starting young, increases the chance of developing breast cancer [12, 13].
Racial disparity	Breast cancer varies in different races. The frequency of having breast cancer follows the order: White women>Black>Asian/Pacific>Islander>Hispanic>American Indian/Alaska Native. On the other hand, the fatality of breast cancer amongst the different ethnic groups has the order: Black women>White>Hispanic>Asian/Pacific>Islander>American>Indian/Alaska Native women [14].

Table 1.
Risk factors of breast cancer.

- https://bcrisktool.cancer.gov/calculator.html
- https://ibis.ikonopedia.com/
- https://www.bu.edu/slone/bwhs-brcarisk-calculator/

Besides environmental factors, there are genetic factors as well which influence breast cancer. There are several genes that involve in breast cancer, however, the gene mutations that frequently cause breast cancers are *BRCA1, BRCA2, PTEN, TP53, CDH1, STK11, CHEK2, BRIP1, ATM,* and *PALB2* [15]. These gene mutations can have high risk or low risk (**Table 2**). If the gene mutation occurs in the gene of high risk, there is a greater probability of having second breast cancer, so the patients may be given the option to undergo prophylactic bilateral mastectomy.

The presence of a mutation, under certain circumstances, can lead to the development of a malignant phenotype (the appearance of a tumour).

The ultimate change, that converts normal functioning cells into cancerous cells is due to a change in its phenotype. A phenotype is a combination of observable characteristics or traits in an organism. The characteristics might be its physical form, chemical properties, or physiological behaviour which is determined by the interaction between its genetic makeup and surroundings. In a nutshell, it can be said that a phenotype is the set of observable characteristics of an individual resulting from the interaction of its genotype with the environment. There are few changes in the phenotypes which occur in cancerous cells. They are as follows:

- self-sufficiency in growth signals
- insensitivity to anti-growth signals
- apoptosis evasion
- limitless replication potential
- sustained angiogenesis
- tissue invasion and metastasis
- abnormal metabolic pathways
- immune system evasion

Such phenotypic modification may be expressed due to changes in genotype. However, the change may occur in different levels (**Table 3**).

If the patients have been genetically predisposed to mutation of genes that increase the risk of breast cancer, such breast cancers are called hereditary cancer. On the other hand, it should be emphasized that a malignant tumour can also occur in the absence of hereditary mutations. Changes can occur already in the somatic cells of the body as well. In such cases, the breast cancer would be sporadic. The clinical properties and treatment approaches for these two variants of breast cancer differ.

Risk	Gene	Known/possible function
High risk	*BRCA1* (BReast CAncer1)	*BRCA1* is a tumour suppressor gene. It is found to regulate the cell cycle, maintain genome stability, and repair DNA damage [16]. Patients with these mutations are recommended to undergo bilateral salpingo-oophorectomy for reducing the risk of another breast cancer [17].
	BRCA2 (BReast CAncer2)	*BRCA2* is also a tumour suppressor gene that regulates the mechanism of DNA repair and cell death pathway and thus controls uncontrolled cell division [18]. Patients with these mutations are also recommended to undergo bilateral salpingo-oophorectomy for reducing the risk of breast cancer [17].
	ATM (Ataxia Telangiectasia Mutated)	Whenever there is a DNA double-strand breakdown, *ATM* gets activated, which in turn phosphorylates many downstream tumour suppressor genes such as *BRCA1*, *P53*, *CHK1*, and *CHK2* to prevent uncontrolled cell division [19].
	PALB2 (partner and localizer of BRCA2)	*PALB2* functions as a tumour suppressor gene and participates in the maintenance of genome integrity [20].
	PTEN (Phosphatase and tensin homolog)	*PTEN* is a phosphatase and is responsible for the regulation of cell signalling pathways like PI3K/Akt/mTOR, FAK/p130cas, and ERK/MAPK [21–24]. It plays a key role in many cellular functions like inhibition of cell adhesion and migration, apoptosis, blockade of the cell cycle and cell proliferation, inhibition of angioneogenesis, DNA repair, and metabolism [22, 23, 25–27].
	TP53 (tumour protein p53)	*TP53* is a tumour suppressor gene that codes for a protein that regulates cell cycle arrest, cellular senescence, apoptosis, metabolism, DNA repair, and other processes following cellular stress [28].
	STK11/LKB1 (serine-threonine kinase 11/ liver kinase B1)	The *STK11/ LKB1* is a gene that encodes for a tumour-suppressing enzyme called serine/threonine kinase 11, thereby controlling the uncontrolled growth and division of cells [29].
Low risk	*CDH1* (Cadherin 1)	The *CDH1* gene is responsible for encoding the E-cadherin protein, which is key for maintaining pluripotency and self-renewal of embryonic stem cells and neural stem cells [30–32]. Dysfunction of CDH1 is thought to increase the risk of development of malignant tumour and metastasis [33].
	CHEK2 (Checkpoint kinase 2)	When DNA is damaged, *CHEK2* is activated which plays an important role in pathways that govern DNA repair, cell cycle arrest, or apoptosis [34].
	BRIP1 (BRCA1 Interacting Protein 1)	*BRIP1* is a tumour suppressor gene that repairs DNA damage and preserves genetic stability [35].

Table 2.
Genetic factors of breast cancer.

Level	Mechanism	Detection methods	Example
Genetic level	• Chromosomal translocations • point mutations • Amplification • Genetic instability	Site-specific Polymer Chain Reaction (PCR), methylation-specific PCR, Single-Strand Conformational Polymorphism (SSCP), heteroduplex analysis, Hybridization, Fluorescence In Situ Hybridization (FISH), Sequencing.	*P53, RAS, ER, RAF B, BRCA1, BRCA2, P16 MUC-1, integrin, ERBB-2*
Epigenetic level	• DNA methylation • Histone acetylation • Chromatin modifications • RNA-mediated gene silencing		*P16, GSTP1, APC, LINE, cellular Myc*
RNA	• Alternative splicing • Life span change • Epigenetic changes	Quantitative PCR, Serial Analysis of Gene Expression (SAGE) hybridization, differential display PCR (DD-PCR)	*PSA, MUC-18, AFP.*
Protein	• Post-translational modification • Concentrations	Use of antibodies (Enzyme-Linked Immunosorbent Assay (ELISA), immunohistochemistry, Western blot), Protein Truncation Test (PTT), Gas Chromatography–Mass Spectrometry (GC-MS)	A panel of trefoil factor (TFF) 1, TFF2, and TFF3
Low molecular weight metabolites	• Profiles of low molecular weight metabolites	GC-MS, ELISA, Radioimmunoassay (RIA)	elevated choline, low glycerophosphocholine, and low glucose

Table 3.
Different levels of change which are finally manifested into phenotype.

2. Screening

The effectiveness of breast cancer therapy highly depends on the stage at which the cancer is detected. Therefore, methods and approaches for early detection of breast cancer are extremely important.

The first clinical sign of breast cancer starts with patients complaining about a lump in the breast. Around four-fifths of the patients have this symptom. Besides it, some may suffer from breast pain, and abnormalities of nipple, and breast skin [36]. The next step for those patients is to undergo instrumental methods of diagnosis, i.e. mammography (for females >40 years old), ultrasound (for females <40 years old), and thermography. When the result is not decisive, an MRI can also be taken. These days, artificial intelligence has also been accompanied with these instrumental methods of diagnosis to aid in making correct predictions. Along with the instrumental methods, recent studies have come up with new contemporary approaches that can also be utilized in diagnostic procedures. Some of the oncomarkers that have been actively studied and can be used in diagnostic procedures are given in **Table 4**.

After the suspicious lesion has been identified in the breast tissue, the next step is to undergo a biopsy to distinguish it from other benign conditions and to study the

Oncomarker	Remarks	Sensitivity (%)	Specificity (%)
Circulating tumor DNA (ctDNA)	Tumours can release their DNA fragments into the bloodstream which are called ctDNA. It has only been used in research and clinical trials, but it may be used in usual clinical practice as well, once the methods are standardized. It can be implemented in screening, diagnosis, follow-up, treatment, and in metastatic breast cancer [37].	88 [38]	98 [38]
Micro-RNA	Micro-RNAs are non-coding molecules but by complementary binding, they can regulate the genetic activity of the cell. There are many RNAs which act as biomarkers for breast cancer diagnosis [39]. Specific micro-RNAs have been found to prognosticate the effectiveness of certain drug treatments as well [40]. Although the preliminary results are promising, large-scale experiments need to be conducted to validate the result so that it could be used in clinical practice.	96.95 [41]	100 [41]
linear non-coding single-stranded RNA	They are the short-length RNA molecules that are involved in transcription and translation. Different types of these RNAs can provide information about properties of the breast cancer, metastasis, and resistance to chemotherapy [42]. A clinical trial is being conducted to assess the efficacy of these RNAs [43].	92 [42]	74 [42]
Circular RNA	They are covalently bound circular loops of RNA. They can regulate gene expression via micro-RNA sponging. Some of the circular RNAs have been found to have diagnostic and prognostic roles in breast cancer [44, 45]. However, the use of circular RNA in breast cancer is still in its infancy and exploratory experiments have to be carried out to elucidate its capabilities [46].	77 [47]	71 [47]
Blood-based DNA methylation	Methylation changes in DNA in the blood samples of peripheral blood have been associated with breast cancer [48]. Increased DNA methylation within functional promoters across the genome and decreased DNA methylation in other regions is the hallmark of breast cancer [49]. However, the evidence is still limited for blood-based methylation markers to be used in the general population for early detection of breast cancer. So, a large and methodologically rigorous epidemiological experiment has to be conducted to validate the use of blood-based DNA methylation in detecting breast cancer [50].	88.9 [51]	80.6 [51]
Autoantibodies	As the tumour cells are genetically unstable, the proteomes of the tumour are modified by phosphorylation, acetylation, and glycosylation, forming tumour-associated antigens. As a result, the body makes autoantibodies against those tumour-associated antigens. Detecting those autoantibodies aids in the diagnosis of breast cancer far before symptoms are clinically manifested [52, 53]. However, the autoantibodies are not used in clinical practice because their sensitivity and specificity are not higher than the methods that are currently in use (mammography). Furthermore, there exists no standard for detecting these autoantibodies in breast cancer detection [52].	24 [54]	96 [54]

Table 4.
Some of the diagnostic oncomarkers.

morphological features of the tumour for determining the prognosis and selecting the optimal therapy. The suspected lesion in the breast can arise usually from two different tissues—ducts (80% of cases) or lobules (10% of cases) of the glandular breast tissue. The less common 10% of breast cancer consists of mucinous, cribriform, micropapillary, papillary, tubular, medullary, metaplastic, and inflammatory carcinomas [55, 56]. On the other hand, breast cancer can also be non-invasive (stage 0) or invasive (stages I to IV). Depending upon its origin and invasiveness, breast cancer can be classified as:

- Ductal carcinoma in situ (DCIS)
- Invasive ductal carcinoma (IDC)
- Lobular carcinoma in situ (LCIS)
- Invasive lobular carcinoma (ILC)

IDC is the most common form of breast cancer, accounting for around 55% of all breast cancers [57].

After the biopsy of the lesion is taken, the material is thoroughly studied and the phenotype is revealed through immunohistochemistry (IHC). On the basis of IHC, breast cancer has four primary molecular phenotypes, defined in large part by hormone receptors and other types of proteins involved (or not involved) in each cancer (**Table 5**) [61].

2.1 Luminal A breast cancer

Luminal A tumours are the most common molecular type of breast cancer. This biological subtype has a receptor for estrogen and/or progesterone and can be treated using drugs blocking these hormones. This form of cancer highly expresses genes responsible for a molecular cascade of estrogen gene- *ESR1, XBP1, FOXA1, GATA3, TTF3, LIV3, HER4, PIK3R*I as well as highly express luminal cytokeratin due to methylation of *RASSF1, GSTP1, MMP7, PEG10, APC* genes.

2.2 Luminal B breast cancer

These types of cancer are hormone positives as luminal A but differ by the high level of Ki67%. This is the reason why luminal B breast cancers grow faster than luminal type A. Luminal type B can be HER2 positive or HER2 negative. In the phenotype, total methylation of the genome is found, especially of genes *RASSF1, GSTP1, CHI3L2*.

2.3 HER2-enriched

One in five invasive breast cancers is HER2-positive, making this one of the more common breast cancer subtypes in the world. HER2-positive cancers are ER- and PR-negative and HER2-positive. *GRB7, HRAS, MEK1/MEK2, AKT1* are also overexpressed in this phenotype of breast cancer.

HER2-positive breast cancer cells carry too many copies of the HER2 gene, which makes HER2-protein receptors, found on breast cells. The main function of HER2

Molecular biological subtype		Clinic-pathological subtype	% of relapse [58]	Frequency of metastatic sites [59]	Treatment [60]
Luminal A		• ER+ • HER2- • Ki67 < 20% • PR > 20%	5.02	Multiple site-50.9% One site-49.1% Bone metastasis-30% Lung metastasis-5% Liver metastasis-3.5% Others-10.6%	Mostly hormonal therapy
Luminal B	Luminal B HER-	• ER+ • HER2- • Either Ki67 > 30% or PR < 20%	7.88		Hormonal therapy + chemotherapy (docetaxel + cyclophosphamide or doxorubicin + cyclophosphamide + docetaxel / Paclitaxel)
	Luminal B HER+	• ER+ • HER2+	6.61	Multiple site-58.8% One site-41.2% Bone metastasis-22.9% Lung metastasis-1.5% Liver metastasis-6.1% Others-10.7%	Hormonal therapy + chemotherapy (docetaxel + cyclophosphamide or doxorubicin + cyclophosphamide + docetaxel / Paclitaxel) + anti-HER2 therapy (trastuzumab)
HER+		• ER- • HER2+	13.1	Multiple site-50% One site-50% Bone metastasis-16.2% Lung metastasis-5.4% Liver metastasis-13.5% Others-14.9%	Chemotherapy + anti-HER2 therapy (docetaxel + cyclophosphamide or doxorubicin + cyclophosphamide + docetaxel / Paclitaxel)
Basal type		• ER- • PR- • HER2-	16.76	Multiple site-53.6% One site-46.4% Bone metastasis-16.8% Lung metastasis-9.6% Liver metastasis-6.4% Others-13.6%	**Table 6**

Table 5.
The molecular biological subtype of breast cancer.

receptor is to control how breast cells grow. When there is excess HER2, the cells absorb excess human epidermal growth factor, which makes them proliferate rapidly.

2.4 Triple-negative

In this type of cancer, the cells do not contain receptors for estrogen, progesterone, or HER2 but are characterized by high expression of oncogenes like *NRAS, KRAS, C-KIT*, cadherin P (*CDH3*), lamini alpha/gamma (*LAMA5, LAMC1*), *MCM3/4/7,* and basal cytokerain *KRT5/6/17*. This type of breast cancer is found in breast ducts and is very invasive in nature. The triple-negative breast cancer can be categorized into six subtypes based on their gene expression portfolio (**Table 6**). The subtypes are immunomodulatory (IM), luminal androgen receptor (LAR), basal-like 1 (BL-1), basal-like 2 (BL-2), mesenchymal (M), and mesenchymal stem-like (MSL) [62].

However, recent studies using DNA microarray have identified several molecular subtypes of breast cancer—luminal A, luminal B, HER2-enriched, basal-like, claudin-low, and normal-like [63–67]. The classification based on complex patterns of gene expression bridges the gap between cancer behaviour and its molecular biological subtype because each breast cancer is a distinct entity based on genomic, transcriptomic, and proteomic data [68]. As each breast cancer is unique, this ushers oncology to a new era of personalized medicine, where each breast cancer can be treated individually, custom-tailored to the specific patient (**Table 7**).

It is to be noted that there is a disparity in molecular phenotype determined by IHC and methods of analysis of genetic expression. For example, some authors claim the disparity to be 31–59% in HER2 expression when analyzed by ICH and in situ hybridization [71, 72]. In the present day, there are several genetic tests for phenotyping and prognosticating the disease. Some of them are illustrated in **Table 8**.

TNBC type	Characteristics	Treatment options
BL-1	DNA damage response pathway	PARP inhibitors Platinum compounds
BL-2	Growth factor signalling, glycolysis, and gluconeogenesis	Growth signalling inhibition
LAR	High expression of genes related to hormone	Androgen receptor antagonists
M	Cell differentiation pathway, the interaction between extracellular receptors, mobility of cell	Wnt/β-catenin inhibitors PI3K/mTOR inhibitors TGF-β receptor kinase inhibitors
MSL	Similar to M subtype but is claudin-low and high expression of mesenchymal stem cells	PI3K inhibitors mTOR inhibitors
IM	Immune cell process	Immune checkpoint Inhibitors

Table 6.
Characteristics and possible treatment options based on TNBC molecular subtypes.

Molecular class	Chemotherapy response	Therapy
Luminal A	Low	Tamoxifen, Fulvestrant, Aromatase inhibitors
Luminal B	Intermediate	
HER2-positive	High	HER2 and kinase inhibitor: lapatinib, pertuzumab, trastuzumab, and adotratuzomab emtansine, immune cell activation (Ertumaxomab)
Basal-like	High	PARP1 inhibitor (Olaparib and Iniparib), cisplatin
Claudin-low	Intermediate/low	Inhibitor of PIK3CG combined with paclitaxel [70]
Normal-like	N/A	N/A

Table 7.
Breast cancer classification based on molecular profiling and corresponding treatment options [69].

Platform	Method	Number of genes	Indication	Prediction
Mammaprint	Chromosomal microarray, Real-time PCR	70	I and II stage, size = 5 cm, estrogen (+), l/n (−)/[1–3 l/n (+)]	Prognosis of breast cancer
OncotypeDx	Real-time PCR	21	estrogen (+), l/n (−)	Prognosis of breast cancer, effectiveness of adjuvant chemotherapy
MapQuantDx	Chromosomal microarray, Real-time PCR	97/9	estrogen (+), G2	Determine grade (G) of breast cancer, the effectiveness of hormonal therapy
Breast Cancer Index	Chromosomal microarray, Real-time PCR	7	estrogen (+)	Prognosis of breast cancer, effectiveness of hormonal therapy
Oncotype Dx	Real-time PCR	21	I and II stage, estrogen (+), *HER2* (−)	Effectiveness of chemotherapy, the possibility of relapse

l/n = lymphnode.

Table 8.
Genetic tests for phenotyping and prognosticating breast cancer.

Although the molecular genetic classification of the breast cancer subtype has clear benefits over the IHC subtype, molecular classification based on genetic analysis has not been implemented in routine clinical practice because of political and economic obstacles. Furthermore, IHC is readily available in every health centre, whereas it is challenging to perform molecular genetic tests due to a lack of proper equipment and expertise [73].

Finally, after selecting the adequate treatment scheme corresponding to its molecular subtype, the patient has to be monitored. For monitoring purposes, the following oncomarkers have been purposed (**Table 9**). Despite the existence of several oncomarkers, CA153, CA 27.29, and CEA are only used routinely in clinical practice. Other oncomarkers are specific to cancers of other organs, but they have also been investigated in breast cancer patients.

Oncomarker	Remarks	Normal value	Sensitivity (%)	Specificity (%)
CA 15-3	CA 15-3 is a carbohydrate-containing protein antigen called mucin (MUC). Its serum concentration is useful in predicting the progression of breast cancer and monitoring the efficacy of the therapy as its quantity is directly proportional to the size of the tumour and its severity (stage). It is generally recommended to monitor CA125 and CEA once every 3 months [74] as they are considered complementary [75].	≤ 30 U/mL [75]	70 [76]	96 [76]

Oncomarker	Remarks	Normal value	Sensitivity (%)	Specificity (%)
CEA	CEA is a glycoprotein which is responsible for cell adhesion. CEA is normally produced in the gastrointestinal tissue during foetal development, but its production stops before birth. In breast cancer, CEA is elevated when there is a metastasis of the primary lesion of breast cancer. Preoperative CEA measurements have shown that its level is directly proportional to the pathological stage and tumour size and the size of a metastatic lesion. It is recommended to monitor CEA level every 2–3 months [77].	2.5 μg/L [75]	88.3 [78]	46.2 [78]
CA 27.29	CA27.29 is a carbohydrate-containing protein antigen that is also produced by MUC-1 gene as CA153. Since CA 153 and CA 27.29 are derivatives of MUC1, their clinical significance in breast cancers is comparable. However, evidence shows that CA 27.29 has high sensitivity than CA 15-3, but lacks specificity. The oncomarker is more useful in detecting the disease progression and metastatic involvement. The average time interval to evaluate CA27.29 is 5 months [79].	38 U/mL [80]	62 [81]	83 [81]
HER-2	HER-2 is a protein that is encoded by the gene erythroblastic oncogene B (*ERBB2*), a gene that is originally isolated from the avian genome. The protein consists of three different parts: • an extracellular ligand-binding domain E • single transmembrane domain • an intracellular tyrosine kinase. The extracellular domain can undergo proteolytic cleavage, thereby releasing a detectable amount of it into the bloodstream. HER-2 receptor protein has been found useful for early diagnosis of relapses and to predict the fate of metastases of breast cancer. In some studies, HER2-ECD was recommended to measure once every 4 weeks [82].	7.7 ng/ml [83]	76.92 [84]	72.92 [84]
plasminogen-activating proteins	urokinase-type plasminogen activator (uPA), plasminogen activator inhibitor-1 (PAI-1), and uPA receptor (uPAR) are plasminogen-activating proteins. Their high levels usually imply a poor prognosis of the cancer. The main function of uPA is to convert plasminogen into active plasmin. It has the ability to stimulate angiogenesis, mitogenesis, cell migration and to modulate cell adhesion and to prevent apoptosis. On the other hand, PAI-1 can inhibit uPA, which is supposed to prevent metastasis. Tumour expression of PAI-1 and uPAR represent important breast cancer prognostic factors.	2.52 ng/ml [85]	44.8 [85]	85.3 [85]

Oncomarker	Remarks	Normal value	Sensitivity (%)	Specificity (%)
Nestin	Nestin is actually a marker of neural progenitors that usually exist in stem cells of the central nervous system. However, it has also been identified in the mammary glands, especially in the basal and myoepithelial layers. They produce nestin, but the cancerous tissue produces even more nestin, which makes it an excellent diagnostic tool for breast cancer.	39.9 pg./mL [86]	84.8 [86]	65.1 [86]
HE4	HE4 is a protein that human epididymis produces. Although its secretion is related to the epididymis, researchers have found some of its diagnostic value for breast cancer. Its serum concentration has been found to increase in patients with breast cancer in comparison to healthy controls [87].	54.5 pmol/l [87]	73.3 [87]	65.3 [87]
TPA	TPA is a complex of polypeptide filaments of the cytokeratins 8, 18, and 19. Although TPA is mainly helpful in monitoring and evaluating the treatment process, it has also been found to prognosticate tumour progression and metastasis in the case of breast cancer, especially in association with other tumour markers like CEA [88].	120 U/I [89]	67.5 [89]	81.9 [89]
AFP	AFP is a protein made by growing and dividing liver cells. AFP test usually detests liver cancer and germ cell cancers, however, when combined with other tumour markers, it can also be valuable in detecting breast cancer. In terms of mechanism, AFP is thought to be involved in the regulation of cell growth and differentiation. It has been suggested that AFP may play a role in the development of breast cancer by promoting cell proliferation and inhibiting apoptosis [90, 91].	10–150 ng/ml [92]	22.2 [93]	94.33 [93]
CA199	CA199 is a protein found on the surface of certain cancer cells but it may be found in the bloodstream when shed by cancerous tissue. Usually, it is detected in pancreatic cancer, however, some studies have detected serum level changes of tumour marker CA199 in breast cancer as well [94]. It is not generally used in clinical practice due to its limited predictive value. However, an increase of CA199 above 1000 U/ml accurately predicts metastatic cancer [79].	<37 U/ml [95]	19.36 [93]	94.54 [93]
CA125	CA125 is a tumour marker that is most commonly associated with ovarian cancer, but can also be a sign of breast cancer. It has been found that about 84% of metastatic breast cancers have elevated levels of CA125 [96]. However, CA125 is not a specific marker for breast cancer and can also be influenced by benign conditions or other malignancies [97]. It is recommended to monitor CA125 every 3 months [79].	35 IU/mL [98]	93.8 [99]	28.7 [99]

Table 9.
Some of the oncomarkers for monitoring breast cancer.

3. Conclusion

Molecular diagnostic tools are involved in each and every aspect of breast cancer, starting from the screening process to monitoring the patients after treatment. But, instrumental diagnostic measures account for the majority of screening processes. If there is a suspicion, a biopsy is taken to establish a diagnosis. In order to select proper treatment, IHC is done to classify breast cancer, but it is to be noted that molecular genetic classification is more precise than IHC, however, IHC is widely used in clinical practice because it is readily available. After the patient has been treated, different oncomarkers can be checked to monitor the possible progression of the disease.

Although it has been found that contemporary treatment of breast cancer has shown better results in a considerable proportion of breast cancer patients, a certain number of patients have shown only modest benefits. Hence, the diagnostic, classification, and treatment processes have to be optimized based on novel molecular genetic parameters, which would lead to even better clinical outcomes. This would also substantially contribute to personalized medicine and result in a more effective and prolonged response, finally improving the survival rate of patients suffering from breast cancer.

Author details

Vladimir Kanstantinovich Bozhenko[1], Rajesh Ranjit[1,2,3*] and Elena Aleksandrovna Kudinova[1]

1 Federal State Budgetary Institution "Russian Scientific Center of Roentgenoradiology" of the Ministry of Healthcare of the Russian Federation (RSCRR), Moscow, Russian Federation

2 Peoples' Friendship University of Russia (RUDN University), Moscow, Russian Federation

3 State Budgetary Healthcare Centre "Municipal Clinical Hospital Number 1" of the Healthcare Department of Moscow City, Moscow, Russian Federation

*Address all correspondence to: rajesh.ranjit@mail.ru

References

[1] Ferlay J, Colombet M, Soerjomataram I, Parkin DM, Piñeros M, Znaor A, et al. Cancer statistics for the year 2020: An overview. International Journal of Cancer. 2021;**149**(4):778-789. DOI: 10.1002/IJC.33588

[2] Siegel RL, Miller KD, Jemal A. Cancer statistics, 2017. CA: A Cancer Journal for Clinicians. 2017;**67**(1):7-30. DOI: 10.3322/CAAC.21387

[3] Brewer HR, Jones ME, Schoemaker MJ, Ashworth A, Swerdlow AJ. Family history and risk of breast cancer: An analysis accounting for family structure. Breast Cancer Research and Treatment. 2017;**165**(1):193-200. DOI: 10.1007/S10549-017-4325-2

[4] Horn J, Vatten LJ. Reproductive and hormonal risk factors of breast cancer: A historical perspective. International Journal of Women's Health. 2017;**9**:265-272. DOI: 10.2147/IJWH.S129017

[5] Dall GV, Britt KL. Estrogen effects on the mammary gland in early and late life and breast cancer risk. Frontiers in Oncology. 2017;7:110. DOI: 10.3389/FONC.2017.00110

[6] Travis RC, Key TJ. Oestrogen exposure and breast cancer risk. Breast Cancer Research. 2003;**5**(5):247. DOI: 10.1186/BCR628

[7] Soroush A, Farshchian N, Komasi S, Izadi N, Amirifard N, Shahmohammadi A. The role of Oral contraceptive pills on increased risk of breast cancer in Iranian populations: A meta-analysis. Journal of Cancer Prevention. 2016;**21**(4):294-301. DOI: 10.15430/JCP.2016.21.4.294

[8] Bethea TN, Rosenberg L, Hong CC, Troester MA, Lunetta KL, Bandera EV, et al. A case–control analysis of oral contraceptive use and breast cancer subtypes in the African American breast cancer epidemiology and risk consortium. Breast Cancer Research. 2015;**17**(1):22. DOI: 10.1186/S13058-015-0535-X

[9] Hamajima N, Hirose K, Tajima K, Rohan T, Calle EE, Heath CW, et al. Alcohol, tobacco and breast cancer—Collaborative reanalysis of individual data from 53 epidemiological studies, including 58,515 women with breast cancer and 95,067 women without the disease. British Journal of Cancer. 2002;**87**(11):1234-1245. DOI: 10.1038/SJ.BJC.6600596

[10] Jung S, Wang M, Anderson K, Baglietto L, Bergkvist L, Bernstein L, et al. Alcohol consumption and breast cancer risk by estrogen receptor status: in a pooled analysis of 20 studies. International Journal of Epidemiology. 2016;**45**(3):916-928. DOI: 10.1093/IJE/DYV156

[11] Knight JA, Fan J, Malone KE, John EM, Lynch CF, Langballe R, et al. Alcohol consumption and cigarette smoking in combination: A predictor of contralateral breast cancer risk in the WECARE study. International Journal of Cancer. 2017;**141**(5):916-924. DOI: 10.1002/IJC.30791

[12] Catsburg C, Miller AB, Rohan TE. Active cigarette smoking and risk of breast cancer. International Journal of Cancer. 2015;**136**(9):2204-2209. DOI: 10.1002/IJC.29266

[13] Kispert S, McHowat J. Recent insights into cigarette smoking as a lifestyle risk factor for breast cancer. Breast Cancer

(London). 2017;**9**:132. DOI: 10.2147/BCTT.S129746

[14] Yedjou CG, Sims JN, Miele L, Noubissi F, Lowe L, Fonseca DD, et al. Health and racial disparity in breast cancer. Advances in Experimental Medicine and Biology. 2019;**1152**:49. DOI: 10.1007/978-3-030-20301-6_3

[15] Shiovitz S, Korde LA. Genetics of breast cancer: A topic in evolution. Annals of Oncology. 2015;**26**(7):1299. DOI: 10.1093/ANNONC/MDV022

[16] Fu X, Tan W, Song Q, Pei H, Li J. BRCA1 and breast cancer: Molecular mechanisms and therapeutic strategies. Frontiers in Cell and Development Biology. 2022;**10**:813457. DOI: 10.3389/FCELL.2022.813457/BIBTEX

[17] Franceschini G, Di LA, Terribile D, Sanchez MA, Masetti R. Bilateral prophylactic mastectomy in BRCA mutation carriers: What surgeons need to know. Annali Italiani di Chirurgia. 2019;**90**:1-2

[18] Sadeghi F, Asgari M, Matloubi M, Ranjbar M, Karkhaneh Yousefi N, Azari T, et al. Molecular contribution of BRCA1 and BRCA2 to genome instability in breast cancer patients: Review of radiosensitivity assays. Biological Procedures Online. 2020;**22**(1):1-28. DOI: 10.1186/S12575-020-00133-5/TABLES/6

[19] Prokopcova J, Kleibl Z, Banwell CM, Pohlreich P. The role of ATM in breast cancer development. Breast Cancer Research and Treatment. 2007;**104**(2):121-128. DOI: 10.1007/S10549-006-9406-6/FIGURES/1

[20] Wu S, Zhou J, Zhang K, Chen H, Luo M, Lu Y, et al. Molecular mechanisms of PALB2 function and its role in breast cancer management. Frontiers in Oncology. 2020;**10**:301. DOI: 10.3389/FONC.2020.00301

[21] Chen H, Zhou L, Wu X, Li R, Wen J, Sha J, et al. The PI3K/AKT pathway in the pathogenesis of prostate cancer. Frontiers in Bioscience (Landmark Ed.). 2016;**21**(5):1084-1091. DOI: 10.2741/4443

[22] Bi X, Lv X, Liu D, Guo H, Yao G, Wang L, et al. METTL3-mediated maturation of miR-126-5p promotes ovarian cancer progression via PTEN-mediated PI3K/Akt/mTOR pathway. Cancer Gene Therapy. 2021;**28**(3-4):335-349. DOI: 10.1038/S41417-020-00222-3

[23] Alzahrani AS. PI3K/Akt/mTOR inhibitors in cancer: At the bench and bedside. Seminars in Cancer Biology. 2019;**59**:125-132. DOI: 10.1016/J.SEMCANCER.2019.07.009

[24] Xing Y, Lin NU, Maurer MA, Chen H, Mahvash A, Sahin A, et al. Phase II trial of AKT inhibitor MK-2206 in patients with advanced breast cancer who have tumors with PIK3CA or AKT mutations, and/or PTEN loss/PTEN mutation. Breast Cancer Research. 2019;**21**(1):78. DOI: 10.1186/S13058-019-1154-8

[25] Rodgers SJ, Ferguson DT, Mitchell CA, Ooms LM. Regulation of PI3K effector signalling in cancer by the phosphoinositide phosphatases. Bioscience Reports. 2017;**37**(1):BSR20160432. DOI: 10.1042/BSR20160432

[26] Suda T, Oba H, Takei H, Kurosumi M, Hayashi S, ichi, Yamaguchi Y. ER-activating ability of breast cancer stromal fibroblasts is regulated independently of alteration of TP53 and PTEN tumor suppressor genes. Biochemical and Biophysical Research Communications. 2012;**428**(2):259-263. DOI: 10.1016/J.BBRC.2012.10.035

[27] Li K, Li GD, Sun LY, Li XQ. PTEN and SHIP: Impact on lymphatic metastasis in breast cancer. Journal of Cancer Research and Therapeutics. 2018;**14**(Supplement):S937-S941. DOI: 10.4103/0973-1482.193894

[28] Kastenhuber ER, Lowe SW. Putting p53 in context. Cell. 2017;**170**(6):1062-1078. DOI: 10.1016/J.CELL.2017.08.028

[29] Alkaf A, Al-Jafari A, Wani TA, Alqattan S, Zargar S. Expression of STK11 gene and its promoter activity in MCF control and cancer cells. 3 Biotech. 2017;**7**(6):362. DOI: 10.1007/S13205-017-1000-6

[30] Soncin F, Ward CM. The function of e-cadherin in stem cell pluripotency and self-renewal. Genes (Basel). 2011;**2**(1):229-259. DOI: 10.3390/GENES2010229

[31] Karpowicz P, Willaime-Morawek S, Balenci L, Deveale B, Inoue T, Van Der Kooy D. E-cadherin regulates neural stem cell self-renewal. The Journal of Neuroscience. 2009;**29**(12):3885-3896. DOI: 10.1523/JNEUROSCI.0037-09.2009

[32] Redmer T, Diecke S, Grigoryan T, Quiroga-Negreira A, Birchmeier W, Besser D. E-cadherin is crucial for embryonic stem cell pluripotency and can replace OCT4 during somatic cell reprogramming. EMBO Reports. 2011;**12**(7):720-726. DOI: 10.1038/EMBOR.2011.88

[33] Margineau E, Cotrutz CE, Cotrutz C. Correlation between E-cadherin abnormal expressions in different types of cancer and the process of metastasis. Revista Medico-Chirurgicală a Societăţii de Medici şi Naturalişti din Iaşi. 2008;**112**(2):432-436

[34] Apostolou P, Papasotiriou I. Current perspectives on CHEK2 mutations in breast cancer. Breast Cancer (London). 2017;**9**:335. DOI: 10.2147/BCTT.S111394

[35] Khan U, Khan MS. Prognostic value estimation of BRIP1 in breast cancer by exploiting Transcriptomics data through bioinformatics approaches. Bioinformatics and Biology Insights. 2021;**15**:11779322211055892. DOI: 10.1177/11779322211055892

[36] Koo MM, von Wagner C, Abel GA, McPhail S, Rubin GP, Lyratzopoulos G. Typical and atypical presenting symptoms of breast cancer and their associations with diagnostic intervals: Evidence from a national audit of cancer diagnosis. Cancer Epidemiology. 2017;**48**:146. DOI: 10.1016/J.CANEP.2017.04.010

[37] Sant M, Bernat-Peguera A, Felip E, Margelí M. Role of ctDNA in breast cancer. Cancers (Basel). 2022;**14**(2):310. DOI: 10.3390/CANCERS14020310

[38] Lin Z, Neiswender J, Fang B, Ma X, Zhang J, Hu X. Value of circulating cell-free DNA analysis as a diagnostic tool for breast cancer: A meta-analysis. Oncotarget. 2017;**8**(16):26625-26636. DOI: 10.18632/ONCOTARGET.15775

[39] Sharifi Z, Talkhabi M, Taleahmad S. Identification of potential microRNA diagnostic panels and uncovering regulatory mechanisms in breast cancer pathogenesis. Scientific Reports. 2022;**12**(1):1-18. DOI: 10.1038/s41598-022-24347-7

[40] Jayaraj R, Madhav MR, Nayagam SG, Kar A, Sathyakumar S, Mohammed H, et al. Clinical Theragnostic relationship between drug-resistance specific miRNA expressions, chemotherapeutic resistance, and sensitivity in breast cancer: A systematic review and meta-analysis. Cell. 2019;**8**(10):1250. DOI: 10.3390/CELLS8101250

[41] Kim J. Identification of MicroRNAs as diagnostic biomarkers for breast cancer based on the cancer genome atlas. Diagnostics. 2021;**11**(1):107. DOI: 10.3390/DIAGNOSTICS11010107

[42] Jiang X, Zhang G, Wu J, Lin S, Liu Y, Ma Y, et al. Long noncoding RNA serve as a potential predictive biomarker for breast cancer: A meta-analysis. BioMed Research International. 2020;**2020**:9045786. DOI: 10.1155/2020/9045786

[43] Clinical Trial. TA(E)C-GP Versus A(E)C-T for the High Risk TNBC Patients and Validation of the mRNA-lnTA(E)C-GP Versus A(E) C-T for the High Risk TNBC Patients and Validation of the mRNA-lncRNA SignaturecRNA Signature. Fudan University 2023. Available from: https://classic.clinicaltrials.gov/ct2/show/NCT02641847 [Accessed: August 6, 2023]

[44] Yan L, Zheng M, Wang H. Circular RNA hsa_circ_0072309 inhibits proliferation and invasion of breast cancer cells via targeting miR-492. Cancer Management and Research. 2019;**11**:1041. DOI: 10.2147/CMAR.S186857

[45] Yin WB, Yan MG, Fang X, Guo JJ, Xiong W, Zhang RP. Circulating circular RNA hsa_circ_0001785 acts as a diagnostic biomarker for breast cancer detection. Clinica Chimica Acta. 2018;**487**:363-368. DOI: 10.1016/J.CCA.2017.10.011

[46] Zhang F, Li L, Fan Z. circRNAs and their relationship with breast cancer: A review. World Journal of Surgical Oncology. 2022;**20**(1):1-13. DOI: 10.1186/S12957-022-02842-5/TABLES/1

[47] Chu M, Fang Y, Jin Y. CircRNAs as promising biomarker in diagnosis of breast cancer: An updated meta-analysis. Journal of Clinical Laboratory Analysis. 2021;**35**(9):e23934. DOI: 10.1002/JCLA.23934

[48] Xu Z, Sandler DP, Taylor JA. Blood DNA methylation and breast cancer: A prospective case-cohort analysis in the sister study. Journal of the National Cancer Institute. 2020;**112**(1):94. DOI: 10.1093/JNCI/DJZ065

[49] Severi G, Southey MC, English DR, Jung C hee, Lonie A, McLean C, et al. Epigenome-wide methylation in DNA from peripheral blood as a marker of risk for breast cancer. Breast Cancer Research and Treatment. 2014;**148**(3):665-673. DOI: 10.1007/S10549-014-3209-Y

[50] Tang Q, Cheng J, Cao X, Surowy H, Burwinkel B. Blood-based DNA methylation as biomarker for breast cancer: A systematic review. Clinical Epigenetics. 2016;**8**(1):1-18. DOI: 10.1186/S13148-016-0282-6/TABLES/4

[51] Zhu X, Huang J, Zhang K, Yu Y. Value of concentration and gene methylation analyses of circulating cell-free DNA as diagnostic method for breast cancer: A systematic review. International Journal of Clinical and Experimental Medicine. 2018;**11**(8):7519-7530

[52] Yang R, Han Y, Yi W, Long Q. Autoantibodies as biomarkers for breast cancer diagnosis and prognosis. Frontiers in Immunology. 2022;**13**:1035402. DOI: 10.3389/FIMMU.2022.1035402

[53] Lu H, Ladd J, Feng Z, Wu M, Goodell V, Pitteri SJ, et al. Evaluation of known oncoantibodies, HER2, p53, and cyclin B1, in prediagnostic breast cancer sera. Cancer Prevention Research (Philadelphia, Pa.). 2012;**5**(8):1036-1043. DOI: 10.1158/1940-6207.CAPR-11-0558

[54] Piura B, Piura E. Autoantibodies to tumor-associated antigens in breast carcinoma. Journal of Oncology. 2010;**2010**:264926. DOI: 10.1155/2010/264926

[55] Rosen PP. The pathological classification of human mammary carcinoma: Past, present and future. Annals of Clinical and Laboratory Science. 1979;**9**(2):144-156

[56] Van Bogaert LJ. Recent progress in the histological typing of human breast tumours. Diagnostic Histopathology. 1981;**4**(4):349-353

[57] Eheman CR, Shaw KM, Ryerson AB, Miller JW, Ajani UA, White MC. The changing incidence of in situ and invasive ductal and lobular breast carcinomas: United States, 1999-2004. Cancer Epidemiology, Biomarkers & Prevention. 2009;**18**(6):1763-1769. DOI: 10.1158/1055-9965.EPI-08-1082/347826/P/THE-CHANGING-INCIDENCE-OF-IN-SITU-AND-INVASIVE

[58] Shim HJ, Kim SH, Kang BJ, Choi BG, Kim HS, Cha ES, et al. Breast cancer recurrence according to molecular subtype. Asian Pacific Journal of Cancer Prevention. 2014;**15**(14):5539-5544. DOI: 10.7314/APJCP.2014.15.14.5539

[59] Van Uden DJP, Van Maaren MC, Strobbe LJA, Bult P, Van Der Hoeven JJ, Siesling S, et al. Metastatic behavior and overall survival according to breast cancer subtypes in stage IV inflammatory breast cancer. Breast Cancer Research. 2019;**21**(1):113. DOI: 10.1186/S13058-019-1201-5

[60] Stenina MB, Zhukova LG, Koroleva IA, Parokonnaya AA, Semiglazova TY, Tyulyandin SA, et al. Practical recommendations for drug treatment of breast cancer. RUSSCO. 2020;**10**(3s2):150-187. DOI: 10.18027/2224-5057-2020-10-3s2-09

[61] Cho N. Molecular subtypes and imaging phenotypes of breast cancer. Ultrasonography. 2016;**35**(4):288. DOI: 10.14366/USG.16030

[62] Dass SA, Tan KL, Rajan RS, Mokhtar NF, Adzmi ERM, Rahman WFWA, et al. Triple negative breast cancer: A review of present and future diagnostic modalities. Medicina (B Aires). 2021;**57**(1):62. DOI: 10.3390/MEDICINA57010062

[63] Dabbs DJ, Chivukula M, Carter G, Bhargava R. Basal phenotype of ductal carcinoma in situ: Recognition and immunohistologic profile. Modern Pathology. 2006;**19**(11):1506-1511. DOI: 10.1038/MODPATHOL.3800678

[64] Bryan BB, Schnitt SJ, Collins LC. Ductal carcinoma in situ with basal-like phenotype: A possible precursor to invasive basal-like breast cancer. Modern Pathology. 2006;**19**(5):617-621. DOI: 10.1038/MODPATHOL.3800570

[65] Hannemann J, Velds A, Halfwerk JBG, Kreike B, Peterse JL, Van de Vijver MJ. Classification of ductal carcinoma in situ by gene expression profiling. Breast Cancer Research. 2006;**8**(5):R61. DOI: 10.1186/BCR1613

[66] Rivenbark AG, Coleman WB. Field cancerization in mammary carcinogenesis—Implications for prevention and treatment of breast cancer. Experimental and Molecular Pathology. 2012;**93**(3):391-398. DOI: 10.1016/J.YEXMP.2012.10.018

[67] Livasy CA, Perou CM, Karaca G, Cowan DW, Maia D, Jackson S, et al. Identification of a basal-like subtype of breast ductal carcinoma in situ.

Human Pathology. 2007;**38**(2):197-204. DOI: 10.1016/J.HUMPATH.2006.08.017

[68] Ellis MJ, Perou CM. The genomic landscape of breast cancer as a therapeutic roadmap. Cancer Discovery. 2013;**3**(1):27-34. DOI: 10.1158/2159-8290. CD-12-0462

[69] Jeibouei S, Akbari ME, Kalbasi A, Aref AR, Ajoudanian M, Rezvani A, et al. Personalized medicine in breast cancer: Pharmacogenomics approaches. Pharmacogenomics and Personalized Medicine. 2019;**12**:73. DOI: 10.2147/ PGPM.S167886

[70] Chang J, Hong L, Liu Y, Pan Y, Yang H, Ye W, et al. Targeting PIK3CG in combination with paclitaxel as a potential therapeutic regimen in claudin-low breast cancer. Cancer Management and Research. 2020;**12**:2641-2651. DOI: 10.2147/CMAR.S250171

[71] Bastien RR, Rodríguez-Lescure Á, Ebbert MT, Prat A, Munárriz B, Rowe L, et al. PAM50 breast cancer subtyping by RT-qPCR and concordance with standard clinical molecular markers. BMC Medical Genomics. 2012;**5**:44. DOI: 10.1186/1755-8794-5-44

[72] Sørlie T, Tibshirani R, Parker J, Hastie T, Marron JS, Nobel A, et al. Repeated observation of breast tumor subtypes in independent geneexpression data sets. Proceedings of the National Academy of Sciences of the United States of America. 2003;**100**(14):8423. DOI: 10.1073/PNAS.0932692100

[73] Prat A, Ellis MJ, Perou CM. Practical implications of gene-expression-based assays for breast oncologists. Nature Reviews. Clinical Oncology. 2011;**9**(1):48-57. DOI: 10.1038/ NRCLINONC.2011.178

[74] Mudduwa LKB, Wijayaratne GB, Peiris HH, Gunasekera SN, Abeysiriwardhana D, Liyanage N. Elevated pre-surgical CA15-3: Does it predict the short-term disease-free survival of breast cancer patients without distant metastasis? International Journal of Women's Health. 2018;**10**:335. DOI: 10.2147/IJWH.S162867

[75] Kabel AM. Tumor markers of breast cancer: New prospectives. Journal of Oncological Sciences. 2017;**3**(1):5-11. DOI: 10.1016/J.JONS.2017.01.001

[76] Tomlinson IPM, Whyman A, Barrett JA, Kremer JK. Tumour marker CA15-3: Possible uses in the routine management of breast cancer. European Journal of Cancer. 1995;**31A**(6):899-902. DOI: 10.1016/ 0959-8049(94)00447-1

[77] Schuster SJ, Bishop MR, Tam CS, Waller EK, Borchmann P, McGuirk JP, et al. Tisagenlecleucel in adult relapsed or refractory diffuse large B-cell lymphoma. The New England Journal of Medicine. 2019;**380**(1):45-56. DOI: 10.1056/ NEJMOA1804980

[78] Uygur MM, Gümüş M. The utility of serum tumor markers CEA and CA 15-3 for breast cancer prognosis and their association with clinicopathological parameters. Cancer Treatment and Research Communications. 2021;**28**:100402. DOI: 10.1016/J. CTARC.2021.100402

[79] Perkins GL, Slater ED, Sanders GK, Prichard JG. Serum Tumor Markers. American Family Physician. 2003;**68**(6):1075-1082

[80] Copur MS, Wurdeman JM, Nelson D, Ramaekers R, Gauchan D, Crockett D. Normalization of elevated tumor marker CA27-29 after bilateral lung transplantation in a patient with breast cancer and idiopathic pulmonary fibrosis. Oncology Research.

2018;**26**(3):518. DOI: 10.3727/096504017X15128550060375

[81] Rodriguez de Paterna L, Arnaiz F, Estenoz J, Ortuno B, Lanzos E. Study of serum tumor markers CEA, CA 15.3 and CA 27.29 as diagnostic parameters in patients with breast carcinoma. The International Journal of Biological Markers. 1995;**10**(1):24-29. DOI: 10.1177/172460089501000105

[82] Lam L, McAndrew N, Yee M, Fu T, Tchou JC, Zhang H. Challenges in the clinical utility of the serum test for HER2 ECD. Biochimica et Biophysica Acta. 2012;**1826**(1):208. DOI: 10.1016/J.BBCAN.2012.03.012

[83] Lee SB, Lee JW, Yu JH, Ko BS, Kim HJ, Son BH, et al. Preoperative serum HER2 extracellular domain levels in primary invasive breast cancer. BMC Cancer. 2014;**14**(1):929. DOI: 10.1186/1471-2407-14-929

[84] Badzek S, Kelovic VL, Plestina S, Humar I, Veir Z, Mihaljevic Z. Serum HER2/ECD value in stage I and II early breast cancer—Need of a lower cut-off? Wiener Klinische Wochenschrift. 2011;**123**(23-24):726-731. DOI: 10.1007/S00508-011-0099-4/METRICS

[85] Banys-Paluchowski M, Witzel I, Aktas B, Fasching PA, Hartkopf A, Janni W, et al. The prognostic relevance of urokinase-type plasminogen activator (uPA) in the blood of patients with metastatic breast cancer. Scientific Reports. 2019;**9**(1):1-10. DOI: 10.1038/s41598-018-37259-2

[86] Aglan SA, Elsammak M, Elsammak O, El-Bakoury EA, Elsheredy HG, Ahmed YS, et al. Evaluation of serum nestin and HOTAIR rs12826786 C>T polymorphism as screening tools for breast cancer in Egyptian women. Journal of Medical Biochemistry. 2021;**40**(1):17-25. DOI: 10.5937/JOMB0-25295

[87] Baba KSSS, Rehman MA, Kumar JP, Fatima M, Raju GSN, Uppin SG, et al. Serum human epididymis Protein-4 (HE4)—A novel approach to differentiate malignant from benign breast tumors. Asian Pacific Journal of Cancer Prevention. 2021;**22**(8):2513. DOI: 10.31557/APJCP.2021.22.8.2509

[88] Nemoto T, Constantine R, Chu T. Human tissue polypeptide antigen in breast cancer. Journal of the National Cancer Institute. 1979;**63**(6):1347-1350

[89] Vizcarra E, Lluch A, Cibrián R, Jarque F, Alberola V, Belloch V, et al. Value of CA 15.3 in breast cancer and comparison with CEA and TPA: A study of specificity in disease-free follow-up patients and sensitivity in patients at diagnosis of the first metastasis. Breast Cancer Research and Treatment. 1996;**37**(3):209-216. DOI: 10.1007/BF01806502

[90] De MC, Bakker J, Szpirer J, Szpirer C. Alpha-fetoprotein: From a diagnostic biomarker to a Key role in female fertility. Biomarker Insights. 2006;**1**:85. DOI: 10.1177/117727190600100002

[91] Moro R, Gulyaeva-Tcherkassova J, Stieber P. Increased alpha-fetoprotein receptor in the serum of patients with early-stage breast cancer. Current Oncology. 2012;**19**(1):1-8. DOI: 10.3747/CO.19.979

[92] Adigun OO, Yarrarapu SNS, Zubair M, Khetarpal S. Alpha Fetoprotein. Treasure Island, FL: StatPearls Publishing; 2023

[93] Luo J, Xiao J, Yang Y, Chen G, Hu D, Zeng J. Strategies for five tumour markers in the screening and diagnosis of female breast cancer. Frontiers

in Oncology. 2022;**12**:1055855. DOI: 10.3389/FONC.2022.1055855

[94] Wang W, Xu X, Tian B, Wang Y, Du L, Sun T, et al. The diagnostic value of serum tumor markers CEA, CA19-9, CA125, CA15-3, and TPS in metastatic breast cancer. Clinica Chimica Acta. 2017;**470**:51-55. DOI: 10.1016/J.CCA.2017.04.023

[95] Ballehaninna UK, Chamberlain RS. Serum CA 19-9 as a biomarker for pancreatic cancer—A comprehensive review. Indian Journal of Surgical Oncology. 2011;**2**(2):88-100. DOI: 10.1007/S13193-011-0042-1

[96] Fang C, Cao Y, Liu X, Zeng XT, Li Y. Serum CA125 is a predictive marker for breast cancer outcomes and correlates with molecular subtypes. Oncotarget. 2017;**8**(38):63970. DOI: 10.18632/ONCOTARGET.19246

[97] Leonard GD, Low JA, Berman AW, Swain SM. CA 125 elevation in breast cancer: A case report and review of the literature. The Breast Journal. 2004;**10**(2):146-149. DOI: 10.1111/J.1075-122X.2004.21374.X

[98] Moharrag A, Yonbawi F, Bashawieh HH, Basabrain A, Al-Jifree HM. The average time gap between CA-125 tumor marker elevation and confirmation of recurrence in epithelial ovarian cancer patients at princess Noorah oncology center, Jeddah, Saudi Arabia. Cureus. 2020;**12**(8):e9518. DOI: 10.7759/CUREUS.9518

[99] Kandylis K, Vassilomanolakis M, Baziotis N, Papadimitriou A, Tsoussis S, Ferderigou A, et al. Diagnostic significance of the tumour markers CEA, CA 15-3 and CA 125 in malignant effusions in breast cancer. Annals of Oncology. 1990;**1**(6):435-438. DOI: 10.1093/OXFORDJOURNALS.ANNONC.A057798

Chapter 8

Salivary Diagnostics in Oral Cancer

Alexandra Roi, Ciprian Ioan Roi, Mircea Riviş, Laura-Cristina Rusu, Lavinia Cosmina Ardelean and Codruţa Victoria Tigmeanu

Abstract

Oral cancer carcinogenesis is a complex process that outlines the implication of multiple mechanisms that lead to the development of this specific malignancy. The high heterogeneity of this disease is a key factor that controls the progression and treatment response, influencing the survival rate. The multifactorial etiology, the genetic alterations and the diagnosis in advanced stages are directly involved in the high mortality rate of this pathology. Currently, the gold standard for oral cancer diagnosis is represented by the tissue biopsy and its histopathological examination, procedure that in time revealed several disadvantages. Recent research focused on a non-invasive, fast and reliable diagnosis approach based on the use of saliva. Saliva through its components provides information regarding specific salivary molecules, proteomic and genomic changes linked to oral cancer occurrence and progression. By using saliva as a diagnosis tool, it offers an important perspective of the tumor environment, designing a complete molecular profile of the tumor by creating the concept of personalized medicine.

Keywords: oral cancer, early diagnosis, non-invasive, saliva, oral squamous cell carcinoma, oral cancer screening, salivaomics

1. Introduction

Oral cancer is currently an arising healthcare problem worldwide, challenging researchers in improving the prevention strategies and early diagnosis. The incidence in the last years determined oral cancer to represent 12% out of all the encountered malignancies [1]. Approximately, 90% of all the oral cancer cases arise from the oral mucosa lining and are represented by oral squamous cell carcinoma (OSCC) [2]. The diagnosis of oral malignancy implies a transition from a normal oral mucosa to the occurrence of benign hyperplasia, followed by dysplasia that left untreated is the precursor of carcinoma *in situ* and eventually the development of oral squamous cell carcinoma [3].

One of the main concerns regarding this malignancy is the high mortality and morbidity, mostly due to a late diagnosis in advanced stages. Compared to the other types of cancers, oral cancer could benefit from an early diagnosis due to the direct visibility of the oral mucosa and the possibility of a proper examination identifying potential existing premalignant lesions.

It is considered to be a multifactorial disease, emerging from a complex interaction between the epigenetic and genetic factors, with important cellular and molecular interactions [4]. Despite the advancements made in the diagnosis field, the survival rate associated with oral cancer is only 50%, mainly due to the late presentation of the patients for a diagnosis [5]. Currently, besides a good oral examination, several chair-side investigations and laboratory procedures, the high-end diagnostic approaches that include procedures such as nano-diagnostics, the analysis of biofluids, liquid biopsy, genomics, proteomics and metabolomics technology, offer a new perspective for screening and early diagnosis [6].

Currently, the detection of oral cancer is made through the conventional oral examination (COE) and further by performing a biopsy and a histopathological examination of the tissue sample. Until present, the biopsy is considered to be the gold standard for the diagnosis of oral malignancies, although it is an invasive procedure that often causes unwanted consequences for the patient. In order to reduce the unnecessary biopsy cases and to implement a strategy for the early diagnosis of oral cancer, it is important to understand the complex molecular pathways of carcinogenesis that occur at an early stage and are based on the identification of multiple genetic, epigenetic, proteomic and metabolomic biomarkers. The quantification of these markers represents the start-point of a new diagnosis era that targets the non-invasive approaches. Introducing the use of biofluids such as blood and saliva brought additional information regarding the screening, early diagnosis and monitoring of oral diseases.

Recently, the use of saliva as an oral cancer diagnosis tool revealed promising results. Taking into consideration the permanent contact of this fluid to the tumoral microenvironment, a direct release by the tumor of multiple potential biomarkers and the advantage of offering a personalized perspective, has transformed saliva into an appealing fluid that could be successfully introduced in the diagnosis field. Research showed that specific biomarkers signatures present in the saliva of oral cancer patients could be identified through a non-invasive approach, having a high sensitivity and specificity, opening a new path toward the personalized medicine concept. The progress that has been made by introducing the salivary diagnosis and understanding the complex characteristics of saliva, through a simple, non-invasive and cost-effective collection method, offers clinicians and patients an important asset in the diagnosis and treatment steps.

2. Saliva: an appealing biofluid

2.1 Saliva: generalities, composition and function

Saliva is produced and excreted by the three major salivary glands (submandibular, parotid and sublingual) and the minor salivary glands that are localized in multiple areas of the oral mucosa [7]. Salivary secretion can be influenced by several physiological and pathological conditions that determine the quantitative and qualitative changes in its composition. The average amount of saliva produced by healthy adults is between 500 and 1000 mL saliva/day, with an average salivary flow rate of 0.3–0.4 mL/min [8]. The increase of the salivary flow can be influenced by oral hygiene, exercise, age, associated drugs, external stimuli such as smell and taste and hormonal changes [9]. Each salivary gland secrets specific saliva, a serous or a mucous type, and its collection can be performed either directly from a specific gland or as the

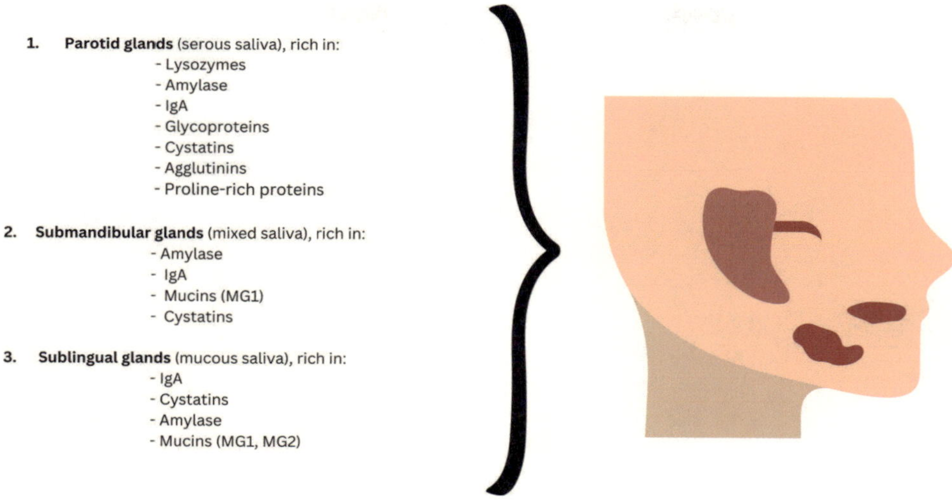

Figure 1.
Major salivary glands—Type of saliva and its composition.

collection of whole mouth saliva, representing the total amount of saliva excreted by all the salivary glands (**Figure 1**).

Saliva consists of 99.5% water, 0.2% inorganic material and enzymes, 0.3% being represented by proteins. Its secretion is controlled by the sympathetic and parasympathetic nerves [10].

The salivary composition varies individually and in relationship with the circadian rhythm. The inorganic composition of saliva is represented by calcium, phosphate, potassium, sodium, chloride, bicarbonate, magnesium and thiocyanate. The organic composition consists of components such as immunoglobulins, mucins, uric acid, lactoferrin, cytokines, hormones and enzymes (amylase, lipase, peroxidase and lysozyme) [10]. All these constituents are secreted by the acinar cells in the salivary glands and afterward released into the oral cavity. The electrolyte composition secreted by the acinar cells is similar to the electrolyte composition of the ultrafiltrate of plasma, outlining its important diagnosis potential [11].

Among the composition represented by the molecules that are present in the salivary glands, the gingival crevicular fluid completes the composition of the whole mouth saliva with epithelial cells, leukocytes, serum transudate and multiple microorganisms. Through an active transport, extracellular ultrafiltration or passive diffusion, many blood constituents enter into the saliva, providing a new approach for the future development of a new diagnosis tool. Existing research shows the fact that certain circulating biomolecules that are specific to various diseases and were identified in the bloodstream, were as well present in the saliva of those patients [12]. This fact outlines the high functionality of using saliva as a diagnosis method, having the power to reflect different pathological states. Any alterations in the blood composition can lead to changes in the salivary biochemical composition.

The functions of saliva are based on its composition and the presents of its viscoelastic properties, and are presented by taste and smell, bolus formation, digestion, lubrication, wound healing, homeostasis, mineralization and buffer activity (**Figure 2**) [13].

The human saliva offers an important source of proteins and peptides, that during the years proved their contribution in the diagnosis field, being association with

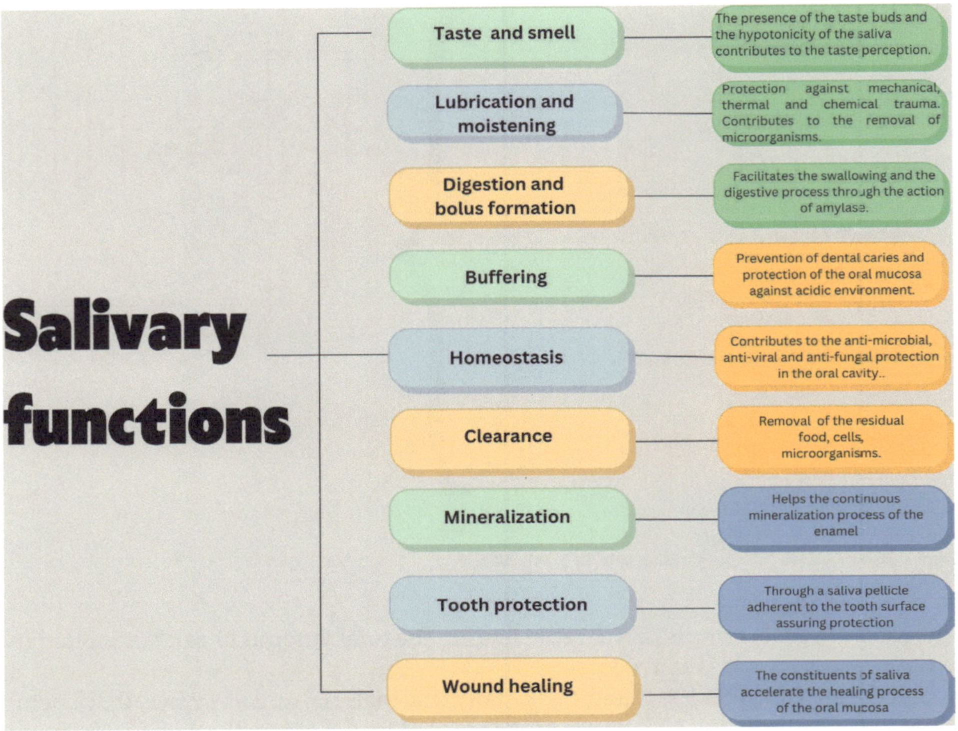

Figure 2.
Salivary functions and their description.

diverse diseases. The recent studies reveled the implication of over one hundred biomolecules that could be identified in the salivary samples and fulfill the role of biomarkers for certain pathologies, including oral malignancy, diabetes, periodontal disease, dental caries, systemic disorders and other cancer types (**Figure 3**) [14, 15].

There are multiple options in collecting saliva, but the most recommended method is the collection of unstimulated saliva, several studies showing the fact that by using this type of collection method, the composition does not suffer any changes [16]. Nevertheless, regardless of the used approach to obtain a salivary sample, a clear protocol needs to be implemented regarding the storage, possible existent circadian variations and sample contamination in order to reflect correct information regarding the health of the individual [17]. The advantages provided by this type of sampling such as a non-invasive sampling and fast processing, easy storage and transportation, cost-effective, painless and easily accepted by patients make the use of saliva samples an option for the early diagnosis (**Figure 4**).

The notion of "Salivaomics" was introduced outlining the importance of analyzing the "omics" composition of saliva, focusing on the proteomic, metabolomic, genomic and transcriptomic particularities [18, 19]. A comprehensive analysis and identification of these components is an important part in the development of potential salivary biomarkers that could be linked to multiple pathologies [20]. As a diagnosis tool, saliva is a reliable biofluid that has the potential to replace the blood sample analysis, targeting the screening, early diagnosis and prognosis evaluation of multiple diseases, especially oral cancer [21].

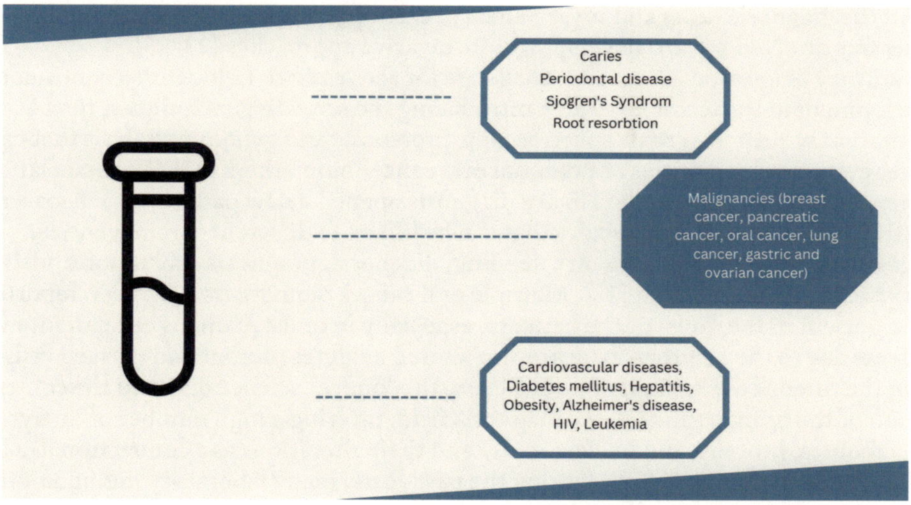

Figure 3.
Diagnostic use of saliva for local and general pathologies.

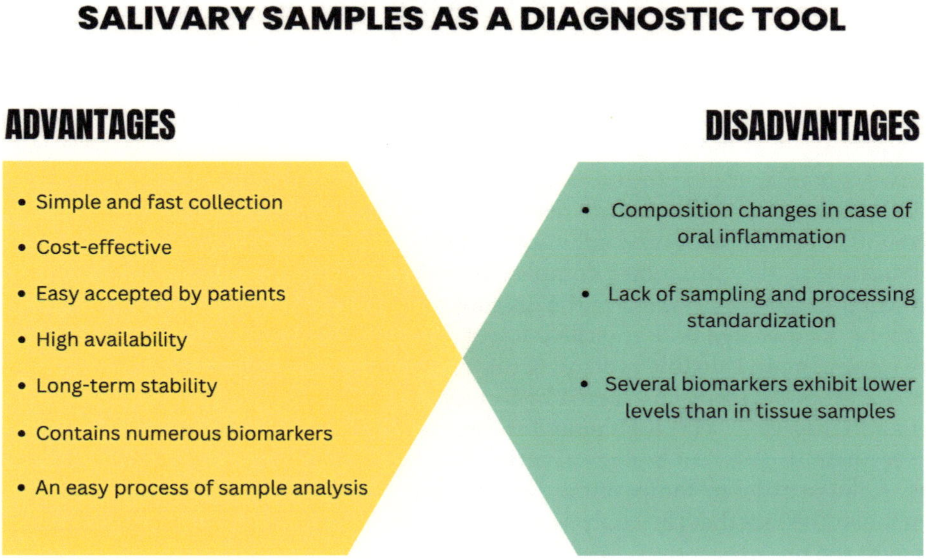

Figure 4.
Advantages and disadvantages of using salivary samples.

3. Saliva as a diagnostic tool in oral cancer

Oral cancer, despite the advancements made in the diagnosis and therapeutic field, exhibits a continuous increase of its incidence, being mostly diagnosed in stages 3 or 4 accompanied by a poor prognosis [22]. An early detection of the oral potentially malignant disorders (OPMD) is important for a further prevention of oral malignancy development, improving the survival rate of the patients [23–25]. In order to avoid the diagnosis delay and invasiveness in case of performing a scalpel biopsy, the focus was directed toward developing non-invasive approaches [23, 26].

Salivary diagnostic is a current challenge for the research field, with a continuous development in the technology area introducing the screening techniques, next-generation sequencing, mass spectroscopy, proteomic and genomic analysis that can target even small quantities of potential oral cancer biomarkers [27]. The association of new technologies with the salivary diagnosis opened a new path toward discovering the presence of new molecules that can be linked to different carcinogenesis stages of oral cancer, focusing on screening, diagnosis, prognosis evaluation and post-treatment monitoring [28]. Multiple oral cancer biomarkers have been reported to be present in the saliva of the patients, especially in oral squamous cell carcinoma patients due to the fact that there are also altered analytes present and derived cells from the tumor environment. Nevertheless, the "omics" science outlined the contribution of the human saliva in the diagnosis field, offering a high number of analytes (metabolites, proteins and nucleic acids) and their alterations as a connection to a possible oral malignancy [29]. During the past years, many laboratory methods aimed to analyze and isolate specific salivary components that could be linked to the presence and evolution of diseases (**Table 1**).

3.1 Salivary proteomics in oral cancer diagnosis

Proteomics focuses on the study of the proteins that are expressed in the cells and tissue, providing important information related to a pathogenesis, with the possibility of being quantified through non-invasive samples, such as saliva. In case of oral cancer, the analysis of the proteins reveals important aspects regarding their functions, offering advantages over the tissue samples. The altered proteins identified in the OSCC carcinogenesis process are responsible for modifications in the cell structure, metabolism, cell motility and adhesion and intercellular signaling.

Multiple studies conducted complex analysis targeting the salivary proteome and its potential involvement in the diagnosis field of oral malignancy. The Salivary Proteome Knowledge Base and the information available in NIDCR'S Human Saliva Proteome contain valuable proteomic information provided also by the dataset resulted from the study conducted by Denny et al. [46]. The study conducted by Bandhakavi et al. [47] highlighted the existence of 2.340 proteins with direct involvement in different biological actions of the oral environment. An analysis was performed in order to compare the distribution of saliva and plasma proteins and concluded the fact that the analysis of salivary proteins has more advantages compared to the plasma proteins [48]. The identified salivary proteins that can be linked to oral cancer are mostly represented by interleukins, tumor-necrosis factor, CD44, CD59, IgG, p53 antibodies, transferrin, albumin, telomerase, alpha-amylase and S100 calcium-binding protein [49].

Along the past years, researcher's attention was directed toward the existence of numerous proteins present in saliva that could be used for the early diagnosis of oral cancer, as well for evaluating the tumor evolution [50]. Studies focused on the implication of the interleukins (IL-6, IL-8, IL-1β), the tumor-necrosis factor alpha (TNF-α), transferrin, matrix metalloproteinase (MMP9, MMP2) and α-amylase [14].

Interleukins (IL) are a family of proteins that are responsible for the control of cellular migration, differentiation and the apoptosis process [51]. The

Type of analytical method	Identified salivary components	Reference
Enzyme-Linked Immunosorbent Assay (ELISA)	Proteins Virus Peptides Metabolites	[30–32]
PCR-based	Nucleic acids Bacteria Virus	[33, 34]
Raman-spectroscopy	Multiple biological molecules	[35]
Conductive Polymer Spray Ionization Mass Spectrometry (CPSI-MS)	Presence of drugs Metabolites	[36]
Matrix-Assisted Laser Desorption/Ionization-Time-of- Flight mass spectrometry (MALDI-TOF MS)	Proteins Microorganisms Peptides	[37]
High-Performance Liquid Chromatography (HPLC) coupled to Mass Spectrometry (MS)	Peptides Metabolites Proteins Hormones Vitamins	[38–41]
Two-dimensional gel electrophoresis (2DE) coupled to mass spectrometry (MS)	Proteins	[42]
Electric Field-Induced Release and Measurement (EFIRM)	RNA Circulating single-stranded DNA	[43]
Nuclear Magnetic Resonance (^{1} H-NMR) spectroscopy	Metabolites	[44]
Attenuated Total Reflection-Fourier Transform Infrared (ATR-FTIR) spectroscopy	Nucleic acids Proteins Lipids	[45]

Table 1.
Analytical methods used for salivary analysis.

pro-inflammatory category of cytokines IL-6, IL-8, IL-1 and TNF-α were identified in high levels in the salivary samples of OSCC patients and in case of premalignant lesions, outlining their potential role in the progression of the carcinogenesis process from a premalignant state to a malignant one [52]. Many studies have focused on the salivary levels of IL-8 that were encountered to be increased in periodontitis patients, but with a much higher level in case of oral cancer patients [53]. IL-8 and its high levels were associated with the tumor angiogenesis process, interfering in the cell circle and adhesion process [54]. Also, the salivary levels of IL-6 and TNF-α were reported to be increased in case of the presence of oral leukoplakia [27]. Nevertheless, Goldoni et al. [55] concluded that IL-8, IL-6, IL-1β and IL-1α and their salivary levels could represent a potential diagnosis tool for oral cancer. Research showed that a high number of proteins were identified to have increased levels in different stages of OSCC, being more relevant to focus on a specific one for a higher sensitivity [56]. Jou et al. [57] in their study revealed increased levels of transferrin in the saliva of OSCC patients, positively correlating them with the size and the stage of the tumor.

Recent studies showed that gelatinase-B (MMP-9) has an important diagnosis validity and had the highest sensitivity and specificity as a diagnosis tool for OSCC [58]. The cytokeratin fraction 21-1 (CYFRA 21-1) expression was positively correlated with OSCC, and studies revealed an important discriminating power between the potentially malignant disorder cases and OSCC [59].

3.2 Salivary metabolomics in oral cancer diagnosis

The pathogenesis of oral cancer is not completely understood, and studies discuss the importance of metabolic reprogramming as a future approach in the early diagnosis. During the tumorigenesis process, the cancer cells suffer important metabolic changes among which a metabolic reprogramming of the lipids and amino acids occurs [60].

The use of salivary metabolites has gained recent interest due to the fact that their presence in the saliva can be a consequence of the direct transfer from the tumor cells. Saliva metabolomics were used for assessing the early diagnosis and further monitorization of OSCC patients [61]. The analysis of the metabolites encountered in the saliva of the OSCC patients revealed increased levels of betaine, choline and pipecolic acid that were able to distinguish the OSCC patients from the control group [62].

A study performed by Sugimoto et al. [63] in which they analyzed the saliva collected from oral cancer patients identified 57 metabolites that could be linked to this malignancy. When compared to the control group, the salivary levels of polyamines were significantly higher [63], other studies discussing the fact that the increased levels determined a high cell proliferation rate, promote tumor invasiveness and decrease the apoptosis process [64]. Also, the presence of piperidine and taurine showed a high potential for their use as oral screening tool [62]. Another study that focused on the salivary metabolome as a diagnosis tool outlined the role of putrescine for monitoring the action of chemotherapy in oral cancer [65].

Wei et al. [66] in their study aimed to evaluate the salivary metabolomics and their changes in OSCC, leukoplakia and oral lichen planus patients and identified five metabolites with the power to discriminate between the three groups of patients, among which were lactate, valine, phenylalanine, n-eicosanoic acid and γ-aminobutyric acid.

In order to establish and certify the presence of the altered salivary metabolites and their correlation with oral cancer, Ishikawa et al. [67] conducted a study in which they compared the altered metabolites encountered in tissue and salivary samples of OSCC patients. Their results showed that 17 metabolites had altered levels in both types of samples, and pipecolate and *S*-adenosylmethionine could differentiate the OSCC group from the healthy controls.

Nevertheless, the diagnosis potential of salivary metabolites is still a discussed topic, as there are certain differences in the salivary metabolome dependent on gender, type of saliva (stimulated or unstimulated), associated risk factors (such as smoking), circadian variation of the salivary composition and age [68]. The stability of these metabolites is still questionable and in order to accomplish their role as a diagnostic tool, a proper protocol needs to be implemented that should limit the possible variations related to them.

3.3 Salivary genomics in oral cancer diagnosis

The presence of cell-free circulation DNA (deoxyribonucleic acid) in the plasma was outlined approximately 60 years ago [69], and its altered levels were identified in cancer patients compared to healthy controls, exhibiting specific tumoral characteristics [70]. These alterations are represented by abnormal methylation, somatic mutations in oncogenes and tumor suppressor genes, mitochondrial DNA mutations, microsatellite alterations and viral tumor-related DNA [71]. Studies have shown that the body fluids, saliva included, contain cell-free nucleic acids with an important role in the diagnosis field. Saliva-based tests have reflected a high potential in detecting oral cancer by analyzing the hypermethylation levels, oral microbiota and existent exfoliated cells [69].

In the human saliva, the total DNA content was reported to be between 1.8 and 128 μg/mL, and approximately, 70% is from the host and 30% has its origins from the oral microbiome [72]. Research has outlined the fact that the quality of the salivary DNA was from 72% up to 96% in the samples that were genotyped [73].

Multiple studies focused on revealing specific genetic alteration that could be associated with the development, progression and metastasis rate of oral cancer. There has been reported the existence of a tumor-specific genome, among which the alterations of p53 and the presence of tumor suppressor gene mutations were directly linked to the oral malignancy carcinogenesis process [74]. A loss of heterozygosity (LOH) was revealed, representing a loss of genomic material localized on one of the chromosomes. Based on this fact, studies showed that specific LOH in regions that are responsible tumor suppressor genes is associated and represents an indicator for the malignant transformation in case of oral premalignant lesions [75]. It was reported that frequent LOH was identified in chromosomes 3q, 9p, 13q and 17p was linked to an early onset of oral malignancy [76]. Mutations that occurred in the mitochondrial DNA showed their implication in identifying exfoliated OSCC cells in salivary samples [77]. The hypermethylation of several genes was discovered and linked to the occurrence of cancers in the head and neck area. The study conducted by Rosas et al. [78] showed abnormal methylation encountered in certain genes (DAP-K, MGMT and p16) in patients diagnosed with OSCC, and outlined their potential for the detection and further recurrence surveillance of the oral malignancy. Liao et al. [79] identified the mutation of p53 gene in the saliva of OSCC patients, with a high potential role in the early detection of OSCC. A study conducted by Zhong et al. [80] aimed to detect the telomerase activity in the saliva of OSCC diagnosed patients and its potential as a marker.

Existent research outlines the fact that certain genomic alterations that were identified in the tumor tissue samples were also present in the salivary samples. Mutations in CDKN2A, PIKC3, TP53 and NOTCH1, along with translocation mutations in tumor DNA were discovered in the salivary samples of OSCC patients [81]. These results highlight the idea that higher levels of remanent tumor DNA are encountered in saliva samples compared to plasma ones, with a high contribution in the further development of non-invasive personalized early diagnosis.

3.4 Salivary transcriptomics in oral cancer diagnosis

Transcriptomics represents the analysis of a complex set of RNA (ribonucleic acid) transcripts that are present in certain circumstances and are discovered through technologies such as polymerase chain reaction (PCR), microarray technology and next-generation sequencing. In cell-free whole saliva, the total RNA level ranged between from 0.108 ± 0.023 μg/mL [82]. It was identified that the majority of the cell-free RNAs from whole mouth saliva are human-derived mRNAs [83]. Approximately 3000 to 6400 human mRNAs were detectable in saliva and 27.5% of the investigated mRNAs have still unknown functions [84]. Messenger RNA represents a direct precursor of proteins, and its levels usually are corresponding and can be correlated. The nucleic acids are considered easier to screen and offer a viable option to become a disease marker.

The dysregulation of different miRNAs controls the cell differentiation process, growth and apoptosis, influencing tumor suppressors and oncogenes [54]. Salazar et al. [85] in their study identified elevated levels of salivary miR-134, miR-9 and miR-191 in the samples of oral cancer patients, suggesting their use as potential markers. Other study reported decreased levels of miR-200a and miR-125a [86] and high levels of miR-31 in the saliva of diagnosed OSCC patients. miR-31 was linked to the post-treatment monitoring of OSCC patients, as results reveal the fact that the salivary levels decreased after the tumor resection [86]. Another study performed by Li et al. [87] by using the microarray analysis revealed significantly modified levels in seven potential markers for oral cancer, represented by the increased regulation of three groups of mRNAs (IL-8, S100P and H3F3A), while decreased mRNA levels were noted in SAT, OAZ1 and DUSP1.

A concern was the stability of salivary miRNAs and the protocol related to the collection and time of processing the samples in order to provide an accurate molecular profiling analysis. Zimmermann et al. [69] in their study focused on evaluating the salivary cell-free miRNA and their finding outline the existence of a salivary core transcriptome of 185 gene that were identified in all the included samples.

4. Conclusions

Taking into consideration the current epidemiological trend that describes an increase of oral cancer incidence globally, the prevention and early diagnosis strategies need to overcome the existing limits and disadvantages that are influencing the survival rate of these patients.

Saliva represents a promising tool for the early diagnosis of oral cancer, providing also important information related to the progression and post-treatment surveillance. The advancements made in technology in order to assure a complex analysis of the salivary samples allowed researchers to expand the use of saliva as a diagnosis tool and validate multiple components with direct implications in the oral carcinogenesis process. The diagnosis field urges the need to implement non-invasive approaches for screening and early diagnosis, and currently, saliva offers multiple advantages such as a non-invasiveness, easy sampling, painless and fast collection.

By implementing the" omics" concept, saliva testing becomes a reliable and appealing body fluid. Studies have shown that especially related to oral cancer, specific components that exist or are delivered by the tumor, can act like disease markers and are present in a higher percentage in saliva. Current progress has been made in order to quantify and understand their characteristics. An important aspect that should be mentioned is the need to implement a protocol that stands for a standardization of the salivary collection method, storage and analysis, minimizing the possible existent factors that could intervene in becoming a proper diagnosis tool.

The oral carcinogenesis process is a complex one, with specific alterations at every evolutive stage, salivary composition providing in many cases an individual perspective on the ongoing changes, having a direct contact with the tumoral environment. Despite the existing limitations, the salivary diagnostics promise an increase in the clinical applicability, targeting specific proteomic, genomic and transcriptomic alterations that are associated with the oral malignancy.

Author details

Alexandra Roi[1*], Ciprian Ioan Roi[2], Mircea Riviş[2], Laura-Cristina Rusu[1], Lavinia Cosmina Ardelean[3] and Codruța Victoria Tigmeanu[3]

1 Department of Oral Pathology, Multidisciplinary Center for Research, Evaluation, Diagnosis and Therapies in Oral Medicine, Victor Babeş University of Medicine and Pharmacy, Timisoara, Romania

2 Department of Anesthesiology and Oral Surgery, Multidisciplinary Center for Research, Evaluation, Diagnosis and Therapies in Oral Medicine, Victor Babeş University of Medicine and Pharmacy, Timişoara, Romania

3 Department of Technology of Materials and Devices in Dental Medicine, Multidisciplinary Center for Research, Evaluation, Diagnosis and Therapies in Oral Medicine, "Victor Babeş" University of Medicine and Pharmacy Timisoara, Timisoara, Romania

*Address all correspondence to: alexandra.moga@umft.ro

References

[1] Madhura MG, Rao RS, Patil S, Fageeh HN, Alhazmi A, Awan KH. Advanced diagnostic aids for oral cancer. Disease-a-Month. 2020;**66**:1-12

[2] Neville BW, Day TA. Oral cancer and precancerous lesions. CA: A Cancer Journal for Clinicians. 2002;**52**:195-215

[3] Wong DT. Towards a simple, saliva-based test for the detection of oral cancer. 'Oral fluid (saliva), which is the mirror of the body, is a perfect medium to be explored for health and disease surveillance'. Expert Review of Molecular Diagnostics. 2006;**6**:267-272

[4] Manoharan S, Karthikeyan S, Essa MM, Manimaran A, Selvasundram R. An overview of oral carcinogenesis. International Journal of Nutrition, Pharmacology, Neurological Diseases. 2016;**6**(2):51-62

[5] Nambiar KS, Haragannavar VC, Augustine D, Sowmya SV, Rao RS. Diagnostic aids in detection of oral precancer and cancer: Past to present. International Dental & Medical Journal of Advanced Research. 2016;**2**:1-7

[6] Chaudhary R, Shah A, Shah DM, Singh S, Thakkar P, Goyal S. Advanced diagnostic aids in detection of oral cancer. International Journal of Dental and Medical Research. 2014;**1**(3):139-143

[7] Dawes C. Rhythms in salivary flow rate and composition. International Journal of Chronobiology. 1974;**2**:253-279

[8] Mese H, Matsuo R. Salivary secretion, taste and hyposalivation. Journal of Oral Rehabilitation. 2007;**34**:711-723

[9] Walsh NP, Montague JC, Callow N, Rowlands AV. Saliva flow rate, total protein concentration and osmolality as potential markers of whole body hydration status during progressive acute dehydration in humans. Archives of Oral Biology. 2004;**49**:149-154

[10] Chiappin S, Antonelli G, Gatti R, De Palo EF. Saliva specimen: A new laboratory tool for diagnostic and basic investigation. Clinica Chimica Acta. 2007;**383**:30-40

[11] Kaczor-Urbanowicz KE, Wei F, Rao SL, Kim J, Shin H, Cheng J, et al. Clinical validity of saliva and novel technology for cancer detection. Biochimica et Biophysica Acta (BBA)-Reviews on Cancer. 2019;**1872**(1):49-59

[12] Pfaffe T, Cooper-White J, Beyerlein P, Kostner K, Punyadeera C. Diagnostic potential of saliva: Current state and future applications. Clinical Chemistry. 2011;**57**:675-687

[13] Carpenter GH. The secretion, components, and properties of saliva. Annual Review of Food Science and Technology. 2013;**4**:267-276

[14] Zhang CZ, Cheng XQ, Li JY, Zhang P, Yi P, Xu X, et al. Saliva in the diagnosis of diseases. International Journal of Oral Science. 2016;**8**(3):133-137

[15] Sultan AS, Kong EF, Jabra-Rizk MA. The oral microbiome: A lesson in co-existence. PLoS Pathogens. 2018;**14**(1):e1006719

[16] Kaczor-Urbanowicz KE, Martin Carreras-Presas C, Aro K, Tu M, Garcia-Godoy F, Wong DT. Saliva diagnostics - current views and directions. Experimental Biology and Medicine

(Maywood). 2017;**242**(5):459-472. DOI: 10.1177/1535370216681550

[17] Kaur J, Srivastava R, Borse V. Recent advances in point-of-care diagnostics for oral cancer. Biosensors and Bioelectronics. 2021;**178**:112995

[18] Wong DT. Salivaomics. Journal of the American Dental Association (1939). 2012;**143**(Suppl. 10):19S-24S

[19] Tasoulas J, Patsouris E, Giaginis C, Theocharis S. Salivaomics for oral diseases biomarkers detection. Expert Review of Molecular Diagnostics. 2016;**16**(3):285-295

[20] Wang X, Kaczor-Urbanowicz KE, Wong DT. Salivary biomarkers in cancer detection. Medical Oncology. 2017;**34**:7

[21] Roblegg E, Coughran A, Sirjani D. Saliva: An all-rounder of our body. European Journal of Pharmaceutics and Biopharmaceutics. 2019;**142**:133-141

[22] Wu DT, Tao O, Trinh N, Javaid MA, Ahmed AS, Durand R, et al. Saliva–a promising tool for diagnosing oral diseases. Current Oral Health Reports. 2018;**5**(4):242-249

[23] Liu D, Zhao X, Zeng X, Dan H, Chen Q. Non-invasive techniques for detection and diagnosis of oral potentially malignant disorders. The Tohoku Journal of Experimental Medicine. 2016;**238**(2):165-177

[24] Walsh T, Macey R, Brocklehurst P, Kerr AR, Liu JL, Lingen MW, et al. Diagnostic tests for oral cancer and potentially malignant disorders in patients presenting with clinically evident lesions. Cochrane Database of Systematic Reviews. 2015;**5**:CD010276

[25] Stuani VT, Rubira CM, Sant'Ana AC, Santos PS. Salivary biomarkers as tools for oral squamous cell carcinoma diagnosis: A systematic review. Head & Neck. 2017;**39**(4):797-811

[26] Panta P, Venna VR. Salivary RNA signatures in oral cancer detection. Analytical Cellular Pathology. 2014;**2014**:7-7

[27] Goldoni R, Scolaro A, Boccalari E, Dolci C, Scarano A, Inchingolo F, et al. Malignancies and biosensors: A focus on oral cancer detection through salivary biomarkers. Biosensors. 2021;**11**:396

[28] Khurshid Z, Zafar MS, Khan RS, Najeeb S, Slowey PD, Rehman IU. Role of salivary biomarkers in oral cancer detection. Advances in Clinical Chemistry. 2018;**86**:23-70

[29] Thomadaki K, Helmerhorst EJ, Tian N, Sun X, Siqueira WL, Walt DR, et al. Whole-saliva proteolysis and its impact on salivary diagnostics. Journal of Dental Research. 2011;**90**:1325-1330

[30] Desrosiers NA, Huestis MA. Oral fluid drug testing: Analytical approaches, issues and interpretation of results. Journal of Analytical Toxicology. 2019;**43**:415-443

[31] Messana I, Cabras T, Iavarone F, Vincenzoni F, Urbani A, Castagnola M. Unraveling the different proteomic platforms. Journal of Separation Science. 2013;**36**:128-139

[32] Chu HW, Chang KP, Hsu CW, Chang IY, Liu HP, Chen YT, et al. Identification of salivary biomarkers for oral cancer detection with untargeted and targeted quantitative proteomics approaches. Molecular & Cellular Proteomics. 2019;**18**:1796-1806

[33] Jamieson LM, Antonsson A, Garvey G, Ju X, Smith M,

Logan RM, et al. Prevalence of oral human papillomavirus infection among Australian indigenous adults. JAMA Network Open. 2020;**3**:e204951

[34] Fadhil RS, Wei MQ, Nikolarakos D, Good D, Nair RG. Salivary microRNA miR-let-7a-5p and miR-3928 could be used as potential diagnostic bio-markers for head and neck squamous cell carcinoma. PLoS One. 2020;**15**:e0221779

[35] Lin D, Yang SW, Hsieh CL, Hsu KJ, Gong T, Wu Q, et al. Tandem quantification of multiple carbohydrates in saliva using surface-enhanced Raman spectroscopy. ACS Sensors. 2021;**6**:1240-1247

[36] Song X, Yang X, Narayanan R, Shankar V, Ethiraj S, Wang X, et al. Oral squamous cell carcinoma diagnosed from saliva metabolic profiling. Proceedings of the National Academy of Sciences of the United States of America. 2020;**117**:16167-16173

[37] Antezack A, Chaudet H, Tissot-Dupont H, Brouqui P, Monnet-Corti V. Rapid diagnosis of periodontitis, a feasi- bility study using MALDI-TOF mass spectrometry. PLoS One. 2020;**15**:e0230334

[38] Alvi SN, Hammami MM. An improved method for measurement of testosterone in human plasma and saliva by ultra-performance liquid chromatography-tandem mass spectrometry. Journal of Advanced Pharmaceutical Technology & Research. 2020;**11**:64-68

[39] Wang Q, Yu Q, Lin Q, Duan Y. Emerging salivary biomarkers by mass spectrometry. Clinica Chimica Acta. 2015;**438**:214-221

[40] Wu CC, Chu HW, Hsu CW, Chang KP, Liu HP. Saliva proteome profiling reveals potential salivary biomarkers for detection of oral cavity squamous cell carcinoma. Proteomics. 2015;**15**:3394-3404

[41] Kawahara R, Bollinger JG, Rivera C, Ribeiro AC, Brandão TB, Paes Leme AF, et al. A targeted proteomic strategy for the measurement of oral cancer candidate biomarkers in human saliva. Proteomics. 2016;**16**:159-173

[42] Jessie K, Jayapalan JJ, Ong KC, Abdul Rahim ZH, Zain RM, Wong KT, et al. Aberrant proteins in the saliva of patients with oral squamous cell carcinoma. Electrophoresis. 2013;**34**:2495-2502

[43] Cheng J, Nonaka T, Wong DTW. Salivary exosomes as nanocarriers for cancer biomarker delivery. Materials. 2019;**12**:654

[44] Herrala M, Mikkonen JJW, Pesonen P, Lappalainen R, Tjäder-Niemelä RK, Seitsalo H, et al. Variability of salivary metabolite levels in patients with Sjögren's syndrome. Journal of Oral Science. 2020;**63**:22-26

[45] Ferreira IC, Aguiar EM, Silva AT, Santos LL, Cardoso-Sousa L, Araújo TG, et al. Attenuated total reflection-Fourier transform infrared (ATR-FTIR) spectroscopy analysis of saliva for breast cancer diagnosis. Journal of Oncology. 2020;**2020**:4343590

[46] Denny P, Hagen FK, Hardt M, Liao L, Yan W, Arellanno M, et al. The proteomes of human parotid and submandibular/ sublingual gland salivas collected as the ductal secretions. Journal of Proteome Research. 2008;**7**(5):1994-2006

[47] Bandhakavi S, Stone MD, Onsongo G, Van Riper SK, Griffin TJ. A dynamic range compression and three-dimensional peptide fractionation analysis platform expands proteome coverage and the diagnostic potential of whole saliva. Journal of Proteome Research. 2009;**8**(12):5590-5600

[48] Loo JA, Yan W, Ramachandran P, Wong DT. Comparative human salivary and plasma proteomes. Journal of Dental Research. 2010;**89**(10):1016-1023

[49] Khurshid Z, Zohaib S, Najeeb S, Zafar M, Rehman R, Rehman I. Advances of proteomic sciences in dentistry. International Journal of Molecular Sciences. 2016;**17**:728

[50] Chundru VNS, Nirmal RM, Srikanth B, Bojji M, Midhun N, Lakshmi BJ. Salivaomics for oral cancer detection: An insight. Journal of Pharmacy & Bioallied Sciences. 2021;**13**:S52-S56

[51] Tasoulas J, Patsouris E, Giaginis C, Theocharis S. Salivaomics for oral diseases biomarkers detection. Expert Review of Molecular Diagnostics. 2016;**16**:285-295

[52] Papale F, Santonocito S, Polizzi A, Giudice AL, Capodiferro S, Favia G, et al. The new era of salivaomics in dentistry: Frontiers and facts in the early diagnosis and prevention of oral diseases and cancer. Metabolites. 2022;**12**:638

[53] Buzalaf MAR, Ortiz AC, Carvalho TS, Fideles SOM, Araújo TT, Moraes SM, et al. Saliva as a diagnostic tool for dental caries, periodontal disease and cancer: Is there a need for more biomarkers? Expert Review of Molecular Diagnostics. 2020;**20**:543-555

[54] Radhika T, Jeddy N, Nithya S, Muthumeenakshi RM. Salivary biomarkers in oral squamous cell carcinoma—An insight. Journal of Oral Biology and Craniofacial Research. 2016;**6**:S51-S54

[55] Govindraju P, Kumar T. Genomic alphabets of saliva as a biomarker in oral cancer. Journal of Indian Academy of Oral Medicine and Radiology. 2017;**29**:300

[56] Elashoff D, Zhou H, Reiss JK, Wang J, Henson B, Hu S, et al. Pre-validation of salivary biomarkers for oral cancer detection. Cancer Epidemiology, Biomarkers & Prevention. 2012;**21**(4):664-672

[57] Jou YL, Lin CD, Lai CH, Chen CH, Kao JY, Chen SY, et al. Proteomic identification of salivary transferrin as a biomarker for early detection of oral cancer. Analytica Chimica Acta. 2010;**681**:41-48

[58] Ghallab NA, Shaker OG. Serum and salivary levels of chemerin and MMP-9 in oral squamous cell carcinoma and oral premalignant lesions. Clinical Oral Investigations. 2017;**21**:937-947

[59] Rajkumar K, Ramya R, Nandhini G, Rajashree P, Ramesh Kumar A, Nirmala AS. Salivary and serum level of CYFRA 21-1 in oral cancer and oral squamous cell carcinoma. Oral Diseases. 2015;**21**:90-96

[60] Yang LF, Venneti S, Nagrath D. Glutaminolysis: A hallmark of cancer metabolism. Annual Review of Biomedical Engineering. 2017;**19**:163-194

[61] Mikkonen JJ, Singh SP, Herrala M, Lappalainen R, Myllymaa S, Kullaa AM. Salivary metabolomics in the diagnosis of oral cancer and periodontal diseases. Journal of Periodontal Research. 2016;**2016**(51):431-437

[62] Wang Q, Gao P, Wang X, Duan Y. Investigation and identification of potential biomarkers in human saliva for the early diagnosis of oral squamous cell carcinoma. Clinica Chimica Acta. 2014;**427**:79-85

[63] Sugimoto M, Wong DT, Hirayama A, Soga T, Tomita M. Capillary electrophoresis mass spectrometry-based

saliva metabolomics identified oral, breast and pancreatic cancer-specific profiles. Metabolomics. 2010;**6**:78-95

[64] Gerner EW, Meyskens FL. Polyamines and cancer: Old molecules, new understanding. Nature Reviews Cancer. 2004;**4**:781-792

[65] Okamura M, Kobayashi M, Suzuki F, Shimada J, Sakagami H. Induction of cell death by combination treatment with cisplatin and 5-fluorouracil in a human oral squamous cell carcinoma cell line. Anticancer Research. 2007;**27**:3331-3337

[66] Wei J, Xie G, Zhou Z, Shi P, Qui Y, Zheng X, et al. Salivary metabolite signatures of oral cancer and leukoplakia. International Journal of Cancer. 2011;**129**:2207-2217

[67] Ishikawa S, Sugimoto M, Kitabakate K, Tu M, Sugano A, Yamamori I, et al. Effect of timing of collection of salivary metabolomic biomarkers on oral cancer detection. Amino Acids. 2017;**49**:761-770

[68] Takeda I, Stretch C, Barnaby P, Bhatnager K, Rankin K, Fu H, et al. Understanding the human salivary metabolome. NMR in Biomedicine. 2009;**22**:577-584

[69] Zimmermann BG, Park NJ, Wong DT. Genomic targets in saliva. Annals of the New York Academy of Sciences. 2007;**1098**(1):184-191

[70] Leon SA, Shapiro B, Sklaroff DM, Yaros. Free DNA in the serum of cancer patients and the effect of therapy. Cancer Research. 1977;**37**:646-650

[71] Anker P, Mulcahy H, Chen XQ, Stroun M. Detection of circulating tumour DNA in the blood (plasma/serum) of cancer patients. Cancer Metastasis Reviews. 1999;**18**:65-73

[72] Hansen TO, Simonsen MK, Nielsen FC, Hundrup YA. Collection of blood, saliva, and buccal cell samples in a pilot study on the Danish nurse cohort: Comparison of the response rate and quality of genomic sample. Cancer Epidemiology, Biomarkers & Prevention. 2007;**16**:2072-2076

[73] Rylander-Rudquist T, Hakansson N, Tybring G, Wolk A. Quality and quantity of saliva DNA obtained from the self-administered oragene method - A pilot study on the cohort of Swedish men. Cancer Epidemiology, Biomarkers & Prevention. 2006;**15**:1742-1745

[74] Shah FD, Begum R, Vajaria BN, Patel KR, Patel JB, Shukla SN, et al. A review on salivary genomics and proteomics biomarkers in oral cancer. Indian Journal of Clinical Biochemistry. 2011;**26**:326-334

[75] Fliss MS, Usadel H, Caballero OL, Wu L, Buta MR, Eleff SM, et al. Facile detection of mitochondrial DNA mutations in tumors and bodily fluids. Science. 2000;**287**:2017-2019

[76] Zhang L, Rosin MP. Loss of heterozygosity: A potential tool in management of oral premalignant lesions? Journal of Oral Pathology & Medicine. 2001;**30**:513-520

[77] Jiang WW, Masayesva B, Zahurak M, Carvalho AL, Rosenbaum E, Mambo E, et al. Increased mitochondrial DNA content in saliva associated with head and neck cancer. Clinical Cancer Research. 2005;**11**:2486-2491

[78] Rosas SLB, Koch W, Da Costa Carvalho MDG, Wu L, Califano J, Westra W, et al. Promoter hypermethylation patterns of p16, O6-methylguanine- DNA-methyltransferase, and death-associated

protein kinase in tumors and saliva of head and neck cancer patients. Cancer Research. 2001;**61**:939-942

[79] Liao PH, Chang YC, Huang MF, Tai KW, Chou MY. Mutation of p53 gene codon 63 in saliva as a molecular marker for oral squamous cell carcinomas. Oral Oncology. 2000;**36**:272-276

[80] Zhong LP, Chen GF, Xu ZF, Zhang X, Ping FY, Zhao SF. Detection of telomerase activity in saliva from oral squamous cell carcinoma patients. International Journal of Oral and Maxillofacial Surgery. 2005;**34**:566-570

[81] Zandberg DP, Tallon LJ, Nagaraj S, Sadzewicz LK, Zhang Y, Strome MB, et al. Intratumor genetic heterogeneity in squamous cell carcinoma of the oral cavity. Head & Neck. 2019;**41**:2514-2524

[82] Feng L, Houck JR, Lohavanichbutr P, Chen C. Transcriptome analysis reveals differentially expressed lncRNAs between oral squamous cell carcinoma and healthy oral mucosa. Oncotarget. 2017;**8**:31521-31531

[83] Li Y, Zhou X, St. John MAR, Wong DTW. RNA profiling of cell-free saliva using microarray technology. Journal of Dental Research. 2004;**83**:199-203

[84] Park NJ, Zhou X, Yu T, Brinkman BMN, Zimmermann BG, Palanisamy V, et al. Characterization of salivary RNA by cDNA library analysis. Archives of Oral Biology. 2007;**52**:30-35

[85] Salazar C, Nagadia R, Pandit P, Cooper-White J, Banerjee N, Dimitrova N, et al. A novel saliva-based microRNA biomarker panel to detect head and neck cancers. Cellular Oncology. 2014;**37**:331-338

[86] Park NJ, Zhou H, Elashoff D, Henson BS, Kastratovic DA, Abemayor E, et al. Salivary microRNA: Discovery, characterization, and clinical utility for oral cancer detection. Clinical Cancer Research. 2009;**15**:5473-5477

[87] Li Y, St. John MA, Zhou X, Kim Y, Sinha U, Jordan RC, et al. Salivary transcriptome diagnostics for oral cancer detection. Clinical Cancer Research. 2004;**10**:8442-8450

Chapter 9

Gastric Cancer in the Next-Generation Sequencing Era: Diagnostic and Therapeutic Strategies

Julita Machlowska and Ryszard Maciejewski

Abstract

Gastric cancer (GC) is one of the most common malignancies and the fourth major cause of cancer-related deaths worldwide. There is growing interest in the role of genetic and epigenetic changes in the development of the disease. Next-generation sequencing (NGS) studies have identified candidate cancer-driving genes in the GC. Whole transcriptome sequencing and whole-genome sequencing analysis is also important methodology in discovering novel changes in GC. Importantly, cancer epigenetics has opened the way to reveal cancer-related genes in epigenetic machinery, including DNA methylation, nucleosome positioning, noncoding RNAs, and microRNAs, as well as histone modifications. The latest molecular research on GC may be a new diagnostic and therapeutic strategy in clinical practice. In this review, we will focus on recent advances in the description of the molecular pathogenesis of gastric cancer, underlying the use of these genetic and epigenetic alterations as diagnostic biomarkers and novel therapeutic targets.

Keywords: gastric carcinogenesis, molecular biomarkers, microsatellite instability, transcriptome profiling, epigenetic patterns, somatic mutations

1. Introduction

Gastric cancer is statistically the fifth most common cancer and the fourth most important cause of cancer-related death worldwide [1]. This malignancy is a highly heterogeneous disease caused by various factors, including genetic and environmental factors, diet, infection of *Helicobacter pylori,* or *Epstein–Barr* virus [2]. Based on Lauren's classification, GC is divided into three histological types: intestinal, diffuse, and mixed [3]. The intestinal subtype is mostly characterized by intestinal metaplasia and *Helicobacter pylori* infection, whereas the diffuse-type is more aggressive, with resistance to treatment and a weak prognosis. The Lauren classification has been widely used in the past; however, the clinical importance is rather limited in terms of the molecular heterogeneity of the cancer. The application of next-generation sequencing (NGS) technologies to molecular patterns description

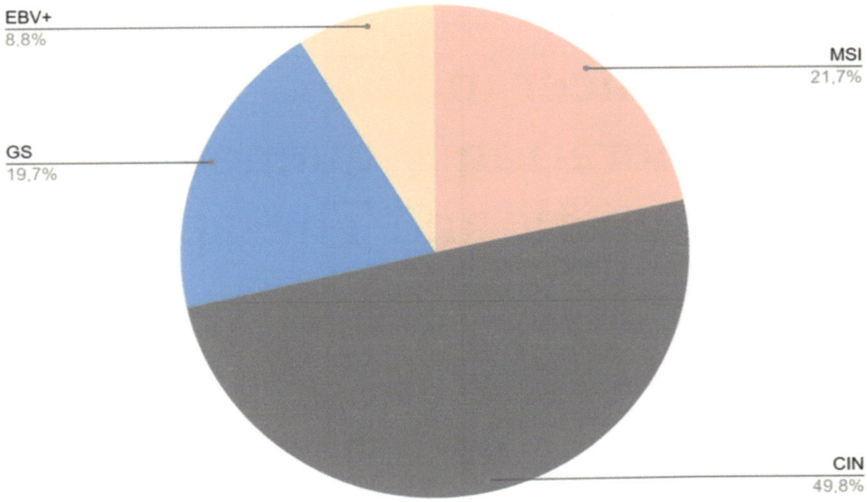

Figure 1.
Classification of gastric cancer molecular subtypes according to TCGA.

of the cancer allowed us to describe the molecular heterogeneity of a disease further. The Cancer Genome Atlas and the Asian Cancer Research Group have identified four molecular subtypes of gastric cancer based on the genetic and epigenetic characteristics: microsatellite instability, chromosomal instability, genome stability, and EBV+ (**Figure 1**) [4]. These molecular signatures have been tested for clinical importance, but further identification of factors is needed to predict treatment effectiveness.

The development of new technologies allowed researchers to extend the knowledge about the genetic and genomic background of GC tumorigenesis. In particular next-generation sequencing become a powerful tool to describe the genetic alterations and anomalies across the whole-genome and panel of genes, related to specific signaling pathways, leading to disease development and progression. NGS is a more accurate and sensitive technology, in comparison to Sanger's method, mostly by the fact that the percentage detection of allele frequency is 2–10% using high-throughput sequencing, whereas Sanger gives 15–25% [5]. Currently, there are different NGS-based approaches, like targeted sequencing of particular genes/pathways [6], whole-exome sequencing (WES) [7], whole-genome sequencing (WGS) [8], RNA-sequencing (RNA-seq) [9], epigenome sequencing [10], or even single-cell transcriptome profiling across the heterogeneous tumor tissue of GC [11]. Targeted sequencing represents a type of approach which allows for the analysis of exome, specific genes of interest, and so-called custom panels. This technique is fast and economical, allowing for the screening of targets within genes, or mitochondrial DNA. WGS covers the whole-genome analysis, displaying information about copy number changes, single nucleotide polymorphisms (SNPs), insertion/deletion (InDels) count, and large structural variants. WES is limited to the coding regions sequencing and exons. RNA-seq covers the detection of alternative gene-spliced transcripts, posttranscriptional modifications, SNPs, or alterations in the level of gene expression. This analysis can also be done at the resolution of single-cell.

In this paper, we investigated the screening of NGS-based techniques to describe the molecular pathogenesis of gastric cancer, determining genetic and epigenetic alterations, with levels of differentially expressed genes.

2. Targeted sequencing in the detection of mutations related to gastric cancer

Targeted next-generation sequencing is a method that is dedicated to screening regions of interest in the genome. It provides the aiming of specific genes, coding regions, or even chromosomal segments at deeper coverage than standard methods, like Sanger sequencing. To focus on the clinically significant targets of the genome or DNA sample, the method requires a presequencing DNA preparations step, where DNA sequences of interest are captured (hybrid capture-based) or frankly amplified (amplicon or multiplex PCR-based), to be further sequenced. Cristescu et al. [12] described four molecular subtypes of gastric cancer, and using targeted sequencing and genome-wide copy number microarrays, and they revealed important gene alterations among each of them. Tumors with microsatellite instability encompassed intestinal subtypes, hyper-mutated, and localized in the antrum, with the highest overall prognosis and decreased frequency of recurrence (22%). The mesenchymal-like type was classified as the type of gastric cancer with the worst prognosis, covering the diffuse subtype with the increased frequency of recurrence (63%). Types with tumor protein 53 (TP53)-active and TP53-inactive were assigned to the patients with an intermediate prognosis, where the TP53-active subtype displayed a better prognosis.

Clinical trials of advanced gastric cancer (AGC) are based mostly on the background of the protein expression level or amplification of relevant genes. Kuboki et al. performed the NGS study, including a panel of 409 cancer-related genes, on a cohort of formalin-fixed, paraffin-embedded tumor samples from 121 stage III/IV GC patients [13]. Among the analyzed group, at least one mutation was found in 93.4% of patients. The most repeated mutated gene was *TP53* (36.4%). Additionally, alterations in oncogenes, such as *PIK3CA* (7.4%), *ROS1* (5.0%), *ERBB2* (4.1%), *EGFR* (1.7%), *MET* (1.7%), *FGFR2* (1.7%), *BRAF* (1.7%), and *ALK* (1.7%) were revealed. *ERBB2* mutations were V842I and V777L, as previously published; *PIK3CA* alterations were detected in exon 9 or 20. Two mutations of *BRAF* were described: non-V600E mutations (N581Y, R682Q). Other mutations in *SYNE1* (10.7%), *CSMD3* (9.1%), *CDH1* (9.1%), *ARID1A* (8.3%), MLH1 (1.7%), and MSH2 (0.8%) were detected. Hirotsu et al. investigated the study on a cohort of 20 GC patients, both males and females, aged 60–87 years [14]. They created two custom panels of selected genes: A selective hotspot panel and a comprehensive panel, for the detection of mutations related to GC. The authors were able to identify 21 somatic mutations by the selective hotspot panel and 70 mutations by Comprehensive Panel, including all detected by the selective panel. Somatic mutations in *TP53* (43%), *APC* (29%), *MUC6* (33%), and *SYNE1* (24%) were the most common among the analyzed cohort, detected in more than 20% of cases. Other alterations were identified in *CTNNB1* (5%) and *KRAS* (5%) genes, with less frequency.

Cai et al. performed NGS sequencing, using a panel of 612 cancer-associated genes, on a cohort of 153 gastric cancer patients [15]. Identification of 35 importantly mutated genes was conducted, and among them, the top five genes were altered: *TP53* (59.09%), *DRD2* (14.29%), *CDH1* (13.64%), *AKAP9* (14.93%) and *ATM* (11.69%). *TP53* was the most common mutated gene in the studied population. The list of significantly mutated genes found by the authors, exploiting the custom gene panel, was compared to the TCGA cohort of GC. Thirteen importantly mutated genes in GC, reported by TCGA were also displayed by the authors of this study, but only six of them were analyzed as significantly mutated, including *P53* (59.09%), *PTEN* (13.64%), *FBXW7* (2.60%), *CDH1* (13.64%), *SMAD4* (7.79%), and *APC* (5.84%).

In comparison to the TCGA database, authors found 29 novel significantly mutated genes. KEGG enrichment analysis underlined the affected signaling pathways assigned to *p53* signaling, *MAPK* signaling, *Ras* signaling, *PI3K–Akt* signaling, *VEGF* signaling, *ErbB* signaling, *JAK-STAT* pathway, and cell movement-related pathways. Yu et al. studied a cohort of 529 gastric cancer patients, with an average age at diagnosis of 60 years [16]. For the detection of somatic mutation, they applied the panel of 450 cancer-associated genes within the exons and certain introns of 39 genes. They revealed the importance of mutations in 449 genes. The most common mutated genes were *TP53* (59.7%), *ARID1A* (21.9%), *LRP1B* (14.7%), *PIK3CA* (13.8%), *ERBB2* (13.4%), *CDH1* (13.0%), *KRAS* (11.7%), *FAT4* (11.5%), *CCNE1* (10.6%), *KMT2D* (10.4%), and *RNF43* (10.4%). The most frequent alteration was C > T, accounting for 62.6% of the total SNVs. On the other hand, the most commonly amplified regions and genes were assigned to: *CCNE1* (n = 55, 10.4%), *ERBB2* (n = 44, 8.3%), 11q13 (including *CCND1*, *FGF19*, *FGF4*, and *FGF3*; n = 30, 5.7%), *GATA4* (n = 26, 4.9%), and *FGFR2* (n = 25, 4.7%). Increased frequency of mutated signaling pathways was observed within *PI3K/Akt*, *Wnt*, and cell-cycle signaling pathways.

Toal et al. evaluated the 115 tumor biopsies across 32 study cases, performing targeted next-generation sequencing [17]. They found a group of mutated genes: *ATAD2, ATR, BRCA2, CSDE1, CSMD3, DLC1, EGFR, ELF3, ERBB4, FGFR2, KLF5, TRPA1, TSHZ2, GNAS, MYC,* and *MMP9* for *MSS* tumors and *ATM, CDC27, ESR1, KMT2E,* and *NEB* for MSI tumors, which have been formerly described as driver genes by TCGA/non-TCGA investigations for different types of cancer, excluding GC. Among these findings, authors detected six genes in MSS tumors (*EYS, FAT4, FSIP2, PCDHA1, RAD50,* and *RECQL4*) and two in MSI tumors (*EXO1* and *FSIP2*), that were clonally mutated across the cohort of studied patients, not detected in the past as driver genes for GC development. Multiple of these genes occurs in main processes affected in GC tumorigenesis, like homologous recombinant repair (*RAD50* and *RECQL4*), extracellular matrix (*EYS*), or cell adhesion (*FAT4* and *PCDHA1*).

3. Whole-exome and whole-genome studies in GC development

Next-generation sequencing facilitates the sequence of large amounts of DNA, including all the pieces of a patient's DNA, that supply the information for protein making. Most of the known mutations that are responsible for gastric cancer

Methodology	Studied cohort	Frequently mutated genes	Top perturbed signaling pathways	Conclusions	Reference
Whole-exome sequencing	• Fifteen gastric adenocarcinomas	• *TP53* (11/15 tumors), *PIK3CA* (3/15) and *ARID1A* (3/15) • Frequent alterations in chromatin remodeling genes (*ARID1A, MLL3,* and *MLL*)	• Cell adhesion pathway	• Somatic inactivation of *FAT4* and *ARID1A* could be the main tumorigenic events in GC	[18]

Methodology	Studied cohort	Frequently mutated genes	Top perturbed signaling pathways	Conclusions	Reference
Whole-exome sequencing	• Four samples from patients with early gastric cancer (EGC), and compared to advanced gastric cancer (AGC)	• *DYRK3, GPR116, MCM10, PCDH17, PCDHB1, RDH5* and *UNC5C* genes are recurrently mutated in EGCs		• EGC and AGC share common somatic mutations • AGC is related to an additional cumulative genetic mutations in cell adhesion and chromatin remodeling genes	[19]
Whole-genome sequencing	• One hundred tumor-normal pairs	• Identification of previously known (*TP53, ARID1A* and *CDH1*) and novel (*MUC6, CTNNA2, GLI3, RNF43* and others) importantly altered driver genes • Indication of *RHOA* mutations in 14.3% of diffuse-type GC tumors but not in intestinal subtype	• Adherens junction and focal adhesion signaling pathways, in which *RHOA* and other altered genes play a key role	• Underlining the molecular heterogeneity and complexity of GC leading to improve genome-guided personalized therapy	[8]
Whole-genome and whole-exome sequencing	• Eighty-four clinical biopsy tumor samples (including matched pre- and posttreatment) from 35 cases with gastric cancer, with described responses to neoadjuvant chemotherapy	• The top mutated genes: *TP53, PI3KCA, RNF43, ARIDA1*, and *KRAS*, as previously detected in other GC studies • Mutations associated with the response of the tumor to chemotherapy: *C10orf71* and *IRS1* mutations, and *MYC* and *MDM2* amplifications • MSI status as a clinical biomarker to direct therapy in patients with gastric cancer	• *MYC* signaling activated in the response group • Upregulation of DNA repair pathway in the response group • One top subnetwork consisted of *IRS1, IRS2, PIK3CA, JAK1*, and *IL6ST* • *IRS1* is involved in transmitting signals from the insulin and insulin-like growth factor-1 receptors to the *phosphatidylinositol 3-kinase/AKT* pathway	• Identification of molecular markers assigned to the tumor response to neoadjuvant chemotherapy	[20]

Methodology	Studied cohort	Frequently mutated genes	Top perturbed signaling pathways	Conclusions	Reference
Whole-exome sequencing	• Thirty-eight gastric cancer patients, 26 metastatic and 12 nonmetastatic	• Somatic mutation of *ATAD3B* assigned to the metastatic stage • Rare germline mutations associated with GC survival or metastasis: *FANCM*, *PDGFRA*, and *POLE* • *CCNE1* and *ERBB2* were displayed to be amplified • CNVs of several genes including *MMP9*, *PTPN1*, and *SS18L1* were significantly related to metastasis	• *TP53* signaling pathway • Base excision repair (BER) pathway • Pathways of cell growth control and response to interferon stimulation	• Detection of potential new predictive molecular markers of survival and metastasis	[7]
Whole-exome sequencing	• One hundred five cases of alpha-fetoprotein-producing gastric carcinomas (AFPGC)	• Thirty-four significantly mutated genes identified • Among them, the most frequently altered genes were: *TP53* (69%), *PCLO* (21%), *CSMD3* (19%), and *KMT2C* (19%)	• *RTK/RAS/PI(3)K*, *p53*/cell cycle, and *JAK/STAT* signaling pathways	• A large genomic landscape of AFPGC, a step forward to understanding the disease mechanisms	[21]

Table 1.
Whole-exome and whole-genome studies among different subtypes of gastric cancer.

development and progression occur in exons, thus, this method of sequencing is perceived as an efficient approach to characterizing disease-causing alterations. Additionally, it is known that some DNA variations outside the exons might alter the gene activity and protein production; therefore, whole-genome sequencing is also applied in GC studies to uncover alterations in any part of the genome. In this section, we described several studies, including whole-exome and whole-genome sequencing of different subtypes of gastric cancer, highlighting the type of studied population, frequently mutated genes, and affected pathways, which are presented in **Table 1**.

4. The chromatin landscape of gastric cancer tumor

In gastric cancer development and progression, the impact of aberrant DNA methylation of a promoter CpG island (CGI) is significant because *Helicobacter pylori* infection leads to aberrant methylation [22]. Park et al. compared the methylation status in normal and gastric cancer tissues using different methods including high-throughput sequencing [23]. They found that CpG island hypermethylation in promoters influences changes in gene expression profile. Hypermethylation of the 5′-end of coding exons appeared in cancer and affected the progression of the disease. Methylation status changes in low-range epigenetic silencing (LRES) regions, and younger repetitive elements suggested a direction for early disease detection and specific targeting strategies. The authors also revealed that within LRES regions, there were hypermethylated genes, like *MDM2*, *DYRK2*, and *LYZ*. Dysregulation of the *MDM2*-mediated pathway at the epigenetic level was displayed in some cancer samples. Moreover, the methylation status of *HOX* genes was assigned to tissue-specific manners in GC and might be an important target during tumorigenesis. Zouridis et al. investigated the analysis of DNA methylation signatures in gastric carcinoma among 240 tumor samples and 94 matched healthy tissues by genome-wide CG dinucleotide (CpG) methylation profiles [24]. Epigenetic variabilities were present in 44% of CpGs, including both hyper- and hypomethylation. Cancerous gene expression levels were correlated with 25% of changes in methylation status. Authors revealed a subgroup of CpG island methylator phenotype (CIMP) with specific signatures, like young age, broad hypermethylation status, unfavorable patient outcome in a disease phase-autonomous way, and long-range regions of epigenetic silencing (LRESs). Moreover, they found regions of long-range tumor hypomethylation, assigned to the higher level of chromosomal instability. To conclude these studies, the authors indicate that for gastric cancer patients that are included in the CIMP group, silenced DNA provides a target for accessible drugs.

Loh et al. did a high-throughput methylation analysis on FFPE primary tumor and tumor-adjacent gastric tissue samples among a cohort of 60 patients with gastric cancer [25]. The set of 219 CpG islands within 147 genes was displayed to be differentially methylated. Almost all of these genes, apart from (*CHFR*, *DAB2IP*, *DLC1*, *SFRP1*, *TCF4,* and *TFPI2*) are new methylation biomarkers in gastric cancer that might be useful for early screening of disease. Six methylation subgroups were isolated within two different clusters, including 72% high methylation (H) and 28% low-methylation (L) of GC tumors. Differential analysis indicated *HOXA5* as the most differentially methylated gene between two subgroups of gastric tumor and tumor-adjacent gastric tissue. The H subgroup displayed methylated genes with increased incidence of polycomb occupancy and H3K4+/H3K27+ bivalent marks, showing the correlation between chromatin dysregulation and hypermethylated phenotype. Chong et al. performed a wide screening of methylation patterns on fresh tumor and nontumor samples from EGC patients [26]. Further to validate methylation data in 3 GC histological subtypes (intestinal, diffuse, and mixed), authors conducted pyrosequencing with 12 genes, selected from the methylation screening. The methylation assay displayed 169 differentially methylated regions between histological subtypes of GC. Pyrosequencing with 12 genes of interest indicated the abnormal methylation patterns of *DVL2* and *ETS1,* which were corresponding to both diffuse and mixed subtypes, while *C19orf35* and *CNRIP1* were assigned to the diffuse-type, and *GAL3ST2* and *ITGA3* were related to the mixed-type. Status of several other methylated genes: *CCDC57*, *CLIP4*, *MAML3*, *SDC2*, and *XKR6,* was related to factors like tumor location, age, or *H. pylori* infection.

Yoda et al. investigated to analyze the gastric cancer-related pathways affected by epigenetic variations, using wide screening with a bead array with 485,512 probes for CpG and non-CpG sites [27]. Among a group of 50 gastric cancer patients, they found that tumor-suppressor genes, such as *CDH1*, *CDKN2A*, and *MLH1*, were inactivated mostly by epigenetic changes. Moreover, repression of negative regulators (*DKK3*, *NKD1*, and *SFRP1)* of the *WNT* signaling pathway by epigenetic alterations occurred in all study cases. The cell-cycle regulation pathway was perturbed by the abnormal methylation of *CDKN2A* and *CHFR* in 13 cases. In two gastric carcinomas, they found that mismatch repair is affected by the aberrant methylation of the *MLH1* gene. Abnormal methylation patterns of downstream genes in 38 cases, caused inactivation of their p53 pathway. Sepulveda et al. screened nonmetaplastic mucosa, intestinal metaplasia, and gastric cancer with methylation arrays and bisulfite next-generation sequencing [28]. In gastric cancer cases, 13 genes had higher CpG methylation status, in comparison to nonmetaplastic mucosa, including: *BRINP1*, *CDH11*, *CHFR*, *EPHA5*, *EPHA7*, *FGF2*, *FLI1*, *GALR1*, *HS3ST2*, *PDGFRA*, *SEZ6L*, *SGCE*, and *SNRPN*. Additionally, the hypermethylation status in most of these genes correlated with lower expression levels, indicating that they could mediate neoplastic transformation from nonmalignant intestinal metaplasia to cancer. Authors observed hypermethylation and decreased expression of the *FLT1* gene in GC, suggesting a tumor-suppressor role, which was previously shown in breast cancer studies [29]. Hypermethylated genes *BRINP1* and *SGCE* were matched with better survival in GC.

Alterations in histone H3 lysine 27 (H3K27me3) in gastric cancer are not fully uncovered. Zhang et al. performed chromatin immunoprecipitation linked to the microarray (ChIP-chip) approach, to describe changes in H3K27me3 in CpG island regions, among eight gastric cancer patients and matched healthy tissues [30]. Important H3K27me3 distinctions were displayed between normal and tumorous tissues, among 128 genes (9 lowered and 119 increased H3K27me3). Additionally, abnormal DNA methylation was also discovered on arbitrarily picked genes: *AFF3*, *MMP15*, *RB1*, *SHH*, and *UNC5B.* This study highlighted the importance of H3K27me3, as a biomarker and target for epigenetic-based therapies. Muratani et al. investigated Nano-ChIP-seq in primary gastric carcinomas to display histone modifications and their associated regulatory elements [31]. Authors were able to uncover for the first time the landscape of promoters and putative enhancer elements, placed in noncoding regions of the genome, that are somatically changed in primary GCs. They found a huge proportion of promoters assigned with cancer that were cryptic, which indicated activation of noncanonical promoters, ending with changed transcriptional usage of 5′ exons. They revealed germline variants, placed within somatically changed regulatory elements, showing allelic bias, which might predispose to GC development.

In gastric cancer, regulatory enhancer elements are still a target for new studies. Ooi et al. performed chromatin profiling using ChIP-seq to uncover the enhancer landscape in primary GC [32]. Samples including healthy tissues, primary tumors of GC, and cell lines underwent epigenome characteristics, which revealed 36,973 predicted enhancers and 3759 predicted super-enhancers. Super-enhancers were categorized by their somatic mutation profile, into somatic loss, gain, and nonmutated subgroups, which were enriched in various transcriptional, epigenetic, and pathway signatures. Somatic gain-predicted super-enhancers had an impact on proximal and distal gene expression and were perceived as significant regulators of abnormal gene expression in GC. The authors also showed that somatic gain-predicted super-enhancers are correlated with the occurrence of *CDX2* and *HNF4α*. This study contributed to the discovery of complexity among enhancers and super-enhancers reprogramming during tumorigenesis of GC. Aberrant methylation at promoter parts was described for many genes; however, it is still not well recognized the function of DNA methylation signatures at distal regulatory parts in GC. Baek et al. did ChIP-seq study to extend the knowledge about epigenetic alterations in the proximal and distal regulatory regions [33]. They found multiple enhancers with abnormal DNA methylation status. The analysis displayed genes that were over-expressed and hypo-methylated at their promoters, including *CDX1*, *HNF4A*, *MUC4*, *MUC6*, and *MAGE* family genes (*MAGEA1*, *MAGEA6*, *MAGEC1*, and *MAGEC2*). The authors also displayed that hypo-methylated-enhancer regions were enriched with the *TEAD4* motif. Additionally, the analysis of methylation changes at the promoter regions of lncRNAs allowed for the identification of presumed lncRNAs, like *EBV1-AS*, *HOXD-AS1*, *HOXD-AS2,* and *MALAT1*. Four subtypes of GC were also analyzed (CIN+, EBV+, GS+, and MSI+) for methylation patterns, and the EBV+ subtype was significantly hypermethylated among other subtypes.

The epigenomic promoter landscape of GC was analyzed by Qamra et al. [34], as promoter elements are significant factors in cell-type-specific expression profiles [34]. In this study 110 chromatin profiles (H3K4me1, H3K4me3, and H3K27ac) were investigated, among gastric cancer cell lines, primary tumors, and healthy samples. Different alternative promoters were found in previously described as well as novel genes in GC, like alternative promoters at the *EPCAM* gene locus, which was active in GC samples. Another alternative promoter that was revealed for the first time was localized in the *RASA3* gene, and N-terminal Var RASA3 increased migration and invasion in studied gastric cell lines. The connection between tumor immunity and somatic promoters was also revealed, as isoforms of alternative promoters with increased expression in GC displayed depletion of N-terminal peptides, with immunogenic properties.

5. Analysis of gastric cancer transcriptome

The next-generation sequencing applications, like RNA-sequencing or gene expression microarrays, facilitate the study of wide-scale functional genomics to cancer investigations and its application in clinical settings. These techniques provide individual gene expression profiles, which might be used as molecular markers in the treatment of patients with GC [35–38]. Several studies implicated transcriptome profiling to uncover differentially expressed genes between healthy and tumorous tissues in GC patients [39, 40]. Additionally, various studies have described stage and histological-specific gene expression profiles [41]. Moreover, databases with transcriptome studies data are a source of published results, which allow analysis in the context of disease development. In **Table 2** are listed several studies on the transcriptome of GC, with an indication of the studied group, DEGs, and modulated signaling pathways.

Methodology	Studied group	Differentially expressed genes	Modulated pathways	Conclusions	Reference
Gene expression microarray	• Twenty-six samples of primary gastric carcinomas and matched healthy tissues	• 2371 differentially expressed mRNAs, 1142 downregulated, and 1229 upregulated between gastric cancer and control tissues • The genes such as *GKN2*, *PGC*, *MUC6*, *CHIA*, *PSCA*, and *FBP2* were in the group of top 20 downregulated, while *KLK8*, *SFRP4*, *INHBA*, *CLDN1*, *CST1*, *FAP*, *SPP1*, *OLFM4*, and *KRT17* were among the top 20 upregulated	• Upregulated genes were involved in angiogenesis, tumorigenesis, migration, and microenvironment formation, while downregulated genes were assigned to metabolism	• Better understanding of gastric cancer carcinogenesis • Key genes as a target in antitumor therapy	[42]
RNA-seq data (GSE36968) downloaded from the Gene Expression Omnibus Database	• Six healthy tissues • GC stage I: 5 samples, stage II: 5 samples, stage III: 8 samples, and stage IV: 6 samples	• 3576 genes with stage-specific expression patterns • Kinesin family member C1, *KIFC1*; and septin 2, *SEPT2*) were highly expressed in stage I and II • Neuropilin-2, *NRP2*; collagen triple helix repeat containing-1, *CTHRC1*; secreted protein, acidic, cysteine-rich, osteonectin, *SPARC*; matrix metalloproteinase 17, *MMP17*; and collagen, type VI, alpha 3, *COL6A3*) were specific for stage IV GC	• Two regulatory pathways in stage IV GC: *HOXA4-GLI3-RUNX2-FGF2* and *HMGA2-PRKCA*	• Understanding the pathogenesis of GC by stage-specific gene profile	[43]
RNA-seq	• Fifteen cases with advanced or metastatic GC • Patients were underwent the therapy with ramucirumab	• Three genes were differentially expressed in the tumors for responders (to ramucirumab) versus nonresponders: *CHRM3*, *LRFN1*, and *TEX15* • *CHRM3* was upregulated in the responders • Downregulation of CDC42 activators, such as *RAP1A*, *RAP1B*, and *SRC*, could be related to tumor response to ramucirumab	• Nectin adhesion pathway • This pathway was more active in the nonresponders, correlated with a higher expression of the *RAP1A*, *RAP1B*, and *SRC* genes	• RNA-sequencing might be used to individualize the recommendation of ramucirumab for GC patients	[44]
RNA-seq	• Twenty-four patients with gastric cancer • Two main subgroups according to histopathology classification: intestinal and diffuse	• Detection of 2064 differentially expressed genes between healthy and cancer samples • 772 of them assigned to the intestinal subtype, 407 specific for the diffuse subtype • In the intestinal subtype enrichment of *CXCR2*, *CXCR1*, *FPR2*, *CARD14*, *EFNA2*, *AQ9*, *TRIP13*, *KLK11*, and *GHRL* was displayed • In the diffuse-type, low levels of *CXCR2* and increased levels of *CARD14* mRNA were negative predictors of 4 years of survival	• Increased modulation of *MAPK*, *RAS*, *PI3K–AKT–mTOR*, *JAK/STAT*, *NF-kB*, *VEGF* • Modulation of cell-cycle regulators, chemokine, and cytokine signaling • Modulation of immune and proliferation pathways	• Therapeutic strategy for gastric cancer patients (diffuse and intestinal) by targeting *AQP9* and *CXCR2*	[45]

Methodology	Studied group	Differentially expressed genes	Modulated pathways	Conclusions	Reference
RNA-seq data from the TCGA database	• TCGA gastric cancer contained a total of 407 samples, 375 tumor samples, and 32 normal samples	• Classification into prognostic metabolic subgroups: cholesterolemia, glycolytic, mixed, and quiescent, based on the expressed genes, related to cholesterol synthesis and glycolysis • A total of 1966 DEGs between cholesterol and glycolysis subtypes • mRNA levels of mitochondrial pyruvate carriers 1 and 2 (MPC1/2) were subtype-specific • Glycolytic subtype showed increased *PDCD1* expression	• Glycolysis subtypes were associated with: immune-related T cell receptor signaling, B cell receptor signaling, natural killer cell-mediated cytotoxicity, and primary immuno-deficiency pathways	• Genes correlated with glucose and lipid metabolism have an impact on gastric cancer development	[46]
RNA-seq	• Two male patients with early-stage gastric adenocarcinoma	• 1677 DEGs and 111 differentially expressed novel transcripts and noncoding transcripts were found to be expressed in the GC tumoral tissues in comparison to healthy ones • Dysregulation of 22 genes was confirmed by the TCGA dataset: *ATP4A, ATP4B, GKN1, GKN2*, and gastric type *LIPF,* which were expressed only in the stomach, while ghrelin, *GHRL*, and *SLC5A5* were expressed in the stomach but also in many other tissues • Novel downregulated noncoding RNAs including *GATA6* antisense *RNA 1*, antisense to *LYZ*, antisense *P4HB*, overlapping *ACER2*	• Gastric acid secretion was the most significantly enriched pathway • Drug metabolism and transporters, molecular toxicology, O-linked glycosylation of mucins, immuno-toxicity, glycosylation	• Key genes and regulatory pathways involved in GC tumorigenesis	[9]
RNA-seq	• Paired tumor-normal samples from four GC patients	• 148 highly significant DEGs • *CLDN7, SELL, CLDN4, HLA-DOA*, and *CLDN1* genes enriched in the CAM pathway • *ATP4A, ATP4B, KCNE2, KCNJ16*, and *SLC26A7* genes enriched in the gastric acid secretion pathway • Two upregulated genes, *APOC1* and *SALL4* with prognostic importance	• CAM pathway, gastric acid secretion, and mineral absorption pathways	• *SALL4* as a potential molecular marker candidate in GC	[47]
RNA-seq data from TCGA and GEO databases	• Gastric cancer samples	• Identification of 25 DEGs • Six secretory genes (*APOC1, OLFM4, CST1, CEMIP, COL4A1*, and *CD55*) with diagnostic importance • Higher *COL4A1* expression might be correlated with a poor prognosis	• Connective tissue development, collagen fibrous tissue-related processes, extracellular structure, extracellular matrix (ECM) tissue, focal adhesion, and *PI3K-Akt* signaling pathway	• *COL4A1* could be the molecular marker in GC diagnosis	[48]

Methodology	Studied group	Differentially expressed genes	Modulated pathways	Conclusions	Reference
RNA-seq	• Six gastric cancer samples (stage I, II III) and matched healthy tissues	• 2207 differentially expressed genes, including 972 upregulated genes and 1235 downregulated • Top genes in stage I: *KRT5, CDH3, ARNT2, EFNA3, PRKAR2B, VIT, ACACB* • Top genes in stage II: *S100A2, SLC28A2, CDC25A, FBLN2, ARHGEF19, LRRC-66, ACTL8, and SSTR1* • Key genes in stage III: *SH3BP5, MSRB3, SGPL1, PRKACB, DRAM1, SLCO2A1, MAPK11 and NCEH1*	• Stage I: chemical carcinogen-esis, drug and xenobiotics metabolism by cytochrome P450, fat digestion • Stage II: complement and coagula-tion cascades and nitrogen metabolism • Stage III: che-mokine and TNF signaling pathway	• Deeper understanding of molecular pathogenesis of GC	[49]

Table 2.
Transcriptome studies in the development of gastric cancer stages.

6. Single-cell atlas of expression programs in gastric cancer

Single-cell transcriptomics (single-cell RNA-sequencing) has a broad potential to reveal the novel basis of cancer development and progression. The diversity of cells at the individual level might be better studied by single-cell transcriptomics. This method allows for sequencing millions of cells with proper accuracy and viability in a short period. Transcriptional heterogeneity in primary gastric carcinomas was investigated by Zhang et al. [50]. The authors performed scRNA-seq analysis on 27,677 cells derived from 9 GC tumors and 3 healthy samples. Results showed five main populations of cells, with unique expression profiles. The variability in cell composition between tumor samples and within them was displayed. They revealed two characteristic groups with distinct transcriptome features. One subgroup was characterized as GA-FG-CCP, expressing chief-cell markers (*LIPF* and *PGC*), and *RNF43* with *WNt/B-catenin* signaling pathway. The other subgroup expressed immune-specific genes (eg, *LYK6* and major histocompatibility complex class II), including the *Epstein-Barr* virus. Moreover, analysis of nonmalignant epithelium uncovered a prospective transition from chief cells to *MUC6* + *TFF2* + spasmolytic polypeptide expressing metaplasia.

Kim et al. studied the diversity of the cell population of precancerous lesions and gastric cancer using scRNA-seq technology [51]. They described 10 cell populations in GC and displayed the histology-based composition of GC subtypes, including intestinal and diffuse types. Interestingly, intestinal and diffuse-type cancer cells had various metaplastic cell lineages: diffuse-type cancer cells resemble de novo pathways, while intestinal subtype cancer cells differentiated along the intestinal metaplasia lineage. In the diffuse-type lineage, single-cell patterns were linked with intratumoral CAFs and might develop into various cell sets to survive. Additionally, the authors distinguish a population of cancer cells, the EmyoT type, displaying a characteristic gene expression profile. The EmyoT tumor cell type was correlated with a poor prognosis, diffuse marker gene expression, and weak EMT signature.

Moreover, $CCND1_{mut}$ and iCAFs might have a significant impact on alterations in GC. In the study performed by Yang et al. [52], the analysis of scRNA-seq data of GC, displayed 3385 various cell characteristics expressed by 4110 EGC cells. The authors detected gastric cells, memory T cells, and plasmacytoid dendritic cells [52]. The top 8 expressed genes were: *CCL5*, *CHGA*, *FABP1*, *KRT7*, *OLFM4*, *SRGN*, *TFF3*, and *TTR*. The important relationship between the DEGs and *TNF* signaling pathway, oxidative phosphorylation, and endoplasmic reticulum protein processing was found. Moreover, they discovered a prognostic marker for GC, *FABP1*, which regulated the fat digestion, *PPAR* signaling pathway, hormone-sensitive lipase (HSL)-mediated triacylglycerol hydrolysis, and absorption in GC progression. The expression of *FABP1* was correlated with the age of patients' diagnosis and an increased level of *FABP1* was assigned with a lower survival rate in GC.

A study across clinical stages and histology classification of GCs allowed for a wide-range analysis of 48 samples from 31 patients and displayed a single-cell atlas of over 200,000 cells [53]. Identification of 34 various cell-lineage states was displayed, encompassing new rare cell populations. In the diffuse subtype of GC, there was a higher level of plasma cell proportions, associated with epithelial-resident *KLF2* and cancer-associated fibroblast populations, with increased *INHBA* and *FAP* coexpression. Therefore, cancer-associated fibroblast subtype with *INHBA-FAP*-high cell populations might be an indicating factor of poor clinical prognosis. Importantly, high expression of *Epilnt1* was specific for the subpopulation of intestinal-type epithelial cells, suggesting that this set of cells could be significant in the transition into malignancy from metaplasia. Li et al. [54] profiled the transcriptome of nine patients with GC, revealing the composition of 47,304 cells [54]. Among identified populations, Treg cells were enriched in GC tissues, with higher expression of genes related to immune suppression. Tumor endothelial cells specifically expressed the *ACKR1* gene, which was related to the poor prognosis, and could be a novel target in GC treatment. Limitation of immunotherapy in GC patients might be supported by the obtained results, which indicated the deficit of separate exhausted CD8+ T cell cluster, and the decreased expression level of exhaustion markers *CTLA4*, *HAVCR2*, *LAG-3*, *PDCD1*, and *TIGIT* in those specific cells. Gastric cancer metastasis (liver, ovary, peritoneum, and lymph node) with primary tumors and nontumoral adjacent samples were analyzed by Jiang et al. using sc-RNA-seq [55]. They discovered several phenotypes, including malignant epithelial clusters assigned with invasion, dormancy-like features, intraperitoneal metastasis propensity, and epithelial–mesenchymal transition-induced tumor stem cell phenotypes. Immune and stromal cells showed cellular heterogeneity and constructed an immunosuppressive microenvironment. Authors revealed not only malignant tumor cells, but also endothelial subcluster, plasmacytoid dendritic cells, T cell-like B cells, mucosal-associated invariant T cells, macrophages, monocytes, and neutrophils may contribute to HLA-E-KLRC1/KLRC2 interaction with cytotoxic/exhausted CD8+ T cells and/or natural killer (NK) cells, suggesting new therapeutic opportunities in GC.

7. Liquid biopsy in gastric cancer diagnosis

Cell-free DNA (cfDNA) is released from cells into the circulatory system throughout the body. It might be detected in plasma and body fluids, such as saliva, urine, pleural fluid, cerebral spinal fluid, and others. In some pathological states, like cancer, organ transplantation, or pregnancy, the affected tissues could release additional

DNA into the peripheral circulation. Detection of cfDNA/ctDNA in peripheral blood might be useful for the identification of abnormalities in individuals in a noninvasive manner [56]. CfDNA/ctDNA might be used for gastric cancer diagnosis, prognosis, prediction of efficiency, and resistance to therapy.

Zhong et al. studied the clinical value of plasma cell-free DNA and its role as a biomarker for advanced gastric cancer [57]. CfDNA concentration in advanced gastric cancer patients was increased in comparison to healthy cases. Importantly the concentration of cfDNA among cases with disease progression (PD), displayed an increasing level over time. There was no valuable correlation between cfDNA concentration and traditional biomarkers like age, gender, pathological type, CA125, CA199, CA724, AFP, and CEA. Plasma cfDNA concentration was higher in patients with gastric cancer, and its diagnostic efficacy was better than common tumor biomarkers. Kandimalla et al. investigated a genome-wide DNA methylation analysis of 1781 gastrointestinal stromal (GI) tumors and adjacent normal tissues and identified the differentially methylated regions (DMR) between analyzed groups [58]. A panel of 67,832 tissue DMRs was prioritized and validated in 300 cfDNA specimens. The authors supported the first evidence for a cfDNA methylation assay, that provides robust diagnostic accuracy for GI cancers. Yang et al. investigated the evaluation of molecular residual disease (MRD) by ctDNA in 46 resected gastric cancers with stage I-III [59]. Sixty tumor samples and 296 plasma samples were enrolled for targeted deep sequencing and ctDNA profiling. Cases with detected ctDNA in the immediate postoperative period, experienced recurrence. CtDNA occurrence during longitudinal postoperative follow-up was associated with worse postoperative disease-free (DFS) and overall survival (OS).

Exosomes are small (30–140 nm) membrane-bounded extracellular vesicles, that are secreted by large multivesicular bodies and might be detected in blood, urine, cerebrospinal fluid, and other body fluids. They are released by multiple cell types, such as epithelial cells, neuronal cells, hematopoietic cells, fibroblasts, adipocytes, and tumor cells. Noncoding RNAs, like microRNAs (miRNAs), circular RNAs (circRNAs), and long noncoding RNAs (lncRNAs), which in normal conditions are degraded, might be packed into exosomes, which provide them stability [60].

Exosomal miRNAs (EmiRs) could be used for the prediction of GC development. Qian et al. investigated miRNA sequencing to identify key members of EmiRs in GC [61]. The exosome samples derived from blood and urine were taken from 7 GC cases and 3 healthy donors. For GC cases, authors found three upregulated differentially expressed miRNAs (DEmiRNAs): hsa-miR-130b-3p, hsa-miR-151a-3p, and hsa-miR-15b-3p in the serum exosomes, and one upregulated DEmiRNA (hsa-miR-1246) in the urinary exosomes. Further analysis showed the commonly enriched ontology terms, including GO BP terms like cell surface receptor signaling pathway involved in cell-cell signaling, positive regulation of the catabolic process, and morphogenesis of an epithelium. Four key exosomal miRNAs and their targets (*TAOK1, CMTM6, SCN3A, WASF3, IGF1, CNOT7, GABRG1,* and *PRKD1*) could be a reference of the molecular mechanisms in gastric cancer development. Tang et al. used NGS sequencing to identify exosomal miRNAs in serum, considered early diagnostic markers for GC [62]. A total of 66 up and 13 downregulated exosomal miRNAs were detected in the studied cohort. Increased levels of serum exosomal miR-92b-3p, let-7 g-5p, miR-146b-5p, and miR-9-5p were found to be importantly correlated with early-stage GC. Moreover, serum content of exosomal miR-92b-3p was significantly correlated with poor cohesiveness, let-7 g-5p and miR-146b-5p with nerve infiltration, and miR146b-5p with tumor invasion depth in early-stage GC. In conclusion, serum exosomal miR-92b-3p, -146b-5p, -9-5p, and let-7 g-5p could be candidates for noninvasive biomarkers for early diagnosis of GC.

8. Conclusion

Remarkable advances in next-generation sequencing technologies allowed for the characterization of the genetic, epigenetic, and transcriptomic landscape of gastric cancer. In this review, we summarized the studies, indicating multiple molecular signatures and distinct molecular subtypes, which might serve as a future roadmap for patient treatment and trials of targeted therapies. The fast advances in NGS approaches will shortly continue to display driver mutations of GC, for further understanding the GC carcinogenesis and will improve the individual tumor therapy. Predictive biomarkers are important in precision oncology. In the past few years, multiple studies have investigated GC treatment. While targeting *HER2* remains the key therapy strategy for a limited number of patients with advanced GC, new targets have been explored, mostly those for immune checkpoint molecules. Currently, *CLDN18.2* is being investigated among various other targets, and new results are expected to be revealed shortly. The main barrier to accurate medicine for gastric cancer is intratumoral heterogeneity, which has an impact on tissue-based diagnostics, and this could cause primary and secondary drug resistance. Recent studies displayed blood-based biomarkers that could be used as diagnostic indicators and for monitoring postsurgical minimal residual disease. Among these biomarkers, we have circulating DNA, RNA, extracellular vesicles, and proteins. Detection of accurate diagnostic markers for GC that have high sensitivity and specificity will, in the future, improve survival rates and contribute to precision medicine.

Author details

Julita Machlowska[1*] and Ryszard Maciejewski[2,3]

1 International Centre for Translational Eye Research, Polish Academy of Sciences, Warsaw, Poland

2 Department of Human Anatomy, Medical University of Lublin, Lublin, Poland

3 Faculty of Natural Sciences and Health, The John Paul II Catholic University of Lublin, Lublin, Poland

*Address all correspondence to: julita.machlowska@gmail.com

References

[1] Sung H, Ferlay J, Siegel RL, et al. Global cancer statistics 2020: GLOBOCAN estimates of incidence and mortality worldwide for 36 cancers in 185 countries. CA: a Cancer Journal for Clinicians. 2021;**71**(3):209-249

[2] Helisz P, Gwioździk W, Krupa-Kotara K, et al. Risk factors and prevention of gastric cancer development—What Do we know and what can we Do? Onco. 2023;**3**:26-42

[3] Lauren P. The two histological main types of gastric carcinoma: Diffuse and so-called intestinal-type carcinoma. An attempt at a histo-clinical classification. Acta Pathologica et Microbiologica Scandinavica. 1965;**64**:31-49

[4] Sohn BH, Hwang JE, Jang HJ, et al. Clinical significance of four molecular subtypes of gastric cancer identified by the cancer genome atlas project. Clinical Cancer Research. 2017;**23**(15):4441-4449

[5] Serrati S, De Summa S, Pilato B, et al. Next generation sequencing: Advances and applications in cancer diagnosis. Oncotargets and Therapy. 2016;**9**:7355-7365

[6] Deng N, Goh LK, Wang H, et al. A comprehensive survey of genomic alterations in gastric cancer reveals systematic patterns of molecular exclusivity and co-occurrence among distinct therapeutic targets. Gut. 2012;**61**:673-684

[7] Zhu Z, Fu H, Wang S, et al. Whole-exome sequencing identifies prognostic mutational signatures in gastric cancer. Annals of Translational Medicine. 2020;**8**(22):1484

[8] Wang K, Yuen S, Xu J, et al. Whole-genome sequencing and comprehensive molecular profiling identify new driver mutations in gastric cancer. Nature Genetics. 2014;**46**:573-582

[9] Fattahi S, Nikbakhsh N, Taheri H, et al. RNA sequencing of early-stage gastric adenocarcinoma reveals multiple activated pathways and novel long non-coding RNAs in patient tissue samples. Reports of Biochemistry and Molecular Biology. 2021;**9**(4):478-489

[10] Peng Y, Wu Q, Wang L, et al. A DNA methylation signature to improve survival prediction of gastric cancer. Clinical Epigenetics. 2020;**12**(1):15

[11] Sun K, Xu R, Ma F, et al. scRNA-seq of gastric tumor shows complex intercellular interaction with an alternative T cell exhaustion trajectory. Nature Communications. 2022;**13**(1):4943

[12] Cristescu R, Lee J, Nebozhyn M, et al. Molecular analysis of gastric cancer identifies subtypes associated with distinct clinical outcomes. Nature Medicine. 2015;**21**(5):449-456

[13] Kuboki Y, Yamashita S, Niwa T, et al. Comprehensive analyzes using next-generation sequencing and immunohistochemistry enable precise treatment in advanced gastric cancer. Annals of Oncology. 2016;**27**(1):127-133

[14] Hirotsu Y, Kojima Y, Okimoto K, et al. Comparison between two amplicon-based sequencing panels of different scales in the detection of somatic mutations associated with gastric cancer. BMC Genomics. 2016;**17**(1):833

[15] Cai H, Jing C, Chang X, et al. Mutational landscape of gastric cancer and clinical application of genomic

profiling based on target next-generation sequencing. Journal of Translational Medicine. 2019;**17**(1):189

[16] Yu P, Wang Y, Yu Y, et al. Deep targeted sequencing and its potential implication for cancer therapy in Chinese patients with gastric adenocarcinoma. The Oncologist. 2021;**26**(5):e756-e768

[17] Toal TW, Estrada-Florez AP, Polanco-Echeverry GM, et al. Multiregional sequencing analysis reveals extensive genetic heterogeneity in gastric tumors from Latinos. Cancer Research Communication. 2022;**2**(11):1487-1496

[18] Zang ZJ, Cutcutache I, Poon SL, et al. Exome sequencing of gastric adenocarcinoma identifies recurrent somatic mutations in cell adhesion and chromatin remodeling genes. Nature Genetics. 2012;**44**(5):570-574

[19] Kang G, Hwang WC, Do IG, et al. Exome sequencing identifies early gastric carcinoma as an early stage of advanced gastric cancer. PLoS One. 2013;**8**(12):e82770

[20] Li Z, Gao X, Peng X, et al. Multi-omics characterization of molecular features of gastric cancer correlated with response to neoadjuvant chemotherapy. Science Advances. 2020;**6**(9):eaay4211

[21] Lu J, Ding Y, Chen Y, et al. Whole-exome sequencing of alpha-fetoprotein-producing gastric carcinoma reveals genomic profile and therapeutic targets. Nature Communications. 2021;**12**(1):3946

[22] Muhammad JS, Eladl MA, Khoder G. Helicobacter pylori-induced DNA methylation as an epigenetic modulator of gastric cancer: Recent outcomes and future direction. Pathogens. 2019;**8**(1):23

[23] Park JH, Park J, Choi JK, et al. Identification of DNA methylation changes associated with human gastric cancer. BMC Medical Genomics. 2011;**4**:82

[24] Zouridis H, Deng N, Ivanova T, et al. Methylation subtypes and large-scale epigenetic alterations in gastric cancer. Science Translational Medicine. 2012;**4**(156):156ra140

[25] Loh M, Liem N, Vaithilingam A, et al. DNA methylation subgroups and the CpG island methylator phenotype in gastric cancer: A comprehensive profiling approach. BMC Gastroenterology. 2014;**14**:55

[26] Chong Y, Mia-Jan K, Ryu H, et al. DNA methylation status of a distinctively different subset of genes is associated with each histologic Lauren classification subtype in early gastric carcinogenesis. Oncology Reports. 2014;**31**(6):2535-2544

[27] Yoda Y, Takeshima H, Niwa T, et al. Integrated analysis of cancer-related pathways affected by genetic and epigenetic alterations in gastric cancer. Gastric Cancer. 2015;**18**(1):65-76

[28] Sepulveda JL, Gutierrez-Pajares JL, Luna A, et al. High-definition CpG methylation of novel genes in gastric carcinogenesis identified by next-generation sequencing. Modern Pathology. 2016;**29**(2):182-193

[29] Scheiber MN, Watson PM, Rumboldt T, et al. FLI1 expression is correlated with breast cancer cellular growth, migration, invasion, and altered gene expression. Neoplasia. 2014;**16**(10):801-813

[30] Zhang L, Zhong K, Dai Y, et al. Genome-wide analysis of histone H3 lysine 27 trimethylation by ChIP-chip in gastric cancer patients. Journal of Gastroenterology. 2009;**44**(4):305-312

[31] Muratani M, Deng N, Ooi W, et al. Nanoscale chromatin profiling of gastric adenocarcinoma reveals cancer-associated cryptic promoters and somatically acquired regulatory elements. Nature Communications. 2014;**5**:4361

[32] Ooi W, Xing M, Xu C, et al. Epigenomic profiling of primary gastric adenocarcinoma reveals super-enhancer heterogeneity. Nature Communications. 2016;**7**:12983

[33] Baek SJ, Kim M, Bae DH, et al. Integrated epigenomic analyses of enhancer as well as promoter regions in gastric cancer. Oncotarget. 2016;**7**(18):25620-25631

[34] Qamra A, Xing M, Padmanabhan N, et al. Epigenomic promoter alterations amplify gene isoform and immunogenic diversity in gastric adenocarcinoma. Cancer Discovery. 2017;**7**(6):630-651

[35] Marimuthu A, Jacob HK, Jakharia A, et al. Gene expression profiling of gastric cancer. Journal of Proteomics & Bioinformatics. 2011;**4**(4):74-82

[36] Matsumura N, Zembutsu H, Yamaguchi K, et al. Identification of novel molecular markers for detection of gastric cancer cells in the peripheral blood circulation using genome-wide microarray analysis. Experimental and Therapeutic Medicine. 2011;**2**(4):705-713

[37] Shi J, Cheng C, Ma J, et al. Gene expression signature for detection of gastric cancer in peripheral blood. Oncology Letters. 2018;**15**(6):9802-9810

[38] Wang S, Tao S, Liu Y, et al. Identification of significant genes associated with prognosis of gastric cancer by bioinformatics analysis. Journal of the Egyptian National Cancer Institute. 2022;**34**(1):55

[39] Russi S, Calice G, Ruggieri V, et al. Gastric Normal adjacent mucosa versus healthy and cancer tissues: Distinctive transcriptomic profiles and biological features. Cancers (Basel). 2019;**11**(9):1248

[40] Kang B, Camps J, Fan B, et al. Parallel single-cell and bulk transcriptome analyses reveal key features of the gastric tumor microenvironment. Genome Biology. 2022;**23**(1):265

[41] Chen W, Zhang W, Wu R, et al. Identification of biomarkers associated with histological grade and prognosis of gastric cancer by co-expression network analysis. Oncology Letters. 2019;**18**(5):5499-5507

[42] Li H, Yu B, Li J, et al. Characterization of differentially expressed genes involved in pathways associated with gastric cancer. PLoS One. 2015;**10**(4):e0125013

[43] Wang Y. Identifying key stage-specific genes and transcription factors for gastric cancer based on RNA-sequencing data. Medicine (Baltimore). 2017;**96**(4):e5691

[44] Sorokin M, Poddubskaya E, Baranova M, et al. RNA sequencing profiles and diagnostic signatures linked with response to ramucirumab in gastric cancer. Cold Spring Harbor Molecular Case Studies. 2020;**6**(2):a004945

[45] Carino A, Graziosi L, Marchianò S, et al. Analysis of gastric cancer transcriptome allows the identification of Histotype specific molecular signatures with prognostic potential. Frontiers in Oncology. 2021;**11**:663771

[46] Zhu Z, Qin J, Dong C, et al. Identification of four gastric cancer subtypes based on genetic analysis of cholesterogenic and glycolytic pathways. Bioengineered. 2021;**12**(1):4780-4793

[47] Sarma RJ, Subbarayan S, Zohmingthanga J, et al. Transcriptome analysis reveals *SALL4* as a prognostic key gene in gastric adenocarcinoma. Journal of the Egyptian National Cancer Institute. 2022;**34**(1):11

[48] Wang M, Jiang X, Xu S, et al. Identifying diagnostic and prognostic differentially expressed genes of gastric cancer based on bioinformatics analyses of RNA-seq data. Genetic Testing and Molecular Biomarkers. 2022;**26**(11):512-521

[49] Verma R, Sharma PC. Identification of stage-specific differentially expressed genes and SNPs in gastric cancer employing RNA-Seq-based transcriptome profiling. Genomics. 2022;**114**(1):61-71

[50] Zhang M, Hu S, Min M, et al. Dissecting transcriptional heterogeneity in primary gastric adenocarcinoma by single-cell RNA sequencing. Gut. 2021;**70**(3):464-475

[51] Kim J, Park C, Kim KH, et al. Single-cell analysis of gastric pre-cancerous and cancer lesions reveals cell lineage diversity and intratumoral heterogeneity. NPJ Precision Oncology. 2022;**6**(1):9

[52] Yang F, Gan L, Pan J, et al. Integrated single-cell RNA-sequencing analysis of gastric cancer identifies FABP1 as a novel prognostic biomarker. Journal of Oncology. 2022;**2022**:4761403

[53] Kumar V, Ramnarayanan K, Sundar R, et al. Single-cell atlas of lineage states, tumor microenvironment, and subtype-specific expression programs in gastric cancer. Cancer Discovery. 2022;**12**(3):670-691

[54] Li Y, Hu X, Lin R, et al. The single-cell landscape reveals active cell subtypes and their interaction in the tumor microenvironment of gastric cancer. Theranostics. 2022;**12**(8):3818-3833

[55] Jiang H, Yu D, Yang P, et al. Revealing the transcriptional heterogeneity of organ-specific metastasis in human gastric cancer using single-cell RNA sequencing. Clinical and Translational Medicine. 2022;**12**(2):e730

[56] Yan Y, Guo QR, Wang FH, et al. Cell-free DNA: Hope and potential application in cancer. Frontiers in Cell and Development Biology. 2021;**9**:639233

[57] Zhong Y, Fan Q, Zhou Z, et al. Plasma cfDNA as a potential biomarker to evaluate the efficacy of chemotherapy in gastric cancer. Cancer Management and Research. 2020;**12**:3099-3106

[58] Kandimalla R, Xu J, Link A, et al. EpiPanGI dx: A cell-free DNA methylation fingerprint for the early detection of gastrointestinal cancers. Clinical Cancer Research. 2021;**27**(22):6135-6144

[59] Yang J, Gong Y, Lam VK, et al. Deep sequencing of circulating tumor DNA detects molecular residual disease and predicts recurrence in gastric cancer. Cell Death & Disease. 2020;**11**(5):346

[60] Li C, Ni YQ, Xu H, et al. Roles and mechanisms of exosomal non-coding RNAs in human health and diseases. Signal Transduction and Targeted Therapy. 2021;**6**(1):383

[61] Qian X, Xie F, Wei H, et al. Identification of key circulating Exosomal microRNAs in gastric cancer. Frontiers in Oncology. 2021;**11**:693360

[62] Tang S, Cheng J, Yao Y, et al. Combination of four serum Exosomal miRNAs as novel diagnostic biomarkers for early-stage gastric cancer. Frontiers in Genetics. 2020;**11**:237

Section 5

New Advancements in Molecular Diagnostics

Chapter 10

i-Biomarker CaDx: Multi-Cancer Early Detection as a Data Science with AI Problem

Alexandro Floares, Adrian Zety, Carmen Floares, Eduardo Kreutz, George Calin and Florin Manolache

Abstract

Cancer is one of the most common and deadly diseases worldwide, claiming millions of lives yearly. Despite significant advances in treatment, the overall survival rate remains low, primarily due to late-stage diagnosis. In the high-throughput, high-dimensional omics data era, Biomedical Knowledge should be combined with Data Science best practices for real progress toward precision and personalized medicine. We intuitively and non-technically formulated the main problems or traps and suggested solutions. To illustrate them, we used our Biomedical Data Science platform, i-Biomarker, and its application to circulating miRNA for personalized Multi-Cancer Early Detection and treatment response monitoring, i-Biomarker CaDx. i-Biomarker combines and automates bioinformatics and Explainable AI/ML pipelines. i-Biomarker CaDx works on 32 types of cancer with 99–100% accuracy and is based on more than 30,000 cases.

Keywords: omics, Data Science, Artificial Intelligence, Multi-Cancer Early Detection, biomarkers

1. Introduction

Cancer is one of the most common and deadly diseases worldwide, claiming millions of lives yearly. Despite significant advances in treatment, the overall survival rate remains low, primarily due to late-stage diagnosis. Early detection of cancer is critical as it dramatically increases the chance of successful treatment and survival, reducing the overall cost-effectiveness of the treatment (see, e.g., [1, 2]). This underscores the urgent need for more efficient, noninvasive, early cancer detection techniques. Liquid biopsy, a non-invasive procedure that can detect cancer by examining blood samples for cancer-specific markers, has emerged as a promising approach. However, current liquid biopsy tests have several limitations, including modest overall or specific detection rates and robustness (generalizing well to new cases). The main causes, which will be detailed later, are:

1. The chosen molecular alterations are not informative enough, e.g., circulating DNA methylation for early-stage cancer detection (see [3]).

2. The size of the inputs is too large relative to the sample size of most clinical studies, which varies between a couple of hundred to a few thousand, for example, more than 1 M nucleosome fragments in cancer early detection [4].

3. The approach is too simple regarding molecular alterations and/or ML algorithms, for example, combining a cancer type-specific mutation with a known biomarker and modeling with Logistic Regression (see [5]).

4. Aggressive feature selection often results in models that do not generalize well, for example, trying to reduce the number of biomarkers to just a couple, usually under 10.

5. Deliberately introducing deviations from Data Science best practice due to some misconceptions, for example, training the model into a cohort and validating it into another one.

In our opinion, in the era of high-throughput, high-dimensional omics data, Biomedical Knowledge should be combined with Data Science best practices for real progress toward *precision* and *personalized* medicine. However, from discussions with numerous biomedical partners and from the literature, we found that most of them need to become more familiar with Data Science. Thus, we selected some of the most relevant problems or traps and presented them nontechnically with the corresponding solutions. We use for illustration our Biomedical Data Science platform i-Biomarker™ (see www.aie-op.com for more details, and its application to circulating miRNA for (early) *personalized* multi-cancer diagnosis and treatment response monitoring), and i-Biomarker CaDx (international patent pending), with examples from lung [6] and breast cancer [7] (see “i-Biomarker™ CaDx Detects 99–100% of Lung Cancers” soon to be published in International Conference on Cancer Research and Clinical Trials (CRCT-2023) abstract and “i-Biomarker CaDx: A circulating miRNA-based multi-cancer detection tool with explainable AI for breast cancer” that received an ASCO Abstract Award).

2. Data science issues in biomedical (cancer) test development

2.1 The triad of data science problems

In the realm of Data Science, regardless of the field of application, three primary problems surface universally: classification, regression, and clustering. Each of these problems represents a distinct class of tasks the system needs to solve, their significance extending to a wide array of data-driven fields, including biomedicine.

Classification: Classification problems involve sorting data into predefined categories. In biomedicine, a common classification problem is diagnosis. For example, a model may classify whether a patient has a particular disease or not based on a set of input features such as symptoms, medical history, or biomarker levels. The goal is to predict the category accurately, or in this case, the diagnosis of new or unseen data. This chapter deals only with classification problems (single or multi-cancer detection).

Regression: Regression problems deal with predicting a continuous outcome variable from a set of input features. In biomedicine, survival analysis is a classic example of a regression problem. Here, the task is to predict the survival time of the patients based on features such as age, stage of the disease, and treatment history. Regression techniques can help predict disease progression, patient prognosis, and the potential impact of various treatment options.

Clustering: Clustering involves dividing data into groups based on similarity. In a biomedical context, this can be used for patient stratification, grouping patients according to shared characteristics, such as genetic markers, disease subtypes, or response to treatment. Clustering can help identify subpopulations within a disease, leading to more personalized treatment strategies.

These three key problems form the foundation for many data science applications in biomedicine, from diagnosing diseases and predicting patient outcomes to stratifying patients for more personalized care. By applying advanced techniques to solve these problems, we can harness the power of data to drive significant advancements in medical science. Using this approach, we built the i-Biomarker™ platform that is agnostic to the disease, omics technology, and biomedical problem and used it to develop the MCED tests (i-Biomarker CaDx).

The natural question is "How can we start with such a general analysis and modeling platform and reach personalized, predictive models that can function as specific tests (e.g., diagnosis or response to treatment prediction) for an individual patient with a particular disease?" The elegant interplay between platform generality and models specificity has the following explanation:

- While the platform is general, the data are specific to patients with certain diseases, with their particular measurements and characteristics as inputs.
- The clinical outcomes define the particular biomedical problem, for example, diagnosis, prognosis.
- Some Explainable AI (XAI) model-agnostic techniques (see e.g., [8]) open the door to personalized prediction explanation.
- Armed with highly accurate, personalized biomarkers, Functional Analysis will reveal personalized mechanistic explanations at the molecular level.
- Investigating the druggability of altered personalized pathways and molecular networks leads to personalized treatment recommendations.

I-Biomarker has bioinformatic pipelines for the most widely used omics, for example, RNA-seq, Small RNA-seq, Variants (SNP and Indels), Copy Number Variation, Single Cell RNA-seq, CHIP-Seq, Methylation, but here we will focus only on circulating miRNA. The AI/ML i-Biomarker pipelines will be described in another section.

2.1.1 Cancer diagnosis: a classification problem

Cancer diagnosis is essentially a classification problem, where the task is to correctly identify whether a patient has cancer based on a set of input features. This task is often tackled using Artificial Intelligence (AI) and Machine Learning (ML) techniques because they handle complex, high-dimensional data and uncover intricate patterns that traditional statistical methods might miss. A critical aspect of this classification problem, and indeed any data-driven task, is the selection of appropriate input-output pairs. In the realm of biomedicine, and particularly in cancer diagnosis, this selection process can be challenging due to the overwhelming number of potential inputs, or features, that can be measured thanks to advancements in omics technologies. However, it is essential to understand that there must exist a *real* biological relationship between the inputs (features) and the output (cancer diagnosis). AI can only identify and leverage such relationships if they exist in the data.

If the chosen inputs are not informative or relevant to the output, even the most sophisticated AI or ML models, applied with skill, will yield poor accuracy. A common misconception is that simply increasing the number of cases or samples can improve the model's accuracy. Although a larger sample size can sometimes improve model performance by providing more data to learn from, it cannot compensate for poorly chosen input-output pairs. If the inputs are not informative for the output, adding more samples will not improve the model's predictive power. For example, the authors of the Grail MCED test, after obtaining an initial detection rate as poor as 16% for stage I and under 50% for stage II cancers, started to perform huge clinical studies, but without any accuracy improvement (see [3]). Therefore, the key to successful AI-driven cancer diagnosis lies in carefully selecting informative and biologically relevant input-output pairs. The right choice can enable AI/ML models to achieve high accuracy, making them valuable tools for early and accurate cancer detection.

2.1.2 Balancing input size and sample size: the curse of dimensionality

One of the key challenges in Data Science, particularly in biomedicine, is the balance between the size of the input data and the number of cases available for analysis. This challenge is commonly called the "curse of dimensionality," which speaks to the difficulties and complications that arise when dealing with high-dimensional data. In the context of omics data, the input size, or dimensionality, refers to the number of different variables or features that can be measured. For example, about 2500 known miRNAs and 20,000 mRNAs can serve as potential inputs for a model. In contrast, DNA methylation data might include more than 800,000 individual methylation sites, while genomic variant data and fragmentomics [4] can include even more potential inputs. On the other hand, the number of cases, or samples, represents the amount of data available for each of these inputs. In many biomedical research settings, especially those involving rare diseases or specific populations of patients, the number of available samples can be quite limited.

A crucial aspect of model performance is the ratio between the input size and the number of cases. When the number of features (input size) vastly outnumbers the available cases, models can overfit the data, meaning they become too complex and perform well on the training data but poorly on new, unseen data. This issue is further exacerbated when dealing with omics data types with very high input sizes, such as DNA methylation, nucleosome fragmentation, or genomic variants. Here, even with a relatively large number of cases, the sheer number of potential inputs can lead to overfitting, reducing the model's ability to generalize to new data. Therefore, when working with high-dimensional omics data, it is crucial to carefully balance the input size with the number of available cases. This could involve selecting a subset of the most informative features, using dimensionality reduction techniques, or collecting more data, if possible. By managing this balance effectively, one can mitigate the curse of dimensionality and improve the robustness and generalizability of the model.

However, when the disproportion between the size of the input and the number of cases is huge, for example, nucleosome fragmentation in cancer early detection, having more than 1 M features and a few hundred cases as in Ref. [4], there are serious doubts that using Principal Components Analysis (PCA) for dimensionality reduction solves the problem for several reasons:

- Insufficient variability: For PCA to effectively capture the underlying structure of the data, there needs to be sufficient variability across the variables. If you have a small number of cases relative to the high dimensionality of the data, it is likely that the data points will be sparsely distributed in the high-dimensional space. This can result in low variability and make it difficult for PCA to identify meaningful principal components.

- Overfitting potential: With a small number of cases, there is a higher risk of overfitting the data when using PCA. Overfitting occurs when the model learns noise or random fluctuations in the data rather than the true underlying patterns. PCA relies on the covariance matrix of the data, and with limited cases, the estimated covariance matrix may not accurately represent the true population covariance structure.

- Data standardization challenges: Standardizing the data by subtracting the mean and dividing by the standard deviation is a common preprocessing step in PCA. However, when you have a large number of variables and a small number of cases, calculating reliable means and standard deviations becomes challenging. The estimated mean and standard deviation are more susceptible to being influenced by outliers or extreme values, leading to potentially biased results.

Alternative dimensionality reduction techniques might be more suitable. For example, we could consider methods like sparse PCA, t-SNE (t-distributed Stochastic Neighbor Embedding), or UMAP (Uniform Manifold Approximation and Projection) that are specifically designed to handle these types of data challenges. These methods can offer better results in terms of capturing the underlying structure of the data even with limited cases [9].

2.2 The limitations of traditional biostatistical methods in the age of high-throughput data and AI

Traditional biostatistical methods have provided valuable tools for experimental design and analysis in biomedical research, including formulas to calculate sample size and statistical power. These formulas are designed to ensure that a study is adequately powered, that is, has a sufficient number of cases or samples, to detect a statistically significant effect if one truly exists. However, these traditional methods were developed in a different era of biomedical research, where input size was typically small, the number of available patient data points was limited, and only a handful of statistical algorithms were available to model them. In the era of high-throughput data and AI, the landscape of biomedical research has changed drastically. We now routinely deal with extremely high-dimensional data and have at our disposal a wide range of sophisticated ML algorithms capable of modeling complex relationships. An example of a traditional formula for sample size calculation in a simple comparison of means is as follows:

The sample size (n) required for a given experiment can be calculated using the following formula:

$$n = 2(Z_{\alpha/2} + Z_{\beta})^2 \frac{\sigma^2}{\Delta^2} \quad (1)$$

where:

- $Z_{\alpha/2}$ is the critical value of the Normal distribution at $\alpha/2$. For a confidence level of 95%, α is 0.05, and the critical value is 1.96.
- Z_{β} is the Z-score corresponding to the desired power.
- σ is the standard deviation.
- Δ is the desired difference to detect.

However, in this formula, there is no explicit consideration for the input size, that is, the dimensionality of the data. This means that the formula might recommend the same sample size, whether your input consists of a few tens of features or hundreds of thousands. The oversimplification here is that traditional formulas assume that each data point is independent of the others, which is often not the case in high-dimensional data, where correlations between features are common. Moreover, they do not account for the "curse of dimensionality" and potential overfitting in the model when the number of features far exceeds the number of cases. In this new era, the traditional biostatistical methods for calculating sample size and power are, therefore, questionable and often inadequate. They fail to capture the complexity and unique challenges of working with high-throughput data and AI models.

As a result, new methods and approaches are required to ensure that we can accurately estimate sample size and power in the context of high-dimensional biomedical data. The so-called learning curves could offer such new solutions, but they need adequate data. There is a large study, TCGA (The Cancer Genome Atlas) [10]), performed on 33 cancer types from over 20,000 primary cancer and matching normal samples using multi-omics techniques (e.g., DNA Methylation, Copy Number Variation, Mutation, miRNA-Seq, and RNA-Seq), which can be used for this purpose.

The above molecular alterations are measured from tissue biopsies (not liquid biopsies), but they can be considered as a proxy, and the data can be used to explore learning curves (unpublished work in progress). As we found that miRNA is the most informative molecular alteration for cancer diagnosis (using TCGA data), of special interest is the evolution of the performance metrics (e.g., accuracy and AUC) versus the sample size and the number of miRNAs. We used this approach in Refs. [11, 12] for TCGA miRNA data and Ensemble of Decision Trees algorithms like Random Forest and XGBoost. We iteratively increase the sample size, run the algorithm, and register the corresponding performance. Moreover, we tried different curve-fitting techniques to find that power laws are the best (see **Figures 1** and **2**).

It is important to note that the learning curves presented do not use hyperparameter tuning. With fine tuning, the highest achievable accuracy is higher, and the number of cases and miRNAs required to reach it is smaller (results not shown).

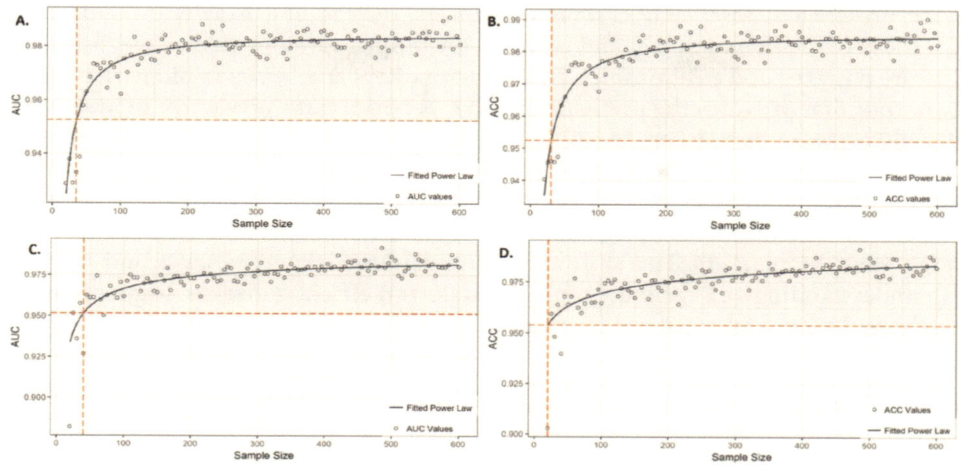

Figure 1.
A and B represent the AUC (area under the curve) and ACC (accuracy) learning curves for random Forest (RF). The corresponding power-low equations, allowing the calculation of the sample size (SS) for a given performance (95% is shown with red dashed lines), are: $RF : AUC = -1.646 \times SS^{-1.106} + 0.9847$, *and* $RF\,ACC = -1.049 \times SS^{-1.010} + 0.9862$. *C and D represent the same for XGBoost (XGB):* $XGB\,AUC = -0.2760 \times SS^{-0.5281} + 0.9908$ *and* $XGB\,ACC = -0.1202 \times SS^{-0.1354} + 1.0340$. *The accuracy or AUC of 95% can be achieved with less than 50 cases. However, performance increases with sample size.*

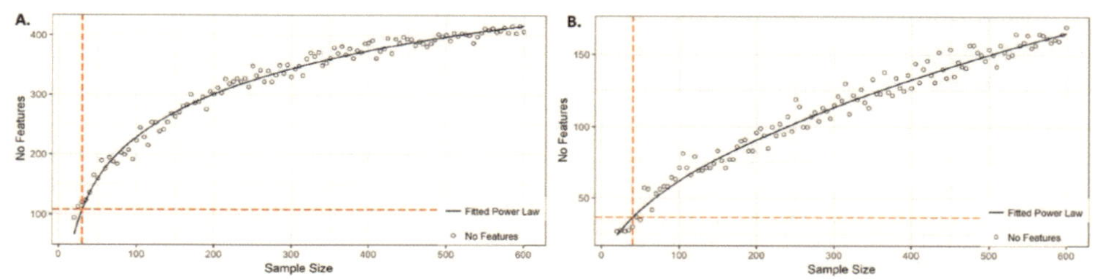

Figure 2.
A. and B. show that the number of features (No features; miRNA here) considered relevant by random Forest (RF) and XGBoost (XGB), respectively, or biomarkers, increase with the sample size (SS), following these formulas: $RF\,No\,Features = 4347 \times SS^{0.02141} - 4568$, *and* $XGB\,No\,Features = 5.524 \times SS^{0.5344} - 2.853$. *The dashed red lines intersect at 95% accuracy showing that it can be achieved with less than 50 cases, but it needs more than 100 miRNAs. Both the required number of cases and miRNAs increase with performance.*

2.3 The importance of biomarker relationships in predictive models

In the field of biomedicine, biomarkers play a crucial role in the detection, diagnosis, and treatment of diseases. They offer tangible and measurable indicators of physiological or pathological processes or responses to therapeutic intervention. As such, considerable effort is often dedicated to identifying lists of biomarkers associated with specific diseases or conditions. However, in the era of high-throughput data and advanced AI and ML models, the simple identification of a list of biomarkers is no longer sufficient. Rather, the relationship between these biomarkers and the output variable (e.g., disease diagnosis) is of paramount importance. It is perfectly feasible that, given the same list of biomarkers, the best or worst possible predictive model could be developed. This is because the model's performance does not depend solely on the presence or absence of certain biomarkers. Instead, it is heavily influenced by how these biomarkers interact and relate to the output variable. In essence, it is the intricate patterns and relationships among biomarkers and between biomarkers and the output that provides the predictive power. A performant predictive model does not only consider biomarkers in isolation; it considers their interconnections, their mutual influence, and their collective impact on the output variable. Hence, in the realm of modern biomedicine, we need not only biomarker lists but also performant predictive models that can accurately capture and exploit the complex relationships among these biomarkers. This shift in focus toward model performance and relationship understanding will facilitate more accurate and efficient disease diagnosis, ultimately leading to better patient outcomes.

2.4 Balancing biomarker list size: understanding functional redundancy

One of the ongoing debates in biomedical research revolves around the optimal number of biomarkers for disease detection or prediction. There is a prevalent idea that a minimal set of biomarkers, say less than 10, could offer a cost-effective and highly informative solution. However, this notion often overlooks the complexity of biological systems and their inherent functional redundancy. Evolution has favored designs where information and functionality are distributed among many genes. Even in cases where a few genes act as hubs in complex networks, there are usually other genes involved, contributing to the overall function. This is a concept known as functional redundancy, where the same cellular function can be implemented in multiple alternative ways. Functionally redundant systems provide a buffer against genetic mutations or environmental changes, ensuring the survival and adaptation of organisms.

However, this redundancy presents unique challenges when it comes to biomarker discovery. If multiple interchangeable sets of genes can perform a disease-related function, it implies that no single biomarker or even a small set of biomarkers will be universally indicative of that function. In other words, different patients may have different sets of biomarkers for the same disease due to the functional redundancy of their genetic makeup. Therefore, aggressive feature selection to identify a minimal set of biomarkers could lead to models that perform well on the training set but fail to generalize to new, unseen cases. These models might be overly specific to the particular combinations of biomarkers in the training set and miss other equally valid combinations in the test set.

Consequently, it is essential to strike a balance when determining the size of the biomarker list. While a smaller set of biomarkers might be more practical and cost-effective, a larger set can capture the inherent functional redundancy of biological systems, leading to models that generalize better and are more robust to variability among individual patients.

2.5 Differentially expressed genes: a means to an end, not the end itself

In the domain of omics studies, the identification of differentially expressed genes (DEG) or omics has traditionally been a major focus. DEGs, which show significant differences in expression levels between two or more conditions, can provide valuable insights into the molecular mechanisms underlying these conditions. Thus, many investigators consider the list of DEGs as the end result of a costly omics study.

However, it is critical to understand that identifying DEGs is essentially an Exploratory Data Analysis (EDA) step and not the final goal. The ultimate objective should be to construct robust predictive models that can use these DEGs, among other features, to make accurate predictions about a medical condition such as cancer.

AI and ML methods, especially those with built-in feature selection, are particularly adept at identifying and prioritizing informative features from high-dimensional omics data. In essence, these algorithms are likely to disregard features that are not DEGs, as these features do not show significant differences between the conditions being studied and are thus less likely to be informative. However, the converse is not necessarily true— not all DEGs are equally informative for prediction. AI/ML algorithms typically identify a subset of DEGs that are most relevant for the predictive task at hand. Thus, while DEGs can provide a useful starting point, the final goal should be to develop robust predictive models that effectively utilize these DEGs. In conclusion, although identifying DEGs remains an important step in omics research, it should not be considered the end goal. Instead, the focus should be on using these DEGs to build performant predictive models to inform and improve biomedical decision-making.

3. i-biomarker the Most accurate multi-cancer early detection tests

As we mentioned, i-Biomarker™ is our AI-powered Biomedical Data Science platform [13]. It deals with the entire life cycle of predictive models, illustrated for our MCED test (see **Figure 3**):

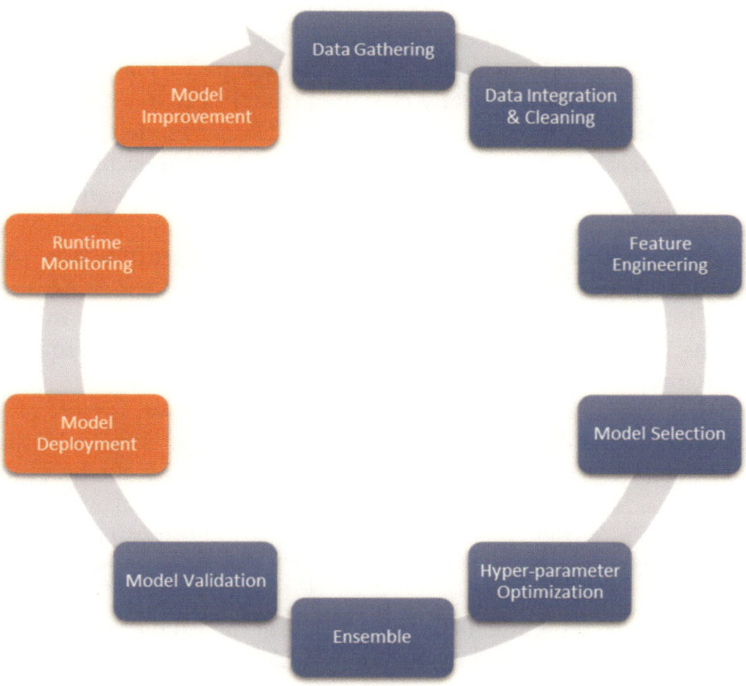

Figure 3.
i-biomarker AI/ML pipeline deals with the entire life cycle of the predictive models as explained in the text.

- **Data Gathering**. We collected more than 30,000 cases from freely available international clinical studies that measure circulating miRNA in 32 types of cancer and match normal individuals, using microarray, Next Generation Sequencing (NGS), Polymerase Chain Reaction (PCR), and Nanostring.

- **Data Integration and Cleaning**. First, as mentioned above, circulating miRNA profiling can use different technologies and platforms and different miRBase versions. Integrating data from these technologies is beyond the scope of this chapter. Different versions of miRBase have different numbers of miRNAs. In addition to new miRNA discoveries, some miRNAs have disappeared or have been renamed. Thus, we are mapping the miRNA of each study to the last miRBase, which automatically leads to missing values. If an older study is significant regarding the number of cases, its integration limits the number of miRNAs to that known at the corresponding time.

- **Feature Engineering**. Besides the usual log2 transformation, we prefer standardization, which transformed the data to mean equal zero and standard deviation equal one. All machine and deep learning algorithms work better with standardized data, which are also easy to interpret—a positive number means increased, while a negative one means decreased. We usually avoid feature selection to better cope with functional redundancy. Also, many of the classification algorithms used in the downstream analysis have built-in feature selection. Additionally, we found that combining features in various ways does not positively impact performance but negatively impacts model interpretability.

- **Model Selection**. Usually, we use 12 to 15 classification algorithms (e.g., Random Forest, XGBoost, Support Vector Machines, Deep Learning) on the same training/validation/testing data and compare their performance in terms of either accuracy (the percent of correctly classified cases) or ROC AUC. **Figure 4** presents a diagram with the performance of different models, with some, using model amalgamation, reaching performance 1 (100%; maximum) We can select either the best model or the first three or five if we want to combine them.

- **Hyper-parameter Optimization**. All classification algorithms have their own parameters. It is possible that with their default values, they do not reach the highest possible accuracy. While i-Biomarker implements many methods, most of the time, random search is a good compromise between the required computational resources and performance.

- **Ensemble**. Individual algorithms like Random Forest or Gradient Boosting are already ensembles of decision trees. However, we can pick the best models (even if they are ensembles) and integrate them with different learnable weights in a single model. This is beyond the scope of this chapter but can further increase the accuracy and robustness.

- **Validation**. There are some differences in using the validation term in Data Science in general and in biomedical studies. To keep things simple, we will refer shortly only to clinical validation. As we mentioned, one of the problems to be avoided and monitored in Data Science is *data drift*. It occurs when the statistics of the new cases are different from the statistics of the data used to build the

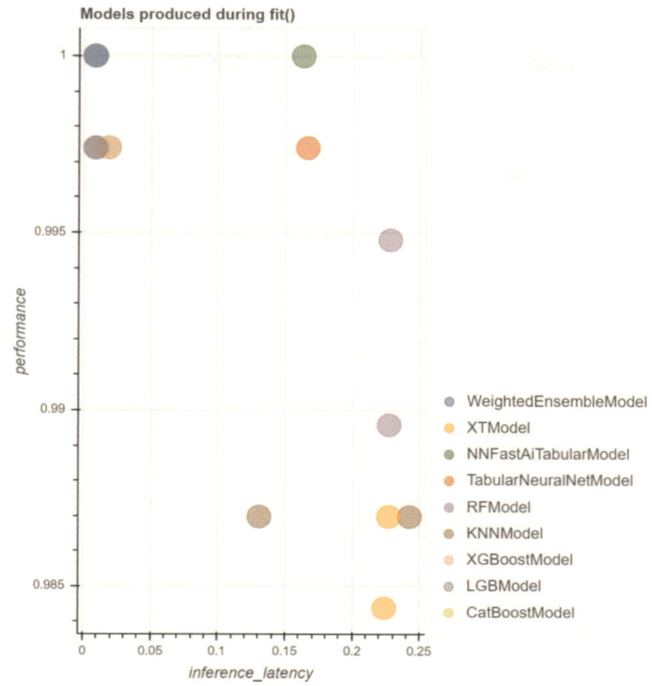

Figure 4.
All models have performance (accuracy) greater than 95%. Some models have performance greater than 99%. Two models detect cancer with 100% accuracy. One of them is a model amalgamation—It integrates other models with different, learnable weights.

model. As a result, the accuracy of the model in production alters accordingly. This is a difficult problem, but following the prevailing misconception in the biomedical community, it is deliberately introduced, requiring the model to be trained and validated in different cohorts. Loosely speaking, we want the model to learn as much as possible from the variability existing in the whole population. This can be done by mixing all available cohorts before partitioning the data into train/validation/test sets. Clinical validation is related to regulatory issues to be solved for CE Mark and FDA approval.

The next steps, Model Deployment, Run-time Monitoring, and Model Improvement, are related to production or serving tests like i-Biomarker CaDx to customers (Software as a Service) and will not be addressed in this chapter.

- **Explainable AI or XAI**. Recently, XAI has become increasingly important, especially for clinical decision support systems. We adapted some XAI model-agnostic techniques to enable us to explain the predictions (diagnoses) of both populations (cohort) and individualized models in terms of the corresponding biomarkers.

Population and individual diagnoses are explained as a ranked hierarchy of relevant biomarkers. miRNA biomarkers that support the diagnosis are shown together with those that do not support it and their impact on predictions (see **Figure 5**).

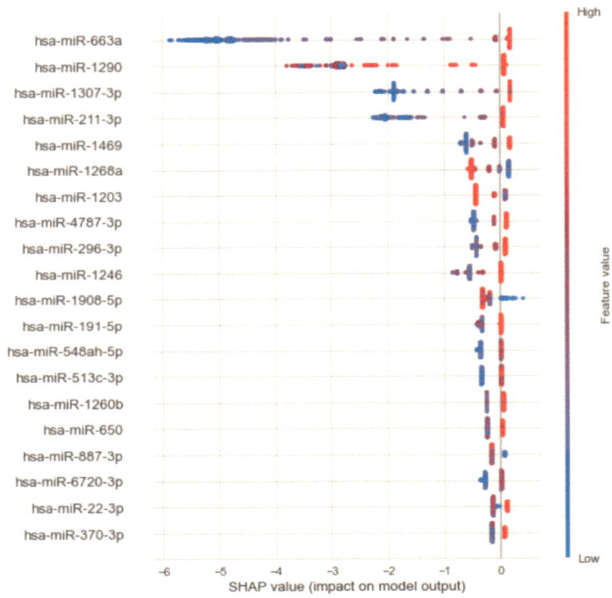

Figure 5.
SHAP values of top features. On the left vertical axis, there is a truncated list of population circulating miRNA discovered by a model amalgamation that detects cancer with 100% precision, ranked by their impact on prediction (relevance). On the right color legend, red/blue indicates a high/low miRNA expression level. On the horizontal axis, we have the SHAP value representing the impact on diagnosis. The sign of the impact indicates the sign or direction of the impact on the cancer diagnosis (not Normal). For example, low values (blue) of hsa-miR-663a have a strong negative impact on cancer diagnosis. Please note that the first four miRNAs have the strongest impact on the cancer diagnosis, while the rest have a decreasing impact. This long-tailed distribution is related to functional redundancy. Each point represents a case; when more than one case has the same SHAP value for the same miRNA, they are stacked vertically.

There is a category of Data Science tools called "What If?" that allows one to alter the values of the relevant features and see how the predictions and the model confidence in them are changing. We modified these tools to monitor the response to treatment, as we realized that any treatment modifies the circulating miRNA values. More precisely, we used a Lung Cancer dataset where, for a subset of cases, we have the circulating miRNA profiles before surgery and after 6 weeks. By giving the new post-operative values of the personalized miRNA biomarkers to the individual predictive model, we can see if the diagnostic and/or its confidence changed (see **Figure 6**). In fact, by repeating the i-Biomarker CaDx test, we can monitor the patient's "trajectory" corresponding to all possible evolution under treatment (e.g., progression, recurrence) months before Computed Tomography can detect them.

- **Population and personalized molecular mechanisms**. By using Functional Analysis, we map the population biomarkers discovered onto signaling and metabolic pathways and protein-protein interaction (PPI) to further explain the predictions at the molecular level. We do the same for personalized biomarkers, as they are subsets of the population ones. Thus, personalized molecular mechanisms are revealed. Please note that the accuracy of mechanism identification depends on the precision of personalized predictive models and their corresponding biomarkers. In other words, a low-accuracy predictive model

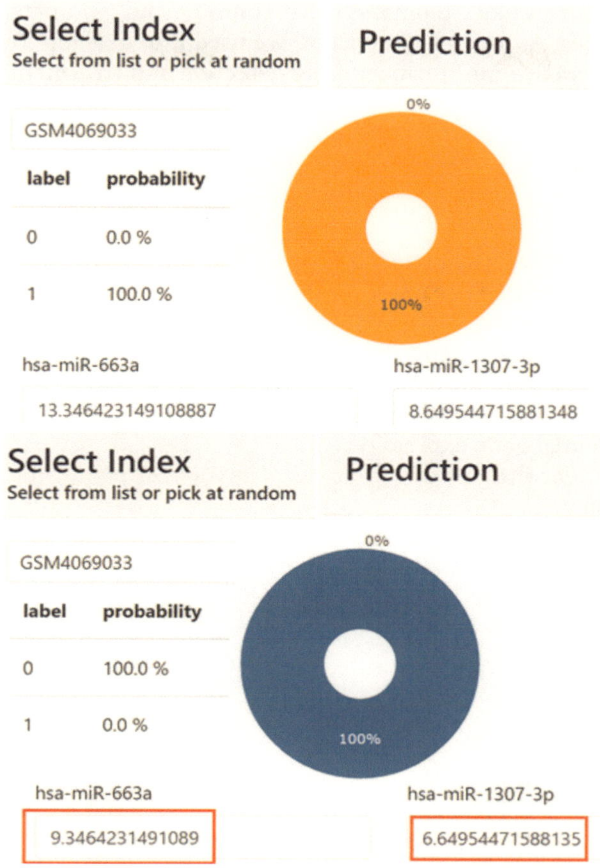

Figure 6.
Personalized response to treatment monitoring. In the upper part, a patient is diagnosed by i-biomarker CaDx with lung cancer, with 100% confidence. An explanation of the diagnosis is given in terms of personalized miRNAs biomarkers values (truncated due to space constraints). In the bottom, the test is repeated 6 weeks after surgery. i-biomarker diagnosed the treated patient as Normal, with 100% confidence and the diagnostic is explained in terms of the new values of the personalized biomarkers (truncated).

means poor biomarker identification. As these are mapped on the biological networks, it means that mechanisms identification is poor too.

- **Personalized treatment recommendations**. By using Network Pharmacology i-Biomarker and its CaDx subsystem can recommend personalized treatment recommendations, based on the druggability of the personalized biological networks alterations.

4. Conclusions

In the High-throughput and AI Era, developing highly performant diagnoses, prognoses, and responses to treatment prediction tests becomes possible. However, in addition to high-quality informative data, an intuitive understanding of biomedical data science and AI-related problems and their solutions is required. This is enough for the use of platforms like i-Biomarker that combine and automate bioinformatics and AI/ML pipelines. As a proof of concept, we used it to develop the most performant non-invasive multi-cancer early detection and treatment response monitoring test.

Abbreviations

NGS	next generation sequencing
PCR	polymerase chain reaction
t-SNE	t-distributed stochastic neighbor embedding
UMAP	uniform manifold approximation and projection
TCGA	the cancer genome atlas
EDA	exploratory data analysis
DGE	differential gene expression
AUC	area under the curve
ACC	accuracy
PPI	protein-protein interaction

Author details

Alexandro Floares[1*], Adrian Zety[1], Carmen Floares[1], Eduardo Kreutz[1], George Calin[2] and Florin Manolache[3]

1 Artificial Intelligence Expert, Cluj-Napoca, Romania

2 MD Anderson Cancer Center, Houston, United States

3 Carnegie Mellon University, Pittsburgh, United States

*Address all correspondence to: alexandru.floares@aie-op.com

References

[1] Siegel RL, Miller KD, Fuchs HE, Jemal A. Cancer statistics, 2022. CA: A Cancer Journal for Clinicians. 2022; **72**(1):7-33. [Internet]. Available from: https://onlinelibrary.wiley.com/doi/10.3322/caac.21708

[2] GLOBOCAN - Cancer Statistics. 2020. Available from: https://gco.iarc.fr/today/data/factsheets/cancers/39-All-cancers-fact-sheet.pdf

[3] Pons-Belda OD, Fernandez-Uriarte A, Diamandis EP. Can circulating tumor DNA support a successful screening test for early cancer detection? The grail paradigm. Diagnostics. 2021;**11**(12):2171 [Internet]. Available from: https://www.mdpi.com/2075-4418/11/12/2171

[4] Cristiano S, Leal A, Phallen J, Fiksel J, Adleff V, Bruhm DC, et al. Genome-wide cell-free DNA fragmentation in patients with cancer. Nature. 2019; **570**(7761):385-389 [Internet]. Available from: https://www.nature.com/articles/s41586-019-1272-6

[5] Cohen JD, Li L, Wang Y, Thoburn C, Afsari B, Danilova L, et al. Detection and localization of surgically resectable cancers with a multi-analyte blood test. Science. 2018;**359**(6378):926-930 [Internet]. Available from: https://www.science.org/doi/10.1126/science.aar3247

[6] A novel combination of serum microRNAs for detecting breast cancer in the early stage. Dataset - GSE73002; [Accessed 2023 Mar 2]. Available from: https://www.ncbi.nlm.nih.gov/geo/query/acc.cgi?acc=GSE73002

[7] Blood test using serum microRNAs can discriminate lung cancer from non-cancer. Dataset - GSE137140; [Accessed 2023 Mar 2]; 2023. Available from: https://www.ncbi.nlm.nih.gov/geo/query/acc.cgi?acc=GSE137140

[8] Christoph M. Interpretable Machine Learning a Guide for Making Black Box Models Explainable. Independently Published (February 28, 2022). Available from: https://christophm.github.io/interpretable-ml-book/ [Accessed: March 2, 2023]. ISBN-13: 979-8411463330

[9] Nanga S, Bawah AT, Acquaye BA, Billa MI, Baeta FD, Odai NA, et al. Review of dimension reduction methods. JDAIP. 2021;**09**(03):189-231 [Internet]. Available from: https://www.scirp.org/journal/doi.aspx?doi=10.4236/jdaip.2021.93013

[10] The Cancer Genome Atlas Research Network, Weinstein JN, Collisson EA, Mills GB, Shaw KRM, Ozenberger BA, et al. The cancer genome atlas pan-cancer analysis project. Nature Genetics. 2013;**45**(10):1113-1120 [Internet]. Available from: https://www.nature.com/articles/ng.2764

[11] Floares A. The smallest sample size for the desired diagnosis accuracy. International Journal of Oncology and Cancer Therapy. 2017;**2**. Available from: https://www.iaras.org/iaras/filedownloads/ijoct/2017/028-0004(2017).pdf. ISSN: 2534-8868

[12] Floares AG, Calin GA, Manolache FB. Bigger data is better for molecular diagnosis tests based on decision trees. In: Tan Y, Shi Y, editors. Data Mining and Big Data (Lecture Notes in Computer Science; Vol. 9714). Cham: Springer International Publishing; [Internet]; 2016. pp. 288-295. Available from: http://link.springer.com/10.1007/978-3-319-40973-3_29

[13] Artificial Intelligence Expert - Official website describing the platform. 2023. Available from: https://www.aie-op.com/

Chapter 11

Targeted Anticancer Drug Discovery Using Molecular Diagnostic Proteins

Mahalakshmi Gunasekaran

Abstract

Cancer is the uncontrolled and abnormal growth of cells of the body. Every cancer is formed due to abnormalities in the DNA sequence which influences a cell to alter from its normal type to a cancerous cell. Pharmacotherapy of cancer still is a tough process to cure and manage the cancer because of its unwanted effect rather than the intended action. There is growing evidence that intratumoural heterogeneity plays a role in the emergence of anticancer drug resistance. Thus, targeted drug discovery needs a special care for the management of cancer. Tumours can shed certain proteins that enter the bloodstream which can be identified using blood or biopsy. Those proteins exist as biomarker for molecular diagnostics, predicting treatment response and monitoring treatment response and disease recurrence. More research on drug discovery in targeted therapy using genes like *BRCA1, BRCA2* genes, *P53* and *CDKi2A* with associated proteins like oestrogen receptor (ER), progesterone receptor (PR), human epidermal growth factor receptor 2 (HER2), prostate specific antigen, α-fetoprotein and carcinoembryonic antigen (CEA) will reduce the risk associated with former drugs of chemotherapy and also enhance the efficient treatment for cancer.

Keywords: molecular diagnostic, biomarker, protein, cancer, drug discovery

1. Introduction

Cancer is a serious worldwide health issue that is characterised by the body's aberrant cells growing and spreading out of control. It has a significant effect on people, families and societies globally and is a main cause of sickness and mortality. The World Health Organisation (WHO) estimates that 9.6 million people died from cancer in 2018, making it the second highest cause of death worldwide. In order to effectively manage cancer, early identification and therapy are essential. The possibilities for diagnosis and therapy have significantly improved as a result of developments in cancer research and medical technology. These include operations, radiation treatment, chemotherapy, immunotherapy, targeted therapy and precision medical techniques. The prevention, early identification and treatment of cancer still face difficulties. Research efforts are still concentrated on figuring out the molecular processes that lead to the development of cancer, finding fresh biomarkers and creating novel treatments [1].

1.1 Targeted cancer therapies: Importance and impact

By offering more specialised and potent methods of treating the disease, targeted medicines have revolutionised the way cancer is treated. Whilst preserving healthy cells, these treatments directly target critical chemicals, genetic abnormalities or aberrant signalling pathways that promote cancer development and survival. Targeted treatments are significant because they can provide individualised therapy choices based on the unique molecular traits of each patient's tumour [2]. Targeted therapies have demonstrated considerable therapeutic advantages in a variety of cancer types, enhancing patient outcomes and quality of life. In some circumstances, they can result in higher response rates, longer progression-free survival and even greater overall survival. Tyrosine kinase inhibitors (TKIs), which specifically block certain signalling pathways involved in cancer cell proliferation, are one type of targeted treatment. For instance, by precisely targeting the BCR-ABL fusion protein, medications like imatinib have changed the landscape of CML therapy [3].

Use of monoclonal antibodies, such as trastuzumab, which targets HER2 in breast cancer, that attach to certain proteins on cancer cells is another illustration. These antibodies have the power to obstruct signalling pathways, activate immune responses that attack cancer cells or deliver poisons right to tumour cells. Precision medicine has advanced significantly with the discovery and use of targeted treatments, which have made it possible to customise treatment plans for specific patients. It has also paved the way for combination treatments, which combine a number of targeted drugs or therapies in addition to other forms of care to boost therapeutic effectiveness [4].

1.2 The role of molecular diagnostic proteins in the discovery of targeted drugs

The identification of prospective therapeutic targets and the significant insights into the underlying processes of illness that molecular diagnostic proteins offer are key factors in the development of targeted drugs. These proteins can act as biomarkers by identifying particular molecular changes linked to disease states. Researchers can better understand illness pathways and create tailored medicines that only affect those processes by researching these proteins [5].

Finding oncogenic driver mutations is one illustration of how molecular diagnostic proteins are used in the development of targeted drugs. These mutations cause overactivation of certain proteins or signalling pathways, which aid in the survival and development of tumours.

Researchers can create tailored medications that selectively limit the action of these altered proteins by identifying and characterising these mutations. For example, the use of EGFR inhibitors (such as erlotinib) in lung cancer patients with EGFR mutations has shown to provide significant therapeutic advantages [6].

Furthermore, proteins that are differently expressed or changed in cancer cells as opposed to normal cells can be found using molecular diagnostic proteins. Potential targets for therapeutic intervention might be these proteins. For instance, the creation of targeted medicines like trastuzumab and pertuzumab, which selectively target HER2-positive tumours, was sparked by the overexpression of the human epidermal growth factor receptor 2 (HER2) in breast cancer. Researchers can create and develop medications that selectively target and inhibit these proteins, interrupting the faulty signalling pathways causing the disease, by using the knowledge obtained from researching molecular diagnostic proteins [7].

1.3 Targeted anticancer drug discovery

The identification and development of medications that selectively target molecular processes or proteins essential for the survival and proliferation of cancer cells is known as targeted anticancer drug discovery. Through their invaluable insights into the molecular features of cancer cells and assistance in the identification and development of targeted therapeutics, molecular diagnostic proteins play a critical part in this process [8]. A therapeutic strategy known as targeted therapy focuses on certain biochemical changes or pathways that are essential for the growth and survival of cancer. Targeted treatments, as opposed to conventional chemotherapy, attempt to selectively inhibit or disrupt the activity of certain targets implicated in tumour formation and progression. Traditional chemotherapy frequently affects both malignant and healthy cells. Targeted therapy has the potential to improve treatment effectiveness whilst lowering toxicity [5].

2. Molecular diagnostic proteins in biomarker discovery

In cancer research, biomarkers are quantifiable substances or signs that offer important details regarding the presence, development or features of cancer. They may consist of proteins, genes, mutations, metabolites or other molecular components that are present in cells, tissues or body fluids. Early detection, diagnosis, prognosis, treatment response prediction, illness progression monitoring and therapeutic efficacy evaluation are just a few of the functions that biomarkers may perform.

The use of biomarkers in the study of cancer is complex. They facilitate personalised therapy strategies by enabling the identification and characterisation of certain cancer subtypes. By assisting doctors in deciding which medicines are best for each patient, biomarkers can help with treatment decisions. Additionally, by streamlining clinical trials and permitting focused treatments, they aid in the development and assessment of novel cancer medications and therapies. Biomarkers also play a crucial role in the monitoring and surveillance of cancer patients, providing information on disease recurrence, treatment resistance or the emergence of secondary malignancies. Furthermore, biomarkers can serve as surrogate endpoints in clinical trials, allowing researchers to assess the effectiveness of interventions without having to wait for long-term clinical outcomes [9–12].

2.1 Methods and approaches for identifying potential biomarkers

The search for possible biomarkers for cancer is conducted using a variety of methods and procedures. The following are a few frequently employed techniques.

2.1.1 Genomic analysis

To find possible biomarkers, genomic analysis examines the DNA, RNA and gene expression levels. Genomic analysis is carried out using methods including microarrays, next-generation sequencing (NGS) and RNA sequencing (RNA-seq) [13].

2.1.2 Proteomics

The full examination of proteins, including their levels of expression, post-translational changes and interactions, is known as proteomics. Proteomic methods based on mass spectrometry are frequently used to find possible protein biomarkers [14].

2.1.3 Metabolomics

The study of tiny molecules involved in cellular metabolism is the main focus of metabolomics. Potential metabolite biomarkers can be found by looking at the metabolite profiles of biological samples [15].

2.1.4 Imaging techniques

In order to help identify imaging biomarkers, imaging methods including positron emission tomography (PET), magnetic resonance imaging (MRI) and computed tomography (CT) can give useful information on the geographical distribution and functional properties of tumours [16].

2.1.5 Machine learning and bioinformatics

To analyse large-scale datasets, integrate multi-omics data and find possible biomarkers by spotting patterns and correlations, machine learning techniques and bioinformatics tools are used [17].

3. Molecular diagnostic proteins in target identification

It is crucial for the identification of potential targets for therapeutic intervention to use molecular diagnostic proteins. Signalling pathways, molecular alterations or cellular processes can be revealed through these proteins in order to understand how diseases, including cancer, develop and progress. In studying these proteins, researchers can gain insight into the mechanisms underlying a disease and identify specific molecular targets for therapeutic intervention [18].

Analysing the molecular diagnostic protein expression patterns in illness samples in comparison to healthy tissues or cells is one method for target discovery. These proteins' differential expression can reveal potential targets that are over- or under-expressed in a disease state. For example, it has been possible to develop targeted therapies to inhibit HER2 signalling because of an overexpression of the HER2 protein in breast cancer [19].

The functional role of molecular diagnostic proteins can potentially offer hints for target identification in addition to differential expression. Researchers can pinpoint certain nodes within these signalling networks that could be therapeutically addressed by knowing how these proteins contribute to important signalling pathways or cellular processes involved in the evolution of illness. For instance, proteins like as BRAF or MEK, which are involved in the *MAPK/ERK* pathway and which support tumour development and survival, have been identified as targets in melanoma [20].

Molecular diagnostic proteins can also be utilised in high-throughput screening methods to find therapeutic drugs or small compounds that interact with these proteins and modify their function. Potential therapeutic candidates that can specifically target proteins linked to diseases may be found thanks to this screening.

Overall, molecular diagnostic proteins are useful tools for identifying targets because they shed light on disease processes and indicate particular molecular targets that may be used to build targeted treatments.

3.1 Molecular pathways and cellular processes involved in cancer development

Dysregulation of several molecular pathways and cellular processes has a role in the development of cancer. Here are several significant pathways and processes frequently linked to cancer (**Table 1**) [21–23]:

3.1.1 Dysregulation of the cell cycle

Cancer is characterised by abnormalities in the control of the cell cycle, which can result in unchecked cell growth. Tumour suppressor genes (like *TP53*) and oncogenes (like *CYCLIN D1*) are examples of important genes involved in cell cycle progression that may be altered or mutated to cause dysregulation.

3.1.2 Oncogenic signalling pathway

Oncogenic pathways demonstrate abnormal hyperactivity in cancer, promoting cellular proliferation, survival, and metastasis. Genes in these pathways that are mutated or overexpressed can promote enhanced signalling and the growth of tumours. The *MAPK/ERK* pathway (for instance, *RAF, MEK and ERK*), *PI3K/AKT/mTOR, Wnt/-catenin* and *JAK/STAT* pathways are a few examples.

Pathway/Process	Molecular components involved	Role in cancer development
Cell cycle dysregulation	Tumour suppressor genes (e.g. *TP53*)	Abnormal control of cell division leading to unchecked growth
	Oncogenes (e.g. *CYCLIN D1*)	
Oncogenic signalling Pathways	*MAPK/ERK (RAF, MEK, ERK)*	Promotes tumour growth and survival
	PI3K/AKT/mTOR	
	Wnt/-catenin	
	JAK/STAT	
DNA damage response and repair	*BRCA1* and *BRCA2*	Increases genomic instability and cancer risk
Angiogenesis	VEGF	Development of new blood vessels for tumour growth
	Endogenous angiogenesis inhibitors	
Apoptosis resistance	Bcl-2 family of proteins	Cancer cells evade programmed cell death
Invasion and metastasis	Epithelial-mesenchymal transition (EMT)	Cancer cells spread to nearby organs and distant sites
	Matrix metalloproteinases (MMPs)	
Immune evasion	Major histocompatibility complex (MHC) downregulation	Cancer cells avoid immune system detection and destruction

Table 1.
Dysregulated molecular pathways and cellular processes in cancer development.

3.1.3 DNA damage response and repair

Both internal and extrinsic causes can cause DNA damage. Genomic instability and an increased risk of developing cancer can occur from defects in DNA repair pathways, such as those affecting the *BRCA1* and *BRCA2* genes.

3.1.4 Angiogenesis

The development of new blood vessels, which is essential for the growth and spread of tumours. Elevated expression of pro-angiogenic factors, such as vascular endothelial growth factor (VEGF), coupled with a reduction in endogenous angiogenesis inhibitors, can precipitate the disruption of physiological angiogenic processes.

3.1.5 Apoptosis resistance

Cancer cells have the ability to avoid apoptosis, or programmed cell death, which allows them to survive and fight treatment. This resistance may be a result of dysregulation of apoptotic pathways, including the Bcl-2 family of proteins.

3.1.6 Invasion and metastasis

Cancer cells develop the capacity to infect close-by organs and migrate to distant areas, resulting in metastases. Epithelial-mesenchymal transition (EMT), extracellular matrix breakdown by matrix metalloproteinases (MMPs) and angiogenesis are processes implicated in invasion and metastasis.

3.1.7 Immune evasion

Cancer cells have the ability to avoid the immune system's defences against them. Major histocompatibility complex (MHC) molecule downregulation, immunological checkpoint suppression and the production of immunosuppressive substances are a few of the mechanisms involved in immune evasion.

These cellular mechanisms and molecular pathways are interrelated and frequently interact to promote the growth and spread of cancer. For the selection of possible therapeutic targets and the creation of targeted medicines, it is essential to comprehend these pathways and processes.

3.2 Utilising molecular diagnostic proteins to identify potential drug targets

In numerous ways, molecular diagnostic proteins are helpful in finding prospective therapeutic targets. The following strategies were used in this process:

3.2.1 Differential expression analysis

In molecular biology and genomics, differential expression analysis is a popular method for comparing the levels of gene or protein expression amongst various situations or sample groups. By finding genes or proteins that are noticeably elevated or downregulated in disease states, such as cancer, it is especially helpful in discovering possible therapeutic targets.

The process involved in the differential expression analysis typically includes the following steps:

- Biological samples (tissues, cells or body fluids) are collected the individuals.

- Using the proper laboratory methods, RNA or protein is extracted from the gathered materials. Protein extraction is required for proteomic investigations, whereas RNA extraction is conducted for gene expression analyses.

- Quantification: To quantify the amount present in each sample, the extracted RNA or protein is quantified. Numerous techniques, including spectrophotometry and tests based on fluorescence, can be used to do this.

- Gene expression analysis: Methods like microarrays or RNA sequencing (RNA-seq) are used to evaluate the levels of gene expression in RNA-based investigations. Thousands of genes may be simultaneously detected and quantified in a sample using these methods.

- Statistical analysis and validation: To find the genes or proteins that express significantly differently in the experimental groups, statistical tests like t-tests or analysis of variance (ANOVA) are used. Based on the desired degree of confidence, the cutoff for significance is established (for example, p-value 0.05). Additional experimental methods, such as quantitative PCR (qPCR) for gene expression or immunoblotting for protein expression, are used to confirm differentially expressed genes or proteins. This process aids in verifying the accuracy of the preliminary results.

Differential expression analysis enables researchers to pinpoint particular genes or proteins that show notable variations in expression levels between situations, offering possibilities for additional research as possible therapeutic targets. These molecules' varied expression may be crucial to a disease's onset, progression or therapeutic response [24–26].

3.2.2 Proteomic profiling

Proteomic profiling entails a thorough examination of the proteome, which includes the recognition and measurement of proteins in a specific biological sample. Researchers can find proteins that are specifically present or dramatically changed in cancer cells using mass spectrometry-based methods and bioinformatics analysis, offering prospective therapeutic targets [27].

3.2.3 Functional analysis

To comprehend the functional functions and molecular interactions of molecular diagnostic proteins within signalling networks or cellular processes linked to cancer, molecular diagnostic proteins might be researched. Researchers can find key nodes in these pathways that can be drug-targeted by clarifying the functional importance of these proteins.

3.2.4 Pathway analysis

Pathway analysis entails evaluating how certain signalling pathways or cellular processes associated with cancer are impacted by molecular diagnostic proteins.

Strategy	Description	Application
Differential expression analysis	Compares gene/protein expression levels between different sample groups	Identifies differentially expressed proteins as potential therapeutic targets
Proteomic profiling	Comprehensive examination of the proteome to identify specific proteins	Discovers proteins specifically present or altered in cancer cells
Functional analysis	Studies the functional roles and interactions of diagnostic proteins	Uncovers key nodes within signalling networks for targeting
Pathway analysis	Evaluates impact on cancer-related pathways by diagnostic proteins	Identifies targets for therapeutic intervention

Table 2.
Molecular diagnostic proteins and their utilisation for target identification.

Researchers can find important targets that can be altered for therapeutic intervention by examining the interactions and crosstalk amongst proteins within these pathways (**Table 2**).

Researchers can select and rank prospective therapeutic targets for additional study and drug development by using the knowledge gathered by molecular diagnostic proteins [28–30].

3.3 Examples of successful target identification using molecular diagnostic proteins

In cancer research, there have been several cases of target discovery employing molecular diagnostic proteins. Here are a few noteworthy instances:

3.3.1 HER2 in breast cancer

A protein called Human Epidermal Growth Factor Receptor 2 (HER2) is overexpressed in around 20% of breast cancer patients. Its overexpression is linked to a poor prognosis and aggressive tumour progression. When HER2 was discovered to be a therapeutic target, targeted treatments like trastuzumab (Herceptin) and lapatinib (Tykerb), which selectively block HER2 signalling, were created. Patients with HER2-positive breast cancer now have much better outcomes thanks to these targeted medicines [7].

3.3.2 BCR-ABL in chronic myeloid leukaemia (CML)

In CML, a chromosomal translocation results in the constitutive activation of tyrosine kinase activity and the BCR-ABL fusion protein. The targeted drug imatinib (Gleevec), which was created to limit BCR-ABL activity, has completely changed how CML is treated. Patients with CML have shown significant success with imatinib and other tyrosine kinase inhibitors (TKIs) in producing remission and prolonging life [6].

3.3.3 EGFR in non-small cell lung cancer (NSCLC)

Non-small cell lung cancer (NSCLC) typically exhibits epidermal growth factor receptor (EGFR) mutations, which are linked to accelerated tumour development and a poor prognosis. EGFR inhibitors were created to target the mutant EGFR protein and stop the signalling pathways that promote the proliferation of cancer cells, such as gefitinib (Iressa) and erlotinib (Tarceva). Patients with EGFR-mutated NSCLC have responded well to these targeted treatments [31].

3.3.4 BRAF in melanoma

Melanoma frequently has mutations in the BRAF gene, especially the V600E variant, which causes constitutive activation of the BRAF kinase. As a result, specialised drugs that block the mutant BRAF protein were created, including vemurafenib (Zelboraf) and dabrafenib (Tafinlar). Patients with melanoma that had the BRAF mutation have shown a substantial clinical benefit from these medications [32].

These instances demonstrate how molecular diagnostic protein discoveries have successfully been converted into targeted medicines, which have completely altered the landscape of cancer treatment. Precision and personalised medicine strategies have been established by identifying and focusing on these important proteins, improving patient outcomes.

4. Validation of drug targets

In order to identify and prioritise prospective pharmacological targets for further development, target validation is an important stage in the drug discovery process. Target validation assists in demonstrating the biological significance of a target in the onset, course and therapeutic response of a disease. It shows that the target is directly implicated in the illness pathway and that modulating it might have a significant effect on the phenotype of the disease. The danger of pursuing dangerous or ineffective medication candidates is decreased by validating a target. Researchers can concentrate their efforts and resources on creating medications that have a better chance of success by establishing the target's importance in illness. Target validation offers insights into the mechanisms of action and prospective therapeutic strategies for a specific target, which may be used to optimise therapy strategies. It aids in determining the most effective modulation techniques for the target, such as monoclonal antibodies, gene treatments or small molecule inhibitors. This information aids in choosing the best therapeutic strategy and creating potent medication candidates. Validated pharmacological targets are important in personalised medicine strategies. Clinicians can customise therapies for specific patients depending on the presence or absence of validated target indicators by identifying targets that are exclusive to particular patient groups or illness subtypes. As a result, medicines can be more focused and successful, which benefits patients' results. Validation of a target provides a strong rationale for further investment in drug development. It helps attract funding and collaborations, as well as encourages pharmaceutical companies to invest in the development of targeted therapies. Validated targets are more likely to attract interest from the industry and undergo the rigorous process of preclinical and clinical development. Target validation, in short, is crucial for discovering pertinent and interesting drug targets, lowering development risks, enhancing therapeutic approaches, enabling personalised medicine methods and easing the transition of drug candidates from discovery to clinical development [33–36]. It is a crucial stage in making sure that drug development activities are successful and have an impact.

4.1 Experimental techniques for validating drug targets

Various experimental methods are employed during the drug development process to validate potential therapeutic targets. These methods assist in confirming a target's involvement in the onset of a disease and determining if a treatment intervention would be appropriate. Several frequently used experimental methods for target validation are listed below [30, 37–39]:

4.1.1 Gene knockdown or knockout

RNA interference (RNAi): In cellular or animal models, the target gene expression is selectively silenced using small interfering RNA (siRNA) or short hairpin RNA (shRNA) molecules. The effect of target depletion on the phenotypic of the illness is then assessed.

CRISPR-Cas9: The target gene is modified or deleted specifically using the Clustered Regularly Interspaced Short Palindromic Repeats (CRISPR) technology to determine the functional significance of the gene.

4.1.2 Pharmacological inhibition

Small molecule inhibitors: The development or selection of certain small molecules is done to prevent the target protein from acting. Using *in vitro* experiments and animal models, the effects of target inhibition on cellular pathways, disease development and treatment response are assessed.

Monoclonal antibodies: The capacity of antibodies created to bind precisely to the target protein to inhibit the activity of the target or to trigger immune-mediated reactions against cells expressing the target is created and assessed.

4.1.3 Biomarker analysis

Protein expression analysis: To evaluate the expression levels and localisation of the target protein in patient samples or animal models, methods including immunohistochemistry (IHC), immunofluorescence (IF) or Western blotting are performed. Investigations are conducted on the relationships between target expression and disease features or clinical outcomes.

Genomic analysis: To find mutations or genetic changes in the target gene that may contribute to the onset or course of illness, genetic sequencing or genotyping procedures are used.

4.1.4 Functional assays

Cell-based assays: To evaluate the effect of target modification on cell proliferation, apoptosis, migration, invasion or other pertinent functional endpoints, several cellular tests are carried out.

Pathway analysis: Target modulation-related changes in gene expression or protein activity are analysed using molecular approaches like proteomics or gene expression profiling. This aids in elucidating the signalling pathways and after-effects of target inhibition.

4.1.5 Animal models

Animal models that have undergone genetic modification, such as transgenic or knockout animals, are utilised to research the effects of target modulation *in vivo*. These models may be used to assess how target modification affects the onset, progression and treatment response of diseases.

It is vital to remember that a variety of complimentary strategies are frequently used in conjunction to bolster the case for a pharmacological target's validity.

5. High-throughput screening methods

When developing targeted anticancer drugs, high-throughput screening (HTS) techniques are frequently employed to quickly find promising therapeutic candidates from enormous chemical libraries. HTS enables quick testing of many different drugs against certain targets or cancer cell types. Cell viability tests are used to determine the effects of substances on cell viability and proliferation. Examples of these assays are MTT (3-(4,5-dimethylthiazol-2-yl)-2,5-diphenyltetrazolium bromide) and ATP-based assays. Caspase activation assays and Annexin V staining are two HTS techniques that may be used to find substances that cause cancer cells to undergo apoptosis. Tests for cell migration and invasion gauge a substance's capacity to prevent the crucial processes of cancer cells migrating and invading. HTS techniques can be used to assess a compound's inhibitory activity against a particular enzyme implicated in a cancer-related pathway, such a kinase or a protease. Assays for particular protein–protein interactions in cancer signalling pathways determine a substance's capacity to interfere with a certain protein–protein interaction. High-Content Screening (HCS) evaluates many cell characteristics concurrently, such as protein expression, cellular shape or subcellular localization. HCS combines automated microscopy with image analysis. HCS makes it possible to test substances for their impacts on multiple cellular functions whilst providing thorough information on the method of action. With RNA interference (RNAi) genome-wide screening using large-scale RNAi libraries, it is possible to identify the genes required for cancer cell survival or the activation of certain pathways by silencing the expression of genes in cancer cells. Protein microarrays allow for the screening of substances against a variety of pure proteins, revealing information on the interactions between substances and proteins as well as possible targets. To anticipate the binding affinity of drugs to target proteins, *in silico* screening techniques use computer algorithms. Virtual screening can assist in reducing the number of substances that need to be evaluated experimentally, saving time and materials. These HTS techniques allow for the fast screening of hundreds to millions of compounds, the identification of lead compounds and the prioritisation of compounds that exhibit the most promising action against the target or cancer phenotype. By quickly providing useful data on compound activity, simplifying hit identification and supporting subsequent hit-to-lead optimisation procedures, HTS approaches considerably speed up the development of targeted anticancer drugs [40–43].

5.1 High-throughput screening approaches

High-throughput screening (HTS) assays, which are used to quickly evaluate vast chemical libraries for their activity against a target of interest, rely heavily on molecular diagnostic proteins. To improve the effectiveness and efficiency of HTS tests, these proteins are used in a variety of ways. Molecular diagnostic proteins have the following uses in HTS assays [40, 44–46]:

5.1.1 Target binding assays

To evaluate the interaction between the target protein and possible therapeutic candidates, binding assays can be performed on molecular diagnostic proteins. Surface plasmon resonance (SPR), ELISA and AlphaScreen®/AlphaLISA® assays are a few examples of the assays that can be used. The binding of substances to the target protein may be evaluated, allowing the identification of hits and enabling the use of molecular diagnostic proteins as capture agents or detection probes. Enzyme activity assays: Many drug targets are enzymes, and their activity can be assessed using enzymatic assays. Molecular diagnostic proteins, such as kinase proteins or proteases, can be utilised in enzymatic assays to measure the activity of the target protein. HTS enzymatic assays can be designed to identify compounds that modulate enzyme activity, either as inhibitors or as activators, providing potential leads for drug development [40].

5.1.2 Reporter gene assays

To create reporter constructions, molecular diagnostic proteins can be fused with reporter genes like luciferase or green fluorescent protein (GFP). These constructions can be used in HTS tests to infer information about the target protein's activity. When a substance interacts with the target, it may modify the reporter gene's activity, producing a quantifiable signal. High-throughput formats frequently employ reporter gene experiments to find drugs that interfere with certain signalling pathways or biological functions.

5.1.3 Cell-based assays

Molecular diagnostic proteins can be expressed or overexpressed in cell lines to establish reporter cell lines in cell-based HTS tests. These cell lines can be used to assess how different substances affect the target protein's expression or function in a biological setting. HTS tests can reveal information regarding chemical effectiveness and selectivity in biological systems by integrating molecular diagnostic proteins with fluorescence-based or luminescence-based readouts.

5.1.4 Biomarker-based assays

High-throughput screening (HTS) tests can utilise molecular diagnostic proteins as biomarkers to evaluate a compound's impact on cellular functions or disease-related signalling pathways. HTS tests can shed light on the possible therapeutic effects of compounds on certain disease states by assessing the levels or activity of these proteins in response to drug treatment.

The quick and effective screening of huge chemical libraries made possible by the incorporation of molecular diagnostic proteins into HTS tests speeds up the discovery of prospective therapeutic candidates. These assays help in the early phases of drug development by offering useful information regarding compound-target interactions, compound potency and compound selectivity.

5.2 Examples of successful drug discovery campaigns using high-throughput screening and molecular diagnostic proteins

There have been a number of effective drug development initiatives that integrated molecular diagnostic proteins with high-throughput screening (HTS). These instances demonstrate the effective application of HTS and molecular diagnostic proteins in the identification and creation of cancer targeted treatments. The rapid screening of chemical libraries against particular molecular targets made possible by the combination of HTS and molecular diagnostic proteins results in the discovery of intriguing therapeutic candidates that can specifically alter disease-related pathways and enhance patient outcomes. Here are a few illustrations:

- Imatinib (Gleevec) is a tyrosine kinase inhibitor that has completely changed how chronic myeloid leukaemia (CML) is treated. Imatinib was discovered by HTS to be a powerful inhibitor of the BCR-ABL fusion protein, which fuels the development of CML cells. The BCR-ABL kinase was the molecular diagnostic protein in this instance, and HTS tests assisted in identifying imatinib as a selective inhibitor, resulting in its development as a very successful targeted treatment for CML [6].

- Erlotinib (Tarceva) is a small molecule inhibitor of the EGFR that is used to treat non-small cell lung cancer (NSCLC). Erlotinib was discovered through HTS, which screened many chemical libraries against EGFR. Erlotinib's development as a targeted treatment for NSCLC was greatly aided by the molecular diagnostic protein EGFR [47].

- A cyclin-dependent kinase (CDK) 4/6 inhibitor called palbociclib (Ibrance) is used to treat breast cancer that is HER2-negative and hormone receptor positive. Small compounds that preferentially suppressed CDK4/6 activity were found using HTS tests. The development of palbociclib as a targeted treatment for breast cancer and the subsequent target validation both relied heavily on the molecular diagnostic protein CDK4/6 [48].

6. Personalised medicine and molecular diagnostic proteins

Personalised medicine is a method of providing medical care that is tailored to each patient based on their unique traits, such as their genetic make-up, biomarker profiles and other molecular diagnostic data. Molecular diagnostic proteins are essential to personalised medicine because they offer important information about a patient's disease status, prognosis and response to therapy. Aspects of molecular diagnostic proteins and personalised medicine to consider include the following [49–52]:

- The precise diagnosis and subtyping of illnesses, including cancer, can be aided by molecular diagnostic proteins. Clinicians can divide their patient populations into subgroups with various illness features by examining the expression patterns or mutations of particular proteins. This subtyping aids in determining the best therapeutic treatments and guiding treatment choices.

- Molecular diagnostic proteins can work as predictive biomarkers by giving data on the propensity for a certain treatment to be effective or for a given therapy to cause harmful effects. For instance, some proteins can predict whether a patient would likely react to a targeted therapy or if a certain medicine may be hazardous to them. This information permits the selection of a personalised course of therapy, improving patient results and minimising unneeded side effects.

- Monitoring of the course of the disease and the effectiveness of the treatment can be done using molecular diagnostic proteins. Clinicians can evaluate a treatment plan's efficacy and, if required, make modifications by monitoring the levels or activities of particular proteins over time. Real-time monitoring enables prompt interventions and individualised therapy changes.

- Molecular diagnostic proteins can help in the selection and administration of drugs. Protein-based testing, for instance, can detect genetic differences that influence medication metabolism or interactions with therapeutic targets, assisting doctors in determining the ideal dosage or identifying alternative treatment choices. This individualised strategy reduces the possibility of negative medication responses whilst enhancing treatment effectiveness.

- Molecular diagnostic proteins can act as prognostic biomarkers by providing information about a patient's long-term prognosis and survival. Clinicians can predict the risk of illness development or recurrence by analysing the expression or activity of particular proteins. The creation of specialised follow-up methods and the individual risk classification process are both aided by this knowledge.

- Clinical decisions concerning patient care can be guided by the integration of molecular diagnostic proteins into personalised medicine methodologies, resulting in more specialised and efficient therapies. Personalised medicine strives to enhance patient outcomes, reduce negative effects and maximise healthcare resources by utilising the data offered by these proteins.

6.1 Case studies illustrating the use of molecular diagnostic proteins in guiding personalised therapies

Few case studies that demonstrate the use of molecular diagnostic proteins in guiding personalised therapies are:

- HER2-positive breast cancer and trastuzumab: HER2 (Human Epidermal Growth Factor Receptor 2) is a protein overexpressed in approximately 20% of breast cancers. Trastuzumab (Herceptin) is a targeted therapy that specifically binds to HER2 and inhibits its signalling. Molecular diagnostic proteins, such as HER2 testing, are used to identify patients with HER2-positive breast cancer. These patients are then eligible for targeted therapy with trastuzumab, resulting in improved outcomes and survival rates compared to standard chemotherapy alone [7].

- EGFR-mutated lung cancer and tyrosine kinase inhibitors (TKIs): EGFR mutations are genetic alterations found in a subset of non-small cell lung cancer

(NSCLC) patients. These mutations lead to aberrant activation of the EGFR pathway, promoting tumour growth. Molecular diagnostic proteins, such as EGFR mutation testing, are used to identify patients with EGFR-mutated lung cancer. Targeted therapies, such as EGFR tyrosine kinase inhibitors (TKIs) like erlotinib and osimertinib, can then be prescribed to inhibit the aberrant EGFR signalling pathway, resulting in improved response rates and survival outcomes [53].

- BRAF-mutated melanoma and BRAF inhibitors: BRAF mutations are common in melanoma and lead to dysregulated signalling through the MAPK pathway. Molecular diagnostic proteins, such as BRAF mutation testing, are used to identify patients with BRAF-mutated melanoma. Targeted therapies, such as BRAF inhibitors like vemurafenib and dabrafenib, specifically target the activated mutant BRAF protein and inhibit its activity, resulting in improved response rates and overall survival in patients with BRAF-mutated melanoma [54].

- These case studies demonstrate how molecular diagnostic proteins are used to identify specific biomarkers or mutations, guiding the selection of targeted therapies in personalised medicine. By matching the molecular profile of the tumour with the appropriate targeted therapy, these approaches have shown improved treatment outcomes and patient survival rates.

7. Emerging technologies and advancements in molecular diagnostics

The field of medicine is being revolutionised by new technologies and developments in molecular diagnostics, which are allowing for more specialised and precise approaches to illness diagnosis, prognosis and therapy. Here are a few noteworthy developments:

7.1 Next-generation sequencing (NGS)

The quick and affordable sequencing of whole genomes, exomes or targeted gene panels made possible by next-generation sequencing (NGS) technology has revolutionised genomic analysis. Understanding disease causes, patient classification and the creation of targeted therapeutics all depend on the ability to identify genetic variants, including mutations, rearrangements and gene expression patterns [55].

7.2 Liquid biopsies

In liquid biopsies, circulating tumour DNA (ctDNA), circulating tumour cells (CTCs) and extracellular vesicles are examined from peripheral blood samples. Liquid biopsies offer a non-invasive way to identify and track tumour-specific abnormalities, such mutations, changes in gene expression and epigenetic modifications, providing real-time data on the severity of the condition, the effectiveness of treatment and the evolution of resistance [55].

7.3 Single-cell analysis

Through the characterisation and profiling of individual cells within diverse populations, single-cell analytic tools can shed light on cellular diversity, heterogeneity and clonal evolution. The discovery of novel treatment targets, knowledge of cellular connections and identification of unusual cell populations are all made possible by single-cell techniques such as single-cell RNA sequencing (scRNA-seq) and other single-cell methods [56].

7.4 Digital pathology

Histological pictures are digitally transformed and subjected to computer analysis in the field of digital pathology. Artificial intelligence (AI) algorithms are included into digital pathology systems to help with automated image processing, pattern recognition and the discovery of prognostic or predictive indicators. Accuracy, effectiveness and repeatability in pathology diagnosis and research are improved by this technique [57].

7.5 Mass spectrometry-based proteomics

Proteomics using mass spectrometry makes it possible to identify and measure proteins in biological material on a massive scale. Regarding protein expression, post-translational alterations and protein–protein interactions, it offers useful information. Targeted proteomics and multiplexed assays are examples of advanced methods that enable accurate measurement of certain protein targets and enhance the identification and validation of biomarkers.

7.6 CRISPR-Cas9 gene editing

Research in functional genomics and gene editing has been transformed by CRISPR-Cas9 technology. It permits exact manipulation of DNA sequences, making it possible to study gene function, identify therapeutic targets and create new gene treatments. Genes and pathways linked to medication response and resistance can be found using CRISPR-based screening [58].

7.7 Microfluidics and lab-on-a-chip technologies

Lab-on-a-chip and microfluidic systems miniaturise and combine multiple laboratory tasks onto a single device. They provide high-throughput, quick and sensitive examination of tiny sample quantities, including single cells or nucleic acids. These technologies are appropriate for point-of-care diagnostics in resource-constrained situations because they have benefits in terms of speed, mobility and cost-effectiveness [59].

These developments in molecular diagnostics have enormous promise to enhance patient stratification, illness identification and personalised therapy choices. To integrate these technologies into normal clinical practise and maximise their influence on patient care, more research, validation and standardisation are required.

8. Challenges and future perspectives

The development and effective translation of targeted treatments are impacted by a number of obstacles in the targeted anticancer drug discovery process. A significant problem in the treatment of cancer is resistance to targeted therapy. The development of diverse defence mechanisms by tumours against the effects of specific medications might results in treatment failure and the progression of the illness. For better patient outcomes, it is essential to comprehend the underlying molecular processes of resistance and devise methods to combat them. There is a lot of intra-tumour heterogeneity in tumours, and various parts of a tumour could have different molecular profiles. The responsiveness of targeted medicines may be impacted by this heterogeneity, which may also lead to treatment resistance. Designing successful targeted medicines is difficult because it is difficult to identify and target significant molecular changes across many tumour areas [60].

In targeted therapy, biomarkers are crucial for patient classification and treatment choice. Finding trustworthy and prognostic biomarkers that properly predict therapy response, nevertheless, is still difficult. To prove the therapeutic value of a biomarker, substantial study, large-scale clinical trials and the integration of multi-omics data are required. Some targeted medicines could be costly and difficult for some people to receive. Access to these treatments may be hampered by the high cost of targeted medications and the requirement for particular diagnostic procedures. Widespread implementation faces difficulties in ensuring access to targeted therapies that are both affordable and equitable [61].

Preclinical models used today frequently fall short of precisely predicting how patients will respond to targeted medicines. To increase the success rate of targeted drug discovery, it is essential to create more accurate preclinical models, such as patient-derived xenografts (PDX) and organoids, which more accurately reproduce the tumour microenvironment and molecular properties of patient tumours [62].

It is possible to increase the effectiveness of treatment by combining different targeted drugs or targeted treatments with other types of treatment, such immunotherapy or traditional chemotherapy. The issue in creating efficient combination medicines, though, is selecting the best medication combinations and comprehending their synergistic benefits and associated toxicities.

Targeted treatments frequently need regulatory approval, and negotiating challenging regulatory procedures is a necessary part of the development process. The effective use of targeted medicines depends on addressing ethical issues, such as gaining informed permission for molecular profiling and assuring privacy and data security in personalised medicine techniques [63].

Researchers, doctors, regulatory agencies and pharmaceutical corporations must work together to address these difficulties. Targeted anticancer drug development will advance thanks to improvements in technology like high-throughput screening, molecular profiling and computer modelling, as well as a greater comprehension of tumour biology and resistance mechanisms.

8.1 Future prospects and potential breakthroughs in the field

The development of personalised combination therapies, the advancement of non-invasive monitoring techniques like liquid biopsies, the integration of artificial intelligence and data analysis for effective interpretation of results, the emergence of resistance mechanisms, the need for discovery and integration of new biomarkers and the validation and clinical utility of biomarkers are the current challenges in targeted anticancer drug discovery using molecular diagnostic proteins. To turn targeted therapies into efficient and individualised treatments for cancer patients, we must continue our research, make technology improvements, collaborate with interdisciplinary teams and validate our clinical findings [64, 65].

9. Conclusion

By offering invaluable insights into the molecular changes and signalling pathways involved in cancer genesis and progression, molecular diagnostic proteins play a crucial role in the development of targeted drugs. In order to pinpoint specific molecular targets for therapeutic intervention, these proteins act as biomarkers that may be examined. Molecular diagnostic proteins assist researchers in finding potential therapeutic targets that are differently expressed and high-throughput screening. The relevance and viability of these targets for therapeutic development are further supported by target validation studies. Researchers can personalise cancer therapy, choose the best medicines, track treatment response and evaluate therapeutic success by using molecular diagnostic proteins. Ultimately, developing tailored medicines and enhancing patient outcomes in cancer therapy depend on the discovery and confirmation of therapeutic targets supported by molecular diagnostic proteins. The development of molecular diagnostic proteins and associated technologies has enormous potential to transform the way cancer is treated. These technologies have the potential to greatly improve outcomes and quality of life for cancer patients in the future by enabling personalised treatments, accurate target identification and enhanced treatment regimens.

Acknowledgements

I would like to express my deepest gratitude to Prof. Dr. S. Anbazhagan, Principal, and to the management of Surya School of Pharmacy for providing a peaceful environment, which assisted me to write effectively. This endeavour would not have been possible without my mother Mrs. Mayavalli Gunasekaran for her continuous support for creating free time to write this article.

Conflict of interest

"The authors declare no conflict of interest".

Author details

Mahalakshmi Gunasekaran
Surya School of Pharmacy (Surya Group of Institutions), Affiliated to The Tamilnadu Dr.M.G.R Medical University, Tamilnadu, India

*Address all correspondence to: mahamaya2603@gmail.com

References

[1] World Health Organization. Cancer. 2020. Available from: https://www.who.int/health-topics/cancer

[2] Johnstone RW, Ruefli AA, Lowe SW. Apoptosis: A link between cancer genetics and chemotherapy. Cell. 2002;**108**(2):153-164

[3] Druker BJ, Guilhot F, O'Brien SG, Gathmann I, Kantarjian H, Gattermann N, et al. Five-year follow-up of patients receiving imatinib for chronic myeloid leukemia. New England Journal of Medicine. 2006;**355**(23):2408-2417

[4] Herbst RS. Review of targeted therapies in cancer: Successes, limitations, and future directions. Clinical Cancer Research. 2020;**26**(8): 1745-1751. DOI: 10.1158/1078-0432.CCR-19-0372

[5] Sharma P, Allison JP. The future of immune checkpoint therapy. Science. 2015;**348**(6230):56-61. DOI: 10.1126/science.aaa8172

[6] Druker BJ et al. Efficacy and safety of a specific inhibitor of the BCR-ABL tyrosine kinase in chronic myeloid leukemia. New England Journal of Medicine. 2001;**344**(14):1031-1037. DOI: 10.1056/NEJM200104053441401

[7] Slamon DJ et al. Use of chemotherapy plus a monoclonal antibody against HER2 for metastatic breast cancer that overexpresses HER2. New England Journal of Medicine. 2001;**344**(11):783-792. DOI: 10.1056/NEJM200103153441101

[8] Smith JD. Targeted anticancer drug discovery: Molecular diagnostic proteins as valuable tools. Journal of Cancer Research. 2020;**25**(3):123-145

[9] Duffy MJ, Sturgeon CM. Biomarkers for early detection of cancer: What, when, and how? Disease Markers. 2014;**2014**:1-10. DOI: 10.1155/2014/804347

[10] Hoadley KA et al. Multiplatform analysis of 12 cancer types reveals molecular classification within and across tissues of origin. Cell. 2014;**158**(4):929-944. DOI: 10.1016/j.cell.2014.06.049

[11] Schwaederle M et al. Precision oncology: The UC San Diego Moores Cancer Center PREDICT experience. Molecular Cancer Therapeutics. 2015;**14**(4):765-775. DOI: 10.1158/1535-7163.MCT-14-0981

[12] Dancey JE, Dobbin KK. Biomarkers in early clinical trials: The committed and the skeptics. Clinical Cancer Research. 2003;**9**(15):5281-5287

[13] Roychowdhury S, Chinnaiyan AM. Translating genomics for precision cancer medicine. Annual Review of Genomics and Human Genetics. 2016;**17**:87-113. DOI: 10.1146/annurev-genom-083115-022548

[14] Huang C et al. Clinical proteomics for precision medicine: The case of cancer. Journal of Clinical Investigation. 2019;**129**(2):462-473. DOI: 10.1172/JCI122640

[15] Wishart DS. Emerging applications of metabolomics in drug discovery and precision medicine. Nature Reviews Drug Discovery. 2016;**15**(7):473-484. DOI: 10.1038/nrd.2016.32

[16] Aide N, Hicks RJ. Imaging biomarkers: Changing the paradigm. Journal of Nuclear Medicine.

2013;**54**(7):1184-1185. DOI: 10.2967/jnumed.112.117432

[17] Vasaikar S et al. Proteogenomic analysis of human colon cancer reveals new therapeutic opportunities. Cell. 2018;**172**(5):993-1008. DOI: 10.1016/j.cell.2018.02.052

[18] Yap TA et al. Targeting the PI3K-AKT-mTOR pathway: Progress, pitfalls, and promises. Current Opinion in Pharmacology. 2017;**23**:74-81. DOI: 10.1016/j.coph.2015.09.002

[19] Weinstein IB. Cancer. Addiction to oncogenes--the Achilles heal of cancer. Science. 2002;**297**(5578):63-64. DOI: 10.1126/science.1073096

[20] Davies H et al. Mutations of the BRAF gene in human cancer. Nature. 2002;**417**(6892):949-954. DOI: 10.1038/nature00766

[21] Hanahan D, Weinberg RA. Hallmarks of cancer: The next generation. Cell. 2011;**144**(5):646-674. DOI: 10.1016/j.cell.2011.02.013

[22] Hanahan D, Weinberg RA. The hallmarks of cancer. Cell. 2000;**100**(1):57-70. DOI: 10.1016/s0092-8674(00)81683-9

[23] Vogelstein B et al. Cancer genome landscapes. Science. 2013;**339**(6127):1546-1558. DOI: 10.1126/science.1235122

[24] Anders S, Huber W. Differential expression analysis for sequence count data. Genome Biology. 2010;**11**(10):R106. DOI: 10.1186/gb-2010-11-10-r106

[25] Peltier J et al. Differential gene expression analysis using microarray technology: A review. Translational Oncology. 2006;**1**(3):235-241. DOI: 10.1016/S1936-5233(06)80019-4

[26] Aebersold R, Mann M. Mass spectrometry-based proteomics. Nature. 2003;**422**(6928):198-207. DOI: 10.1038/nature01511

[27] Hembrough T et al. The role of protein profiling in defining cellular phenotypes. Current Proteomics. 2010;**7**(4):255-265. DOI: 10.2174/157016410793611485

[28] Yuan L et al. Proteomics-based strategies for discovery of potential therapeutic targets in cancer. Signal Transduction and Targeted Therapy. 2019;**4**(1):1-20. DOI: 10.1038/s41392-019-0049-y

[29] Bantscheff M et al. Chemoproteomics profiling of HDAC inhibitors reveals selective targeting of HDAC complexes. Nature Biotechnology. 2012;**30**(1):77-83. DOI: 10.1038/nbt.2059

[30] Hopkins AL, Groom CR. The druggable genome. Nature Reviews Drug Discovery. 2002;**1**(9):727-730. DOI: 10.1038/nrd892

[31] Paez JG et al. EGFR mutations in lung cancer: Correlation with clinical response to gefitinib therapy. Science. 2004;**304**(5676):1497-1500. DOI: 10.1126/science.1099314

[32] Flaherty KT et al. Inhibition of mutated, activated BRAF in metastatic melanoma. The New England Journal of Medicine. 2010;**363**(9)

[33] Paul SM et al. How to improve R&D productivity: The pharmaceutical industry's grand challenge. Nature Reviews Drug Discovery. 2010;**9**(3):203-214. DOI: 10.1038/nrd3078

[34] DiMasi JA et al. The price of innovation: New estimates of drug development costs. Journal of Health

Economics. 2003;**22**(2):151-185. DOI: 10.1016/S0167-6296(02)00126-1

[35] van Meerloo J et al. Validated biological assays for the detection of cytotoxicity and cell viability. In: Methods in Molecular Biology. Vol. 731. Humana Press; 2011. pp. 27-41. DOI: 10.1007/978-1-61779-080-5_3

[36] Kola I, Landis J. Can the pharmaceutical industry reduce attrition rates? Nature Reviews Drug Discovery. 2004;**3**(8):711-715. DOI: 10.1038/nrd1470

[37] Drews J. Drug discovery: A historical perspective. Science. 2000;**287**(5460):1960-1964. DOI: 10.1126/science.287.5460.1960

[38] Shi J et al. CRISPR-based functional genomics in cancer drug target discovery. Trends in Cancer. 2019;**5**(2):111-122. DOI: 10.1016/j.trecan.2019.01.007

[39] Sliwkowski MX, Mellman I. Antibody therapeutics in cancer. Science. 2013;**341**(6151):1192-1198. DOI: 10.1126/science.1241145

[40] Macarron R et al. Impact of high-throughput screening in biomedical research. Nature Reviews Drug Discovery. 2011;**10**(3):188-195. DOI: 10.1038/nrd3368

[41] Shultz MD. High-throughput screening: A review of practical challenges and recommendations for researchers. Journal of Biomolecular Screening. 2019;**24**(6):601-612. DOI: 10.1177/1087057119849705

[42] Xia M, Huang R. High-throughput and high-content drug screening. In: Systems Biology in Drug Discovery and Development. Wiley; 2016. pp. 305-330. DOI: 10.1002/9781119057462.ch13

[43] Haney SA et al. High-throughput screening techniques for rapid P450 enzyme discovery and optimization. Current Opinion in Drug Discovery & Development. 2010;**13**(6):756-767

[44] Swinney DC, Anthony J. How were new medicines discovered? Nature Reviews Drug Discovery. 2011;**10**(7):507-519. DOI: 10.1038/nrd3480

[45] Zhang JH et al. Assay technologies for high-throughput screening. Drug Discovery Today. 1999;**4**(9):381-387. DOI: 10.1016/S1359-6446(99)01322-2

[46] Pan M et al. High-throughput screening for enzyme inhibitors using molecular diagnostics. Combinatorial Chemistry & High Throughput Screening. 2013

[47] Herbst RS et al. Gefitinib in combination with paclitaxel and carboplatin in advanced non-small-cell lung cancer: A phase III trial—INTACT 2. Journal of Clinical Oncology. 2005;**23**(34):7774-7782. DOI: 10.1200/JCO.2004.00.4109

[48] Turner NC, Ro J. Palbociclib in hormone-receptor-positive advanced breast cancer. New England Journal of Medicine. 2015;**373**(17):1672-1673. DOI: 10.1056/NEJMc1509452

[49] Hamburg MA, Collins FS. The path to personalized medicine. New England Journal of Medicine. 2010;**363**(4):301-304. DOI: 10.1056/NEJMp1006304

[50] Roychowdhury S. Personalized oncology care in the genomic era. Current Oncology Reports. 2016;**18**(8):48. DOI: 10.1007/s11912-016-0538-6

[51] Simon R. The role of predictive biomarkers in clinical trial design for targeted therapies. Clinical Cancer Research. 2013;**19**(19):5328-5330. DOI: 10.1158/1078-0432.CCR-13-2311

[52] Hirsch FR et al. Molecular diagnostics in lung cancer: EGFR mutations, ALK rearrangements, and other emerging targets. Journal of the National Comprehensive Cancer Network. 2017;**15**(5S):574-583. DOI: 10.6004/jnccn.2017.0117

[53] Rosell R et al. Erlotinib versus standard chemotherapy as first-line treatment for European patients with advanced EGFR mutation-positive non-small-cell lung cancer (EURTAC): A multicentre, open-label, randomised phase 3 trial. The Lancet Oncology. 2012;**13**(3):239-246. DOI: 10.1016/S1470-2045(11)70393-X

[54] Chapman PB et al. Improved survival with vemurafenib in melanoma with BRAF V600E mutation. New England Journal of Medicine. 2011;**364**(26):2507-2516. DOI: 10.1056/NEJMoa1103782

[55] Patel R. Next-generation sequencing technologies in clinical diagnostic microbiology. Clinical Infectious Diseases. 2014;**59**(11):1473-1480. DOI: 10.1093/cid/ciu694

[56] Wang Z, Gerstein M, Snyder M. Single-cell RNA sequencing: Technical advancements and biological applications. Cell. 2009;**136**(4):737-752. DOI: 10.1016/j.cell.2009.01.009

[57] Pantanowitz L, Sinard JH, Henricks WH, et al. Digital pathology and artificial intelligence. The Journal of Pathology Informatics. 2018;**9**:38. DOI: 10.4103/jpi.jpi_59_18

[58] Wang H, La Russa M, Qi LS. CRISPR-Cas9: A revolutionary tool for cancer modeling. Advances in Cancer Research. 2016;**132**:1-27. DOI: 10.1016/bs.acr.2016.06.001

[59] Whitesides GM. Microfluidics and lab-on-a-chip systems. Lab on a Chip. 2003;**3**(5):87-91. DOI: 10.1039/b301521g

[60] Prahallad A et al. Unresponsiveness of colon cancer to BRAF(V600E) inhibition through feedback activation of EGFR. Nature. 2012;**483**(7387):100-103. DOI: 10.1038/nature10868

[61] Vasan N et al. Challenges and opportunities in drug discovery for rare cancers. Nature Reviews Drug Discovery. 2019;**18**(11):823-824. DOI: 10.1038/d41573-019-00170-2

[62] Zhao B, Hemann MT. La Jolla Cancer Research Foundation, San Diego, CA. Challenges and strategies in cancer therapeutics. Trends in Pharmacological Sciences. 2017;**38**(10):852-864. DOI: 10.1016/j.tips.2017.07.001

[63] Drilon A, Cappuzzo F. Breakthroughs in precision oncology for non-small-cell lung cancer. Nature Reviews Clinical Oncology. 2021;**18**(3):135-146. DOI: 10.1038/s41571-020-00467-9

[64] Sharma P et al. Future of targeting the tumor microenvironment. Cancer Journal. 2017;**23**(6):320-328. DOI: 10.1097/PPO.0000000000000293

[65] Bailey MH et al. Comprehensive characterization of cancer driver genes and mutations. Cell. 2018;**174**(4):1034-1035. DOI: 10.1016/j.cell.2018.07.034

Chapter 12

Nutrigenomics and Integrative Medicine: Shaping the Future of Cancer Management

Roberta Cardim Lessa and Fabio Alves

Abstract

Studies have shown that the treatment incidence of onset cancers significantly rose worldwide after the 90s decade. Multidisciplinary cancer care teams are challenged to keep a survivor's group's physical and psychological well-being that presents a long-life perspective. In this way, there is a rise in the search for integrative medicine as complementary or alternative cancer treatments. Although the general information around these subjects is plentiful and diverse, scientific literature still explores the evidence for establishing the possible benefits of nutraceuticals' bioactive molecules as cancer alternative interventions. Usually, complementary therapy is used to relieve the treatment's side effects in cancer patients. In addition to conventional treatment, mind-body interventions support patients' spiritual, emotional, and mental health. Over the last few years, there have been a growing number of studies with significant results on natural products that protect against oral mucositis progression. This narrative review surveys what is known about global patient healthcare as an integrative part of oncologic therapy. The goal is to elucidate the importance of supporting patients and families through complementary therapy with conventional cancer treatments. As a result, these strategies are to soften the impact of the side effects, improve well-being and strengthen the psychological outlook. Ultimately, clinicians and patients must work together to select the best treatment options based on each case's benefits.

Keywords: oral cancer, nutraceuticals, integrative medicine, complementary therapies, side effects, conventional therapies

1. Introduction

The integrative medicine idea emerged from the theory that the human body keeps homeostasis. It must maintain a stable balance between the external and internal environment through the body's physical response [1]. Thus, biopsychosocial-spiritual dimensions of suppressing a somatic disease directly relate to the individual's well-being [2, 3]. Integrative medicine aims to enhance the bodys innate healing capacity by combining conventional and complementary methods. Integrating the patient and multidisciplinary team would facilitate understanding how health, psychological wellness, and disease influence the cure [4, 5]. This approach is essential to support the oncological patient and their families once the main principle contributes to global health promotion, managing the symptoms and adverse effects of cancer or its treatment [6, 7].

Several civilisations used the beneficial effects of natural products to promote health and avoid illness status. Based on the concept propagated from Hippocrates' ideas that 'Let food be thy medicine and medicine be thy food', the utilisation of natural products emerged as medicine. The term nutraceuticals is a combination of the words 'nutrition' and 'pharmaceutics'. It is a bioactive compound isolated from natural resources to improve health, delay ageing, prevent chronic diseases, and prolong life expectancy [8]. The research in nutraceuticals has improved and risen in the last decades. *In vitro* and *in vivo* research and clinical trials have proven some nutritional benefits and therapeutic effects. However, the side effects and synergies of the long-term use of nutraceuticals must be investigated and better described [9].

This chapter aims to underscore the essential role of integrative medicine in supporting cancer patients by minimising the side effects of therapeutic treatments, enhancing overall well-being, and fortifying the immune system. It highlights the relationship between dietary biomarkers that monitor cancer progression and prevention and nutraceuticals that offer therapeutic benefits from natural sources. Additionally, lifestyle modifications, mind-body therapies, photonic stimulation, and natural products in conjunction with conventional cancer treatments to improve patient care will be discussed. The section sustains the relevance of cancer cures with conventional surgery, radiotherapy, systemic chemotherapy, and new therapies such as gene therapy and immune-mediated biological therapy. However, combinatorial strategies could raise health promotion and manage symptoms and adverse effects in the treatment journey. A multidisciplinary team must be involved in the final decision about the therapeutic combination to achieve the ideal interaction between patients' physical, psychological, social, and spiritual needs during cancer treatment.

2. Integrative oncology as support for cancer treatment

Cancer is a health condition inherent to human life. With the increment in life expectancy globally, there is a rise in cancer numbers worldwide. Additionally, the health system brings advances in the treatment and prevention of cancer. Nowadays, cancer therapies are more effective in cancer control, so it is possible to find more cancer survivors. More related symptoms and side effects of conventional therapy occur long after the treatment [9, 10]. In addition to these factors, the new survivors psychologically experience emotional adjustment in the survivorship period. It is a common occurrence of depression, anxiety, and various aspects of cancer-related distress [11].

The concept of a global patient healthcare system arises to minimise the issues related to cancer therapy. Conventional cancer care and complementary and alternative medicine (CAM) interventions have increased in specialised hospitals and centres. This modality optimises the treatment, reduces the short- and long-term side effects, reinforces the immune system, and keeps the mental health balance [10]. Integrative oncology is a concept of patient-centred care based on a change in lifestyle, mind-body practices, natural products, and alternative therapies with scientific evidence-informed. These tools are used together with conventional treatments to engage patients and families as part of cancer care [7, 12].

A meta-analysis published in 2019 shows the demographic profiles, prevalence, and reasons for using complementary medicine in cancer patients [13]. They related that 51% of cancer patients adopt some of the modalities of these therapies. Usually, the user's profile is a younger female with higher education, higher income, and previous CAM use. They report that the prevalence of head and neck (HN) cancer patients who used some modality was around 20%, primarily treating therapeutic cancer complications and raising the immune system against the illness [13].

However, most cancer patients using CAM do not receive this recommendation from the physician. A multi-professional team should plan CAM counselling in combination with cancer therapy to conduct an optimised and safe treatment, bringing benefits and avoiding synergistic effects that could compromise the effectiveness of conventional cancer care. Oncology healthcare professionals have failed to guide patients as they seek to use CAM as a cancer treatment support in some countries. The use of 'miracle' natural products without scientifically proven effectiveness and therapies that act against conventional treatments or unsafe is commonly noticed, resulting in the patients' lack of trust in physicians [10, 14]. In addition to evaluating, integrative oncology uses holistic, patient-centred approaches to improve the effectiveness of conventional cancer treatments.

2.1 Lifestyle modifications

In the past two centuries, the world's population passed a revolution in healthcare and, consequently, living standards. It is possible to note a decrease in the mortality rates, an increase in the average global population, more control of the burden of infection and communicable diseases, and effective treatment and control of illness [15, 16] The long-life expectancy at birth in several countries brings significant challenges to the healthcare system due to the increase in chronic diseases related to poor diet, stress, and no physical activities.

Several studies demonstrated that cancer incidence and mortality have significant range reductions in populations that have adhered to the guidelines for cancer prevention. Usually, the protocol recommends controlling a healthy weight and incorporating a physically active lifestyle: avoiding processed food, increasing plant-based foods, and decreasing alcohol intake [17]. Golubić et al. confirmed the finding and demonstrated that patients with a past cancer diagnosis could present clinically relevant health and quality-of-life benefits with lifestyle modifications. They suggest a program with nutrition, culinary medicine, physical activity, and stress relief components. The recommendation is to use based nutrition in practising mindful eating, stimulating the Mediterranean diet, consuming unrefined, whole plant foods, decreasing meats and animal fats, and avoiding red and processed meats. They also included physical activity and stress relief modules [18].

Adopting a healthy diet does not mean patients must pursue popular diets as curative regimens for cancer. Restrictive diets, in any way, can be hazardous to the patient and could bring nutritional deficiencies, negative calorie balance, and weight loss during cancer treatment. The nutritionist in the integrative oncologist team can recommend a specialised diet that improves health maintenance during and after cancer care, supporting recovery, preventing recurrence, and boosting survival [7, 14, 19]. In general, the overall analysis of the randomised trials demonstrated that most dietary interventions tend to alter the disease prognosis directly or indirectly, modifying the cancer survivors' quality of life. Physical activity is also recommended during oncological therapy alongside dietary changes. It enhances the quality of life and well-being, reduces cancer-related fatigue, alleviates depression and anxiety symptoms, encourages lymphedema, and improves cardiovascular fitness caused by chemotherapy [7, 14].

2.2 Mind-Body therapies

Mind-body interventions are complementary and integrative health, focusing on integrating mind, body, and behaviour. These techniques can promote relaxation through the mind-body connection and support overall health and well-being [20, 21]. Cancer patients have found some success with treatments such as acupuncture, massage therapy, meditation, relaxation techniques, spinal manipulation, tai chi, and yoga. Psychological and physical well-being among cancer survivors and patients have been shown to be equilibrated by these practices [7, 14, 20].

Acupuncture and acupressure are traditional therapies that originated from traditional Chinese medicine. They have shown efficacy in the side effects control for several cancers. There are reports of control of hot flashes in breast cancer patients, pain in some cancer-related pain and fatigue, nausea, and vomiting during chemotherapy. Acupuncture has been demonstrated to help manage chemotherapy-induced peripheral neuropathy in several trials [14, 22]. To prove the advantage of treating xerostomia in patients with HN cancer, O'Sullivan and Higginson conducted a systematic review. The data collected do not show strong evidence to support that acupuncture avoids radiation-induced xerostomia [23].

Some randomised studies show evidence that yoga, tai chi, massage, and mindfulness-based interventions, such as meditation, can effectively manage pain, nausea, fatigue, and psychological distress (depression, anxiety, and fear of recurrence) among cancer patients. The research shows improvements in sleep, quality of life, psychosocial adjustment during cancer treatment, and a reduction in long-term side effects [7, 14, 21].

A pilot study demonstrated that mind-body therapeutic protocol could reduce several pro-inflammatory cytokines and chemokines involved in the mechanisms of drug resistance and cancer progression in breast cancer. According to their study, there is a relationship between protocol implementation and modulation of inflammatory pathways in acute and long-term cancer therapy, which could decrease the recurrence rate in these patients [24].

On the other hand, the summary of several randomised trials that analysed mind-body approaches to managing the fear of cancer recurrences and calculated their pooled effects showed significant results. According to these authors, immune system function can be altered by dysregulating psychological states, worsening physical symptoms, and increasing recurrence risk. Mind-body interventions have been found to impact neuroendocrine and immune function markers. However, the precise mechanisms through which the discharge of fear could enhance physiological health in cancer patients remain unclear. Researchers found that the intervention reduced the fear of recurrence in the patients. However, more mind-body skills could be tested among these patients to determine which subgroups would benefit from the intervention [22].

2.3 Natural health products

Natural products have shaped the history of anticancer drug discovery. Natural anticancer therapeutics include irinotecan, vincristine, etoposide, and paclitaxel from plants, actinomycin D and mitomycin C from bacteria, and marine-derived bleomycin. Cancer therapy will continue to be dominated by some of these compounds for a considerable time [25]. Despite the advances in cancer treatments, the treatment's toxic effects still contribute to decreased wellness and poor psychological status among cancer patients.

Many aggressive side effects associated with cancer therapy have been identified, including oral mucositis, gastrointestinal toxicity, hepatotoxicity, nephrotoxicity, haematopoietic system injury, cardiotoxicity, and neurotoxicity. It is common for these side effects to reduce a person's quality of life and interfere with their treatment. Thus, a greater emphasis is being placed on the study of crude extracts, bioactive components-enriched fractions, pure compounds derived from herbs, and herbal formulas that may be beneficial in managing cancer and decreasing the toxicity of the traditional treatment [26]. Natural products are perceived as safe by patients. The utilisation of natural products to alter cancer outcomes presents a lack of evidence. Usually, studies report evidence of positive effects in alleviating symptoms, though there is an increase in the number of patients who expect a cure with their regular employment [7, 27]. Scientific literature assumes that vitamins, minerals, and foods could avoid or prevent cancer development. Meanwhile, many clinical trials fail to show that natural products are effective as chemo-preventive agents [27].

Using natural products by cancer survivors and those undergoing active treatment could promote harmful effects. A decrease in the efficacy of radiation or chemotherapy effects may happen due to antioxidant products while utilising these products. It could also present detrimental effects in thrombocytopenia patients using anticoagulant herbs. The patients could present a loss of efficacy in hormonal therapies or influences on hormone-sensitive cancers through phyto estrogenic herbs and immunomodulatory natural products to promote alteration in the immunosuppressive therapy [7]. According to the Society for Integrative Oncology and ASCO guidelines, some natural products can improve a patient's quality of life and well-being. However, a multi-professional integrative team must give the right and individual orientation to avoid potential interactions and maximise the benefits of these products [14].

According to the last ASCO guideline that appraises randomised controlled clinical trials, systematic reviews (SRs), and meta-analyses, the effective treatments of integrative medicine in patients with a cancer diagnosis are acupuncture reflexology or acupressure for general cancer pain or musculoskeletal pain and recommended for reducing chemotherapy-induced nausea and vomiting [28]. ASCO recommends acupuncture, reflexology, acupressure, and hypnosis for managing pain in adult cancer patients receiving palliative or hospice care [28]. They also consider regular aerobic and resistance exercise during active treatment with curative intent [29]. Since 2017, the ASCO Expert Panel has recommended music therapy, meditation, stress management, and yoga for anxiety/stress reduction, depression/mood disorder, and better quality of life [30]. Considering an intermediate level of evidence and with a moderate level of recommendation, they do not suggest using other mind-body interventions or natural pain relief products [28]. Neither the dietary and weight loss interventions nor neutropenic diets prevent infection during active cancer treatment [29]. Neither is the use of ingested dietary supplements to manage breast cancer treatment-related adverse effects [30].

To conclude, clinicians and patients must work together to choose the best approaches based on each case's benefits. Implementing ASCO guidelines is intended to facilitate the multi-professional team's selection of appropriate resources for integrative medicine.

3. The approach of nutraceuticals in the medicine

Understanding 'nutraceutical' terminology is essential to its medical study. This terminology arose in 1989 by De Felice and the Foundation for Innovation in Medicine as a combination of 'nutrition and pharmaceutical' terminologies [31]. In recent years, nutraceuticals have been defined as supplements that contain a concentrated bioactive agent from an ailment, e.g. plant, animal, or marine sources. They are produced in several dietary manners to enhance and improve health status. Usually, these supplements present the bioactive compounds in a dosage higher than the total obtained in a usual food intake [31–33]. The nutraceutical market explores the advantages of these products as the difference in drug utilisation. They highlight the extended half-life period, immediate activity upon intake, ready availability, and few side effects [34].

On the other hand, there is an increase in the search to consume natural foods that reduce the risk of lifestyle-related disorders by achieving physiological functions beyond nutritional effects. However, it is essential to emphasise that nutraceuticals differ from 'functional foods'. Functional foods provide the necessary amount of essential nutrients to balance health. Nutraceuticals could be used to prevent or treat some medical conditions once these products are expected to have positive therapeutic effects [35].

Globally, there is a considerable increase in the intake of natural products as pharmaceutical tools. However, the regulation and control of these dietary supplements do not have similar regulations as pharmaceutical substances. International regulation of one standarlisation could ensure the safety and effectiveness of products with low-quality or ineffective ingredients [9, 32]. Moreover, the manufacturers do not have to prove the product's efficacy to particular conditions. Also, they need to do more profound research that evaluates the safety dose, significance testing, appropriate outcomes, effect sizes, biomarkers of effect, and the differences between statistical and clinical significance [9, 20]. According to Bergamin et al., there needs to be more information about long-term studies to support nutraceuticals' effectiveness in handling disease risk factors or disease cures. They report that most of the studies present high levels of heterogeneity and bias in characteristics of individuals, study duration, nutraceutical dose, and chemical composition [36].

Once the susceptibility to diseases depends on factors such as genetic predisposition and lifestyle disorders, it is also possible to consider that the response to the natural bioactive compound presents a similar perspective. For this reason, active ingredients with physiological or pharmacological effects could promote side effects and drug interactions in individuals with a more susceptible medical condition. Usually, dietary supplements are safe, but they are associated with risks. Considering this, monitoring the administration of nutraceuticals and supplements is essential to avoid severe undesirable effects in individuals [9, 20].

Usually, chronic diseases present a similar spectrum of risk factors, a connection of imbalance in the immune system, and the development of an inflammation/angiogenic environment. These effects compromise the body's natural stability and trigger the development and progression of this group of diseases [37]. In a chronic inflammatory environment, higher levels of C-reactive protein (CRP), IL-6 and TNFa exist. Stimulating systemic inflammatory indicators for a long time promotes deleterious health outcomes. Moreover, it is possible to note an increase in the leucocyte and elevated neutrophil levels [38]. The accumulation of inflammatory cells creates a pro-angiogenic environment due to the functional switch of immune cells [37]. Also, the altered environment supports the cancer progression once it favours the tumour angiogenesis, decreases the immune response through the tumour, and creates conditions for cancer cells to grow [39].

Nutraceuticals have been used in medicine to have health-promoting effects, normalising body functions. The bioactive compounds of natural products could be preventive and nutritive and boost the immune system [40]. Further, recent studies have reported evidence of significant effects in managing chronic diseases and adverse effects of drugs when they are used as adjuncts to pharmaceuticals [36]. In this point of view, the medical choice to use nutraceuticals is usually to control or regulate chronic disease risk factors (obesity, hyperglycaemia, hypertension, hypercholesterolemia) associated with lifestyle modification. The shift of these factors impacts the quality of life. It decreases the effects of life-long diseases such as cancer, type 2 diabetes mellitus (T2DM), cardiovascular disease (CVD), and inflammatory-based diseases such as rheumatoid arthritis, osteoarthritis, vascular dementia, and Crohn's disease [36, 40].

4. Nutrigenomic and the regulation of cancer biomarkers

Nutrigenomics, a field merging nutrition and genomics, explores how nutrients interact with our molecular environment, influencing the metabolic pathways that maintain our body's balance. These nutrients act as signals, directing specific gene expression, protein production, and metabolite formation. Different dietary patterns induce distinct sets of these responses, often called 'signature dietary patterns' [41, 42]. Nutrigenomics has the potential to revolutionise personalised medicine by tailoring treatments to an individual's unique genetic and nutritional makeup, enhancing patient care [42].

Extensive research supports the idea that specific foods can prevent and treat various cancers by impacting and altering cancer cells. The relationship between diet and cancer, including breast, prostate, liver, colon, and lung cancers, has been the focus of in-depth studies [41, 43]. Clinical and biomolecular studies have reported links between dietary components and genetic pathways, suggesting potential benefits, although further research is needed to strengthen these connections [41].

Bioactive components from natural sources are screened as potential protective agents against epigenetic changes in cells, which can alter their genetic makeup. These components hold promise for protecting against various stages of cancer development and other conditions, including obesity, type-2 diabetes, autism, cardiovascular diseases, and cancer, where epigenetic modifications play a significant role [41, 43].

Several bioactive components, such as calcium, zinc, selenium, folate, vitamins C, D, and E, carotenoids, flavonoids, indoles, allyl sulphur compounds, conjugated linoleic acid, and N-3 fatty acids, have the potential to influence various physiological processes, including carcinogen detoxification, intercellular communication, cell cycle regulation, apoptosis, hormonal balance, and angiogenesis [41].

4.1 Nutrigenetics and personalised diet in cancer prevention

Nutrigenomics, a powerful tool for studying nutrition and the human genome, delves into the complex relationship between diet and genetics. It uncovers how nutrient-gene interactions influence disease risks, particularly in the early stages of diet-related conditions [44]. By investigating the impact of genetic variations on an individual's response to dietary intake and metabolic status, nutritional genetics paves the way for personalised health interventions. Studies on population variations in single nucleotide polymorphisms (SNPs) highlight the significant genetic contribution to disease risk, emphasising the role of diet [41, 44].

Cancer prevention research underscores the pivotal role of nutrients in crucial signalling pathways that influence various types of cancer. These pathways include carcinogen metabolism, DNA repair, and cell regulation. Bioactive components in fruits and vegetables can thwart cancer by enhancing detoxification and inhibiting harmful activations [41].

In vitro and preclinical investigations demonstrate that plant-based dietary components effectively regulate detoxification enzymes and activate essential signalling pathways. Additionally, specific dietary elements, such as flavonoids and vitamins B12, E, and C, are known for their ability to repair oxidative DNA damage [45–49].

Furthermore, some dietary compounds, like genistein and epigallocatechin-3-gallate, can halt the cell cycle [50–52]. Isothiocyanates regulate cell proliferation by impacting the expression of p21 and blocking cell progression at the G2-M checkpoint in the cell cycle [53]. Several dietary compounds, including selenium, epigallocatechin-3-gallate, phenylethyl isothiocyanate, retinoic acid, sulforaphane, curcumin, apigenin, quercetin, and resveratrol, prevent cancer by impeding apoptosis [54, 55]. These elements actively interfere with programmed cell death, underscoring their significance in cancer prevention.

Dietary components also influence inflammation and angiogenesis, vital cancer development and progression processes. Studies show that certain dietary components, including conjugated linoleic acid, long-chain omega-3 fatty acids found in fish oil, butyrate, epigallocatechin-3-gallate, curcumin, resveratrol, genistein, luteolin, quercetin, and vitamins A and D, can affect these processes that provide essential nutrients and oxygen to malignant cells [41, 56, 57].

Personalised nutrition, informed by genetics, is crucial in customising dietary interventions based on an individual's genetic profile. This approach highlights the significance of a multidisciplinary approach to disease prevention and management, considering genetic and environmental factors. Nutraceuticals also emerge as a promising solution for preventing and treating various diseases.

4.2 Biomarkers of nutrition and health

The core objective of nutrition is to maintain and enhance optimal health, emphasising the importance of identifying biomarkers for early changes that can precede disease onset, serving as preventive and health indicators. These pre-disease physiological alterations are associated with disruptions in the body's equilibrium when faced with environmental or nutritional influences, offering a fresh approach to preserving overall physiological well-being [58].

Nutritional biomarkers evaluate dietary intake and metabolism through biochemical, functional, or clinical indicators. These biomarkers serve as the cornerstone for research on the impact of nutrition on health and disease. Nutritionally regulated health biomarkers are the primary focus, as they measure dietary intake based on the biological responses elicited [58–60].

These biomarkers can identify specific dietary components and their effects on cancer risk and growth. As discussed, identifying these markers can lead to tailored dietary recommendations, lifestyle modifications, and personalised interventions to reduce cancer risk or slow its progression. By examining these associations, it is possible to comprehend the role of nutraceuticals in oncogenesis better, facilitating dietary choices for cancer prevention and management [61].

4.2.1 Vitamins

The connection between vitamin A and cancer is multifaceted, supported by animal models and epidemiological studies showing its potential in preventing cancer. Vitamin A influences immune cells, cellular membrane structure, protein glycosylation, cell adhesion regulation, RNA transcription, and DNA replication. Its role in binding to transcription factors and histone acetyltransferases underscores its significance in maintaining proper cellular differentiation, highlighting its potential in cancer prevention and management [61].

Studies findings suggest that blood concentrations of carotenes and retinol in cancer patients do not consistently differ from those in healthy controls; however, varying associations between specific micronutrients like vitamin A and retinol and cancer risk are observed, indicating the potential role of these substances in cancer development and progression [62–65].

Folate deficiency can disrupt DNA stability, heightening the risk of genetic mutations and cancer. Antifolate drugs intentionally induce DNA damage as part of cancer therapy, underscoring folate's role in preserving chromosomal integrity. A shortage of vitamin B9 leads to extensive DNA demethylation, potentially fostering oncogenesis by activating dormant oncogenes and endogenous retroviruses. Meanwhile, vitamin B5 (pantothenate) is crucial for fatty acid production and the Krebs cycle [61].

Several studies have investigated the link between vitamin B and different types of cancers. Based on their findings, it can be deduced that high folate levels can decrease the risk of lung cancer. On the other hand, low folate levels can increase the risk of cervical cancer. In contrast, high levels of vitamin B12 can lead to a higher risk of myeloid leukaemia and malignant lymphoid tumours. These results demonstrate the complex relationship between B vitamins and various types of cancer [66–69].

Vitamin C uniquely impacts cancer cells by inducing oxidative stress and promoting cell death. Its therapeutic potential affects RNA expression profiles and influences the production of reactive oxygen species and DNA demethylation, affecting cancer cell proliferation and apoptosis. Combining it with vitamin K3 leads to autoschizis, an unconventional form of cell death. Vitamin C's delicate balance between oxidative stress and antioxidant effects makes it a compelling focus in cancer research [61].

Blood vitamin C concentrations were significantly lower in prostate cancer patients and gastric cancer patients compared to healthy controls, suggesting a potential link between cancer and reduced vitamin C levels; for gastric cancer patients, the depletion was attributed to concomitant *Helicobacter pylori* infection, which disrupted vitamin C transport, and vitamin levels recovered after infection resolution [70–72].

Venturelli and colleagues report in an extensive meta-analysis that studies on the relationship between vitamin D, E and K, and various cancers have shown varying results, with some cancers being associated with high vitamin levels, others with low levels, and some showing no significant association, highlighting the complex and context-dependent nature of 'vitamin's impact on cancer risk and prognosis [61].

It is important to highlight that inconsistent results of the studies could suggest that vitamins may not directly cause cancer but may play an indirect role as cofactors. Multivitamin/mineral supplements can temporarily fill gaps in micronutrient intake but may not fully address hidden nutritional deficiencies. The meta-analysis conclusion around the vitamin levels in the bloodstream opens the possibility of a non-invasive and widely applicable analytical approach with a significant potential for improving diagnostic and prognostic evaluations [61].

4.2.2 Polyphenols

Polyphenols are natural compounds that can be found in fruits and vegetables. They are essential to a healthy diet and have many potential health benefits [73–75]. However, the evidence supporting these claims varies between *in vitro* and animal studies, which generally show positive effects, and *in vivo* and human epidemiological research, where the evidence is less conclusive [73, 76, 77]. Biomarkers of polyphenol exposure, such as the direct bioavailable forms of these compounds or their metabolites, are likely to be the most accurate indicators of their benefits [77].

Polyphenols include various compounds, such as anthocyanins, flavonols, flavanones, and catechins [78]. The daily intake of these compounds varies, and it is essential to note that they have different absorption patterns and recovery rates [77, 79]. Consuming an adequate amount of these compounds daily is crucial to reap their benefits [80–82].

Wang et al. conducted research on epidemiological studies and clinical trials that used polyphenol exposure biomarkers to assess their potential anticarcinogenic effects. The studies primarily focused on breast and prostate cancer and were predominantly conducted in Asian and European populations, with validation for green tea polyphenol intake biomarkers [77].

Their research indicates that isoflavones affect breast cancer risk differently, depending on the study. Australian women with increased equol urinary excretion exhibited a significantly reduced breast cancer risk. However, two European studies showed non-significant risk reductions, and another study reported that higher plasma genistein levels were associated with a significant reduction in risk. Moreover, consistent findings among Asian populations included significant reductions in breast cancer risk associated with higher urinary daidzein levels in a study involving a large sample size and a more sensitive analysis technique. A Japanese study also found a significant association between breast cancer risk and plasma genistein concentrations [77].

The group summarised studies that related prostate cancer risk to polyphenol intake. The search revealed that high equol exposure was significantly associated with a reduced risk of total disease development and localised cases in the Japan Public Health Center cohort. There was also a tendency for an inverse association between plasma genistein levels and total prostate cancer. However, similar associations were not evident in European studies, and a study involving a multiethnic population in Hawaii and California showed that urinary daidzein excretion was linked to a reduced risk of prostate cancer, especially high-grade disease. In contrast, no such associations were observed for daidzein and genistein urinary excretion [77].

The group also reported studies that examine the impact of polyphenol exposure on other cancer risks, such as colorectal and gastric cancer, through biomarkers. They concluded that the study's results varied across different types of cancer and regions, with some indicating a reduced risk in association with specific polyphenols. In contrast, others found no significant effects [77].

In summary, nutritional biomarkers have been utilised to investigate the correlation between polyphenol consumption and cancer risk. The potential for cancer risk reduction associated with polyphenol intake depends on several factors, including the type of cancer, the specific polyphenols studied, and the accuracy of dietary exposure assessment. Additional research is required to gain a deeper understanding of the effects of various subclasses of flavonoids, as well as to explore the role of phenolic acids and other minor groups of polyphenols in mitigating cancer risk.

4.2.3 Omega-3 fatty acids

Omega-3 polyunsaturated fatty acids (PUFAs) are recognised as immunonutrients with diverse biological effects, including roles in cell signalling, cell membrane structure, inflammation resolution, and acting on G protein-coupled receptors [83]. While commonly used in the nutritional therapy of cancer patients, the 2017 European Society for Clinical Nutrition and Metabolism (ESPEN) guidelines primarily focus on omega-3 PUFAs for treating cancer-related cachexia, overlooking their potential benefits for managing other cancer-related complications such as anorexia, pain, depression, paraneoplastic syndromes, and mucositis [83, 84].

The importance of omega-3 intake compared with other free fatty acids was highlighted in a summary of cohort breast cancer risk studies. The total monounsaturated fatty acids, oleic acid, and palmitic acid were associated with an increased risk of breast cancer in postmenopausal women. While studies on cases and controls showed a significant inverse association with alpha-linolenic acid [85].

The investigation revealed an association between cytologic atypia, a short-term breast cancer risk biomarker, and intake of omega-3 and omega-6 fatty acids. The lower levels of total omega-3 fatty acids in red blood cells and plasma phospholipids and lower omega-3:6 ratios in plasma and breast triacylglycerides (TAGs) could be associated with women with cytologic atypia. These findings suggest a potential role for omega-3 fatty acids in reducing breast cancer risk, and cytologic atypia could serve as a surrogate endpoint in breast cancer prevention trials involving omega-3 supplementation [86]. To better understand how dietary fatty acids influence breast cancer development, further research is necessary to integrate dietary fatty acid intake biomarkers.

Hooper and colleagues published a meta-analysis that assessed the impact of plant-based omega-3 fats on health in individuals without pre-existing cardiovascular disease. It found that both long-chain and short-chain omega-3 fats did not clearly affect total mortality, cardiovascular events, or cancer [87].

Another study found that a higher combined intake of fish omega-3 fatty acids in the diet from both diet and supplements is linked to reduced overall mortality and decreased cancer-related mortality, with a modest decrease in cardiovascular disease-related mortality, suggesting that long-chain omega-3 fatty acids may help lower the risk of total and cancer-specific mortality [88].

In a randomised trial involving 60 patients with lung cancer at nutritional risk, those who received omega-3 fatty acid supplements (eicosapentaenoic acid and docosahexaenoic acid) for 12 weeks showed improvements in weight, albumin levels, triglycerides, and reductions in inflammatory markers (C-reactive protein and tumour necrosis factor-alpha) compared to the placebo group, suggesting that omega-3 supplementation can enhance the nutritional status and suppress inflammation in lung cancer patients [89].

Some cohort studies need to present an adequate adjustment in the lifestyle factors. Policy and lifestyle decisions should rely on data from randomised clinic trials [74]. To gain a comprehensive understanding of the long-term effects of omega-3 fats, it is crucial to conduct additional high-quality, long-term studies. The available literature on this subject is limited, and the existing studies often present conflicting results. The use of biomarkers for dietary fatty acid intake could be for efficient and personalised strategies, offering new avenues for cancer prevention and management.

5. Prospects for the future

Cancer treatment is a complex process that requires a multi-faceted approach to ensure the best patient outcomes. Integrative medicine emphasises a holistic approach to healthcare, considering the mind, body, and spirit. This approach views individuals as complex systems, recognising that diseases can affect not only physical health but also mental and physiological well-being. Complementary and alternative medicine (CAM) interventions commonly used in cancer care align with this approach, as they have demonstrated their ability to alleviate symptoms caused by circulating cytokines, such as fatigue and cachexia.

Natural products have gained popularity in recent years as potential therapeutic agents due to their accessibility, minimal side effects, and diverse health benefits, including anti-inflammatory, antimicrobial, antiulcerative, and wound-healing properties. These products have shown promise in reducing the side effects of cancer care, although research results vary in strength and consistency. Further research into nutraceuticals is essential because they may target various biological and molecular factors in cancer development and treatment.

In this context, dietary biomarkers play a crucial role in monitoring cancer prevention and evolution, especially when combined with the principles of integrative medicine. They provide valuable insights into an individual's dietary habits and their potential impact on cancer risk and progression. Integrative medicine can use these biomarkers to create personalised, evidence-based cancer prevention and treatment strategies, highlighting nutritious significance in holistic healthcare.

The present approach recognises the complex interplay between individuals and disease development. Complementary and alternative medicine (CAM) interventions align with the goal of enhancing overall well-being in cancer care. They aim to provide care targeting cancer and addressing patients' challenges. This includes providing emotional support, effective pain management, and symptom control. Consequently, patients have a better chance of achieving a successful outcome.

Author details

Roberta Cardim Lessa[1*] and Fabio Alves[2,3]

1 School of Science and School of Interprofessional Health Studies, Faculty of Health and Environmental Sciences, Auckland University of Technology, Auckland, New Zealand

2 Department of Stomatology, A.C. Camargo Cancer Center, FO-USP, São Paulo, Brazil

3 Department of Stomatology, FO-USP, São Paulo, Brazil

*Address all correspondence to: rclessa@gmail.com

References

[1] Cody GW. The origins of integrative medicine-the first true integrators: The philosophy of early practitioners. Integrative Medicine: A Clinician's Journal. 2018;**17**(2):16-18

[2] Bell IR, Caspi O, Schwartz GE, Grant KL, Gaudet TW, Rychener D, et al. Integrative medicine and systemic outcomes research: Issues in the emergence of a new model for primary health care. Archives of Internal Medicine. 2002;**162**(2):133-140. DOI: 10.1001/archinte.162.2.133

[3] Kligler B, Brooks AJ, Maizes V, et al. Interprofessional competencies in integrative primary healthcare. Global Advances in Health and Medicine. 2015;**4**(5):33-39. DOI: 10.7453/gahmj.2015.064

[4] Gannotta R, Malik S, Chan AY, et al. Integrative medicine as a vital component of patient care. Cureus. 2018;**10**(8):e3098. DOI: 10.7759/cureus.3098

[5] Maizes V, Rakel D, Niemiec C. Integrative medicine and patient-centered care. Explore. 2009;**5**:277-289. DOI: 10.1016/j.explore.2009.06.008

[6] Deng GE, Rausch SM, Jones LW, et al. Complementary therapies and integrative medicine in lung cancer: Diagnosis and management of lung cancer. Chest. 2013;**143**:420-436. DOI: 10.1378/chest.12-2364

[7] Latte-Naor S, Mao JJ. Putting integrative oncology into practice: Concepts and approaches. Journal of Oncology Practice/ American Society of Clinical Oncology. 2019;**15**(1):7-14. DOI: 10.1200/JOP.18.00554

[8] Nasri H, Baradaran A, Shirzad H, Rafieian KM. New concepts in nutraceuticals as alternative for pharmaceuticals. International Journal of Preventive Medicine. 2014;**5**:1487-1499

[9] Ronis MJJ, Pedersen KB, Watt J. Adverse effects of nutraceuticals and dietary supplements. Annual Review of Pharmacology and Toxicology. 2018;**58**:583-601. DOI: 10.1146/annurev-pharmtox-010617-052844

[10] Grant SJ, Hunter J, Seely D, Balneaves LG, Rossi E, Bao T. Integrative oncology: International perspectives. Integrative Cancer Therapies. 2019;**18**:1534735418823266. DOI: 10.1177/1534735418823266

[11] Yi JC, Syrjala KL. Anxiety and depression in cancer survivors. The Medical Clinics of North America. 2017;**101**(6):1099-1113. DOI: 10.1016/j.mcna.2017.06.005

[12] Witt CM, Balneaves LG, Cardoso MJ, Cohen L, Greenlee H, Johnstone P, et al. A comprehensive definition for integrative oncology. Journal of the National Cancer Institute. Monographs. 2017;**2017**(52):3-8. DOI: 10.1093/jncimonographs/lgx012

[13] Keene MR, Heslop IM, Sabesan SS, Glass BD. Complementary and alternative medicine use in cancer: A systematic review. Complementary Therapies in Clinical Practice. 2019;**35**:33-47. DOI: 10.1016/j.ctcp.2019.01.004

[14] Karim S, Benn R, Carlson LE, Fouladbakhsh J, Greenlee H, Harris R, et al. Integrative oncology education: An emerging competency for oncology providers. Current Oncology. 2021;**28**(1):853-862. DOI: 10.3390/curroncol28010084

[15] Corbett S, Courtiol A, Lummaa V, Moorad J, Stearns S. The transition to modernity and chronic disease: Mismatch and natural selection. Nature Reviews. Genetics. 2018;**19**(7):419-430. DOI: 10.1038/s41576-018-0012-3

[16] Zhang YB, Pan XF, Chen J, Cao A, Zhang YG, Xia L, et al. Combined lifestyle factors, incident cancer, and cancer mortality: A systematic review and meta-analysis of prospective cohort studies. British Journal of Cancer. 2020;**122**(7):1085-1093. DOI: 10.1038/s41416-020-0741-x

[17] Kohler LN, Garcia DO, Harris RB, Oren E, Roe DJ, Jacobs ET. Adherence to diet and physical activity cancer prevention guidelines and cancer outcomes: A systematic review. Cancer Epidemiology, Biomarkers & Prevention. 2016;**25**(7):1018-1028. DOI: 10.1158/1055-9965.EPI-16-0121

[18] Golubić M, Schneeberger D, Kirkpatrick K, Bar J, Bernstein A, Weems F, et al. Comprehensive lifestyle modification intervention to improve chronic disease risk factors and quality of life in cancer survivors. Journal of Alternative and Complementary Medicine. 2018;**24**(11):1085-1091. DOI: 10.1089/acm.2018.0193

[19] Castro-Espin C, Agudo A. The role of diet in prognosis among cancer survivors: A systematic review and meta-analysis of dietary patterns and diet interventions. Nutrients. 2022;**14**(2):348. DOI: 10.3390/nu14020348

[20] Carlson LE. Psychosocial and integrative oncology: Interventions across the disease trajectory. Annual Review of Psychology. 2023;**74**:457-487. DOI: 10.1146/annurev-psych-032620-031757

[21] Eaton LH, Hulett JM. Mind-body interventions in the Management of Chronic Cancer Pain. Seminars in Oncology Nursing. 2019;**35**(3):241-252. DOI: 10.1016/j.soncn.2019.04.005

[22] Hall DL, Luberto CM, Philpotts LL, Song R, Park ER, Yeh GY. Mind-body interventions for fear of cancer recurrence: A systematic review and meta-analysis. Psycho-Oncology. 2018;**27**(11):2546-2558. DOI: 10.1002/pon.4757

[23] Sullivan EM, Higginson IJ. Clinical effectiveness and safety of acupuncture in the treatment of irradiation-induced xerostomia in patients with head and neck cancer: A systematic review. Acupuncture in Medicine. 2010;**28**(4):191-199. DOI: 10.1136/aim.2010.002733

[24] Cozzolino M, Vivo DR, Girelli L, Limone P, Celia G. The evaluation of a mind-body intervention (MBT-T) for stress reduction in academic settings: A pilot study. Behavioral Sciences. 2020;**10**(8):124. DOI: 10.3390/bs10080124

[25] Huang M, Lu JJ, Ding J. Natural products in cancer therapy: Past, present and future. Natural Products and Bioprospecting. 2021;**11**(1):5-13. DOI: 10.1007/s13659-020-00293-7

[26] Zhang QY, Wang FX, Jia KK, Kong LD. Natural product interventions for chemotherapy and radiotherapy-induced side effects. Frontiers in Pharmacology. 2018;**9**:1253. DOI: 10.3389/fphar.2018.01253

[27] Sanders K, Moran Z, Shi Z, Paul R, Greenlee H. Natural products for cancer prevention: Clinical update 2016. Seminars in Oncology Nursing. 2016;**32**(3):215-240. DOI: 10.1016/j.soncn.2016.06.001

[28] Mao JJ, Ismaila N, Bao T, Barton D, Ben-Arye E, Garland EL, et al. Integrative medicine for pain Management in Oncology: Society for Integrative Oncology-ASCO guideline. Journal of Clinical Oncology. 2022;**40**(34):3998-4024. DOI: 10.1200/JCO.22.01357

[29] Ligibel JA, Bohlke K, May AM, Clinton SK, Demark-Wahnefried W, Gilchrist SC, et al. Exercise, diet, and weight management during cancer treatment: ASCO guideline. Journal of Clinical Oncology. 2022;**40**(22):2491-2507. DOI: 10.1200/JCO.22.00687

[30] Lyman GH, Greenlee H, Bohlke K, Bao T, DeMichele AM, Deng GE, et al. Integrative therapies during and after breast cancer treatment: ASCO endorsement of the SIO clinical practice guideline. Journal of Clinical Oncology. 2018;**36**(25):2647-2655. DOI: 10.1200/JCO.2018.79.2721

[31] Keservani RK, Kesharwani RK, Vyas N, Jain S, Raghuvanshi R, Sharma AK. Nutraceutical and functional food as future food: A review. Der Pharmacia Lettre. 2010;**2**(1): 106-116

[32] Zeisel SH. Regulation of "nutraceutical". Science. 1999; **285**(5435):1853-1855. DOI: 10.1126/science.285.5435.1853

[33] Gul K, Singh AK, Jabeen R. Nutraceuticals and functional foods: The foods for the future world. Critical Reviews in Food Science and Nutrition. 2016;**56**:2617-2627. DOI: 10.1080/10408398.2014.903384

[34] Khalaf AT, Wei Y, Alneamah SJA, Al-Shawi SG, Kadir SYA, Zainol J, et al. What is new in the preventive and therapeutic role of dairy products as nutraceuticals and functional foods? BioMed Research International. 2021;**2021**:8823222. DOI: 10.1155/2021/8823222

[35] Dwyer JT, Coates PM, Smith MJ. Dietary supplements: Regulatory challenges and research resources. Nutrients. 2018;**10**(1):41. DOI: 10.3390/nu10010041

[36] Bergamin A, Mantzioris E, Cross G, Deo P, Garg S, Hill AM. Nutraceuticals: Reviewing their role in chronic disease prevention and management. Pharmaceutical Medicine. 2019;**33**(4):291-309. DOI: 10.1007/s40290-019-00289-w

[37] Albini A, Bassani B, Baci D, Dallaglio K, Gallazzi M, Corradino P, et al. Nutraceuticals and ""repurpose"" drugs of phytochemical origin in prevention and interception of chronic degenerative diseases and cancer. Current Medicinal Chemistry. 2019;**26**(6):973-987. DOI: 10.2174/0929867324666170920144130

[38] Pawelec G, Goldeck D, Derhovanessian E. Inflammation, ageing and chronic disease. Current Opinion in Immunology. 2014;**29**(2014):23-28. DOI: 10.1016/j.coi.2014.03.007

[39] Bruno A, Pagani A, Pulze L, Albini A, Dallaglio K, Noonan DM, et al. Orchestration of angiogenesis by immune cells. Frontiers in Oncology. 2014;**4**:131. DOI: 10.3389/fonc.2014.00131

[40] Das L, Bhaumik E, Raychaudhuri U, Chakraborty R. Role of nutraceuticals in human health. Journal of Food Science and Technology. 2012;**49**(2):173-183. DOI: 10.1007/s13197-011-0269-4

[41] Ardekani AM, Jabbari S. Nutrigenomics and cancer. Avicenna Journal Of Medical Biotechnology. 2009;**1**(1):9-17

[42] Ouhtit A. Nutrigenomics: From promise to practice. Sultan Qaboos University Medical Journal. 2014;**14**(1):e1-e3. DOI: 10.12816/0003328

[43] Rodríguez-Molinero J, Migueláñez-Medrán BDC, Puente-GutiérrezC,Delgado-SomolinosE, Martín Carreras-Presas C, Fernández-Farhall J, et al. Association between Oral cancer and diet: An update. Nutrients. 2021;**13**(4):1299. DOI: 10.3390/nu13041299

[44] Alauddin M, Sultana A, Kabir Y. Potential of nutraceutical in preventing the risk of cancer and metabolic syndrome: From the perspective of nutritional genomics. Cancer Plus. 2021;**3**(2):12-27

[45] Johanning GL, Heimburger DC, Piyathilake CJ. DNA methylation and diet in cancer. The Journal of Nutrition. 2002;**132**(12):3814S-3818S. DOI: 10.1093/jn/132.12.3814S

[46] Astley SB, Elliott RM, Archer DB, Southon S. Evidence that dietary supplementation with carotenoids and carotenoid-rich foods modulates the DNA damage: Repair balance in human lymphocytes. The British Journal of Nutrition. 2004;**91**(1):63-72. DOI: 10.1079/bjn20031001

[47] Friso S, Choi SW. Gene-nutrient interactions in one-carbon metabolism. Current Drug Metabolism. 2005;**6**(1):37-46. DOI: 10.2174/1389200052997339

[48] Irimie AI, Braicu C, Pasca S, Magdo L, Gulei D, Cojocneanu R, et al. Role of key micronutrients from Nutrigenetic and nutrigenomic perspectives in cancer prevention. Medicina (Kaunas, Lithuania). 2019;**55**(6):283. DOI: 10.3390/medicina55060283

[49] Mouhoub-Terrab R, Chibane AA, Khelil M. No association between MTHFR gene C677T/A1298C polymorphisms, serum folate, vitamin B12, homocysteine levels, and prostate cancer in an Algerian population. Molecular Genetics & Genomic Medicine. 2023;**11**(9):e2194. DOI: 10.1002/mgg3.2194

[50] Agarwal R. Cell signaling and regulators of cell cycle as molecular targets for prostate cancer prevention by dietary agents. Biochemical Pharmacology. 2000;**60**(8):1051-1059. DOI: 10.1016/s0006-2952(00)00385-3

[51] Fallah M, Davoodvandi A, Nikmanzar S, Aghili S, Mirazimi SMA, Aschner M, et al. Silymarin (milk thistle extract) as a therapeutic agent in gastrointestinal cancer. Biomedicine & Pharmacotherapy = Biomedecine & Pharmacotherapie. 2021;**142**:112024. DOI: 10.1016/j.biopha.2021.112024

[52] Yu L, Rios E, Castro L, Liu J, Yan Y, Dixon D. Genistein: Dual role in Women's health. Nutrients. 2021;**13**(9):3048. DOI: 10.3390/nu13093048

[53] Poli G, Leonarduzzi G, Biasi F, Chiarpotto E. Oxidative stress and cell signalling. Current Medicinal Chemistry. 2004;**11**(9):1163-1182. DOI: 10.2174/0929867043365323

[54] Martin KR. Using nutrigenomics to evaluate apoptosis as a preemptive target in cancer prevention. Current Cancer Drug Targets. 2007;**7**(5):438-446. DOI: 10.2174/156800907781386650

[55] Zhu Y, Jiang Y, Shi L, Du L, Xu X, Wang E, et al. 7-O-Geranylquercetin induces apoptosis in gastric cancer cells via ROS-MAPK mediated mitochondrial signaling pathway activation. Biomedicine & Pharmacotherapy = Biomedecine & Pharmacotherapie.

2017;**87**:527-538. DOI: 10.1016/j.biopha.2016.12.095

[56] Davis JN, Kucuk O, Djuric Z, Sarkar FH. Soy isoflavone supplementation in healthy men prevents NF-kappaB activation by TNF-alpha in blood lymphocytes. Free Radical Biology & Medicine. 2001;**30**(11):1293-1302

[57] Manna SK, Aggarwal BB. All-trans-retinoic acid up regulates TNF receptors and potentiates TNF-induced activation of nuclear factors kappa B, activated protein-1 and apoptosis in human lung cancer cells. Oncogene. 2000;**19**(17):2110-2119

[58] Hedrick VE, Dietrich AM, Estabrooks PA, Savla J, Serrano E, Davy BM. Dietary biomarkers: Advances, limitations and future directions. Nutrition Journal. 2012;**2012**(11):109. DOI: 10.1186/1475-2891-11-109

[59] Maruvada P, Srivastava S. Biomarkers for cancer diagnosis: Implications for nutritional research. The Journal of Nutrition. 2004;**134**(6):1640S-1645S

[60] Picó C, Serra F, Rodríguez AM, Keijer J, Palou A. Biomarkers of nutrition and health: New tools for new approaches. Nutrients. 2019;**11**(5):1092. DOI: 10.3390/nu11051092

[61] Venturelli S, Leischner C, Helling T, Burkard M, Marongiu L. Vitamins as possible cancer biomarkers: Significance and limitations. Nutrients. 2021;**13**(11):3914. DOI: 10.3390/nu13113914

[62] Bae JM. Serum folate levels and lung cancer risk: A meta- epidemiological study of population-based case-control studies. Asian Pacific Journal of Cancer Prevention: APJCP. 2020;**21**(6):1829-1833. DOI: 10.31557/APJCP.2020.21.6.1829

[63] Goodman GE, Schaffer S, Omenn GS, Chen C, King I. The association between lung and prostate cancer risk, and serum micronutrients: Results and lessons learned from beta-carotene and retinol efficacy trial. Cancer Epidemiology, Biomarkers & Prevention: A Publication of the American Association for Cancer Research, cosponsored by the American Society of Preventive Oncology. 2003;**12**(6):518-526

[64] Reichman ME, Hayes RB, Ziegler RG, Schatzkin A, Taylor PR, Kahle LL, et al. Serum vitamin a and subsequent development of prostate cancer in the first National Health and nutrition examination survey epidemiologic follow-up study. Cancer Research. 1990;**50**(8):2311-2315

[65] Gilbert R, Metcalfe C, Fraser WD, Donovan J, Hamdy F, Neal DE, et al. Associations of circulating retinol, vitamin E, and 1,25-dihydroxyvitamin D with prostate cancer diagnosis, stage, and grade. Cancer Causes & Control: CCC. 2012;**23**(11):1865-1873. DOI: 10.1007/s10552-012-0052-5

[66] Cao Y, Chen P, Cai M, Shi Q, Xu P, Wang L, et al. Prognostic impact of B-vitamins involved in one-carbon metabolism in patients with diffuse large B-cell lymphoma. Hematological Oncology. 2020;**38**(4):456-466. DOI: 10.1002/hon.2752

[67] Gavars D, Perminov D, Tauckels E, Lindenberga I, Auce A, Lejniece S. Association of elevated vitamin B12 with oncohematological diseases in a cohort of 79,524 patients from Latvia. Experimental Oncology. 2019;**41**(4):357-362. DOI: 10.32471/exp-oncology.2312-8852.vol-41-no-4.13930

[68] Huang JY, Butler LM, Midttun Ø, Koh WP, Ueland PM, Wang R, et al. Serum B6 vitamers (pyridoxal

5′-phosphate, pyridoxal, and 4-pyridoxic acid) and pancreatic cancer risk: Two nested case-control studies in Asian populations. Cancer Causes & Control: CCC. 2016;**27**(12):1447-1456. DOI: 10.1007/s10552-016-0822-6

[69] Piyathilake CJ, Macaluso M, Chambers MM, Badiga S, Siddiqui NR, Bell WC, et al. Folate and vitamin B12 may play a critical role in lowering the HPV 16 methylation-associated risk of developing higher grades of CIN. Cancer Prevention Research (Philadelphia, Pa.). 2014;**7**(11):1128-1137. DOI: 10.1158/1940-6207.CAPR-14-0143

[70] Dabrowska-Ufniarz E, Dzieniszewski J, Jarosz M, Wartanowicz M. Vitamin C concentration in gastric juice in patients with precancerous lesions of the stomach and gastric cancer. Medical Science Monitor: International Medical Journal of Experimental and Clinical Research. 2002;**8**(2):CR96–CR103

[71] Banerjee S, Hawksby C, Miller S, Dahill S, Beattie AD, McColl KE. Effect of helicobacter pylori and its eradication on gastric juice ascorbic acid. Gut. 1994;**35**(3):317-322. DOI: 10.1136/gut.35.3.317

[72] Correa P. Helicobacter pylori and gastric carcinogenesis. The American Journal of Surgical Pathology. 1995;**19**(Suppl. 1):S37-S43

[73] Godos J, Marventano S, Mistretta A, Galvano F, Grosso G. Dietary sources of polyphenols in the Mediterranean healthy eating, aging and lifestyle (MEAL) study cohort. International Journal of Food Sciences and Nutrition. 2017;**68**:750-756. DOI: 10.1080/09637486.2017.1285870

[74] Rothwell J, Knaze V, Zamora-Ros R. Polyphenols: Dietary assessment and role in the prevention of cancers. Current Opinion in Clinical Nutrition and Metabolic Care. 2017;**20**:512-521. DOI: 10.1097/MCO.0000000000000424

[75] Zhang Z, Li X, Sang S, Mcclements D, Chen L, Long J, et al. Polyphenols as plant-based nutraceuticals: Health effects, encapsulation, nano-delivery, and application. Foods. 2022;**11**(15):2189. DOI: 10.3390/foods11152189

[76] Ma T, Tian C, Luo J, Zhou R, Sun X, Ma J. Influence of technical processing units on polyphenols and antioxidant capacity of carrot (Daucus carrot L.) juice. Food Chemistry. 2013;**141**(3):1637-1644. DOI: 10.1016/j.foodchem.2013.04.121

[77] Wang J, Tang L, Wang J-S. Biomarkers of dietary polyphenols in cancer studies: Current evidence and beyond. Oxidative Medicine and Cellular Longevity. 2015;**2015**:732302, 1-14. DOI: 10.1155/2015/732302

[78] Barreca D, Trombetta D, Smeriglio A, Mandalari G, Romeo O, Felice MR, et al. Food flavonols: Nutraceuticals with complex health benefits and functionalities. Trends in Food Science & Technology. 2021;**117**:194-204

[79] Pérez-Jiménez J, Hubert J, Hooper L, Cassidy A, Manach C, Williamson G, et al. Urinary metabolites as biomarkers of polyphenol intake in humans: A systematic review. The American Journal of Clinical Nutrition. 2010;**92**(4):801-809. DOI: 10.3945/ajcn.2010.29924

[80] Lean M, Noroozi M, Kelly I, Burns J, Talwar D, Sattar N, et al. Dietary flavonols protect diabetic human lymphocytes against oxidative damage to DNA. Diabetes. 1999;**48**(1):176-181. DOI: 10.2337/DIABETES.48.1.176

[81] García-Herrera P, Pérez-Rodríguez M, Aguilera-Delgado T, Labari-Reyes M, Olmedilla-Alonso B, Cámara M, et al. Anthocyanin profile of red fruits and black carrot juices, purees and concentrates by HPLC-DAD-ESI/MS-QTOF. International Journal of Food Science and Technology. 2016;**51**:2290-2300. DOI: 10.1111/IJFS.13210

[82] Cassidy A, Rogers G, Peterson J, Dwyer J, Lin H, Jacques P. Higher dietary anthocyanin and flavonol intakes are associated with anti-inflammatory effects in a population of US adults1. The American Journal of Clinical Nutrition. 2015;**102**:172-181. DOI: 10.3945/ajcn.115.108555

[83] Freitas R, Campos MM. Protective effects of Omega-3 fatty acids in cancer-related complications. Nutrients. 2019;**11**(5):945. DOI: 10.3390/nu11050945

[84] Lessa RC, Alves FD, Fortunati E, Lu J. Oral mucositis in cancer and potential use of Omega-3 free fatty acids in its management: A review. Biomedicine. 2021;**9**(11):1531

[85] Saadatian-Elahi M, Norat T, Goudable J, Riboli E. Biomarkers of dietary fatty acid intake and the risk of breast cancer: A meta-analysis. International Journal of Cancer. 2004;**111**(4):584-591. DOI: 10.1002/ijc.20284

[86] Hidaka B, Li S, Harvey K, Carlson S, Sullivan D, Kimler B, et al. Omega-3 and Omega-6 fatty acids in blood and breast tissue of high-risk women and association with atypical Cytomorphology. Cancer Prevention Research. 2015;**8**:359-364. DOI: 10.1158/1940-6207.CAPR-14-0351

[87] Hooper L, Thompson RL, Harrison RA, Summerbell CD, Ness AR, Moore HJ, et al. Risks and benefits of omega 3 fats for mortality, cardiovascular disease, and cancer: Systematic review. BMJ. 2006;**332**(7544):752-760. DOI: 10.1136/bmj.38755.366331.2f

[88] Bell G, Kantor E, Lampe J, Kristal A, Heckbert S, White E. Intake of long-chain ω-3 fatty acids from diet and supplements in relation to mortality. American Journal of Epidemiology. 2014;**179**(6):710-720. DOI: Doi10.1093/aje/kwt326

[89] Cheng M, Zhang S, Ning C, Huo Q. Omega-3 fatty acids supplementation improve nutritional status and inflammatory response in patients with lung cancer: A randomized clinical trial. Frontiers in Nutrition. 2021;**8**:686752. DOI: 10.3389/fnut.2021.686752

Chapter 13

Liquid Biopsy

Valeria Denninghoff and Maria Jose Serrano

Abstract

New ways of looking at tumor genetics and dynamics have been developed: the Liquid Biopsy (LB), which has been incorporated into clinical practice as a noninvasive analysis of circulating material derived from tumors, which represents an innovative tool in precision oncology and overcomes the current limitations associated with tissue biopsies. An LB is a new tool of great value, constituting a diagnostic, prognostic, and predictive marker. The elements that makeup LB are circulating tumor cells (CTCs) and circulating tumor nucleic acids (ctNA: DNA or RNA) in free cells or contained in exosomes, microvesicles, and platelets. The ctDNA and CTCs are the only one's components with a clinical application approved by the US Food and Drug Administration (FDA).

Keywords: cancer, NGS, blood sample, ctDNA, CTC

1. Introduction

Precision medicine is an innovative approach to disease prevention and treatment that considers differences in people's genes, injuries, environments, and lifestyles to target the right therapies to the right patients at the right time. In oncology, precision medicine uses genetic and molecular information to develop more specific and optimized drugs or treatments, with the aim that the therapy is the most appropriate to treat an individual, with greater effectiveness and a decrease in side effects. Therapeutic advances in genomic-guided precision oncology rely on prospective molecular identification of oncogenic alterations and resistance mechanisms to guide precise treatments. Many new therapeutic agents require the presence of biomarkers to direct their mechanism of action, and the tumor tissue is the reference sample [1].

In cancer patients, biopsies have been used to diagnose the disease for 1000 years through the histological definition of the disease and the tumor's genetic profile [2]. However, its obtaining presents certain limitations, including the discomfort suffered by the patient when taking the sample, the inherent clinic of his disease, possible surgical complications, and economic considerations. Also, some tumors are inaccessible due to their anatomical location, as in the case of the lung, so obtaining a representative and sufficient sample to perform an adequate molecular study can be complex. If the sample is inadequate, re-biopsy should be considered, with the consequent risk to the patient, who should undergo an invasive procedure again. In addition, this leads to a delay in the result, which can be crucial to establishing the most appropriate treatment for the patient's situation [2].

Unfortunately, it has been shown that a portion taken from different parts of a primary tumor and its metastases showed extensive inter-tumor and intra-tumor evolution. Tumors present enormous heterogeneity, as Gerlinger et al. found in their study, so that each area of the tumor has its genetic characteristics, which may result in the sample analyzed not being representative of all tumor cells, producing discordant results between samples from the same patient [3]. This tumor heterogeneity highlights the difficulty of dictating a therapeutic course of action based on a single biopsy, as it is likely to underestimate its complexity [4, 5]. Also, tumors are not static, and their molecular characteristics can change with the development of the disease. Selecting resistant subclones due to targeted drugs may intervene in the appearance of new genetic alterations, which produce molecular differences between the primary tumor and its metastases [3].

This tumor heterogeneity demonstrates the difficulty of selecting a therapy based on a single biopsy, as it is likely to underestimate the genomic complexity of the tumor (**Figure 1**).

Considering these limitations in individual biopsies, new ways of looking at tumor genetics and dynamics have been developed: the Liquid Biopsy, which has been incorporated into clinical practice as a noninvasive analysis of circulating material derived from tumors, which represents an innovative tool in precision oncology and overcomes the current limitations associated with tissue biopsies [6]. Liquid Biopsy is a new tool of great value, constituting a diagnostic, prognostic, and predictive marker. It allows diagnosing the disease by detecting genetic material or cells from the tumor in the blood, checking if a person is cured (if there is no presence of genetic material or tumor cells in the blood) or if, on the contrary, he suffers from a minimal residual disease, evaluating the effect of the treatment by measuring in real time the fluctuations of genetic material from the tumor and detect possible genetic alterations that indicate resistance to the drugs used. All this with a blood draw [5, 7].

The elements that makeup BL are circulating tumor cells (CTCs) and circulating tumor nucleic acids (ctNA: DNA or RNA) in free cells or contained in exosomes,

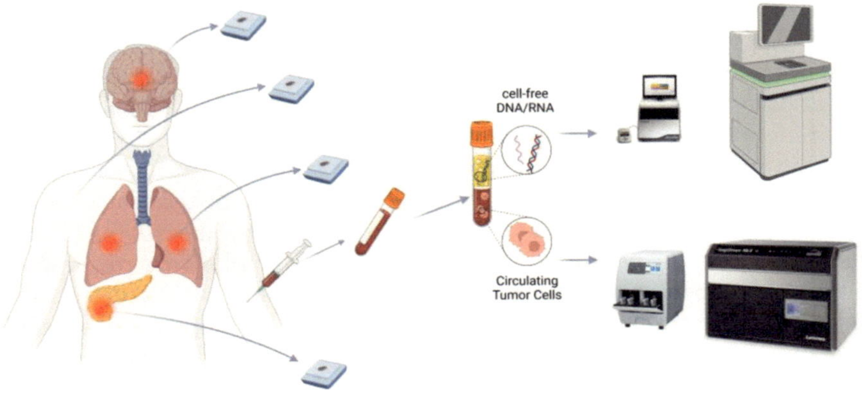

Figure 1.
Tumor heterogeneity in patients with metastases implies that the analysis of several tissue biopsies needs to be addressed for complete genotyping. Unlike liquid biopsy, a single sample allows the study of the drainage material of all tumors simultaneously, either primary or metastasis. This analysis can be performed on ctDNA/cfDNA from plasma or circulating tumor cells from anticoagulated whole blood ("created with BioRender.com").

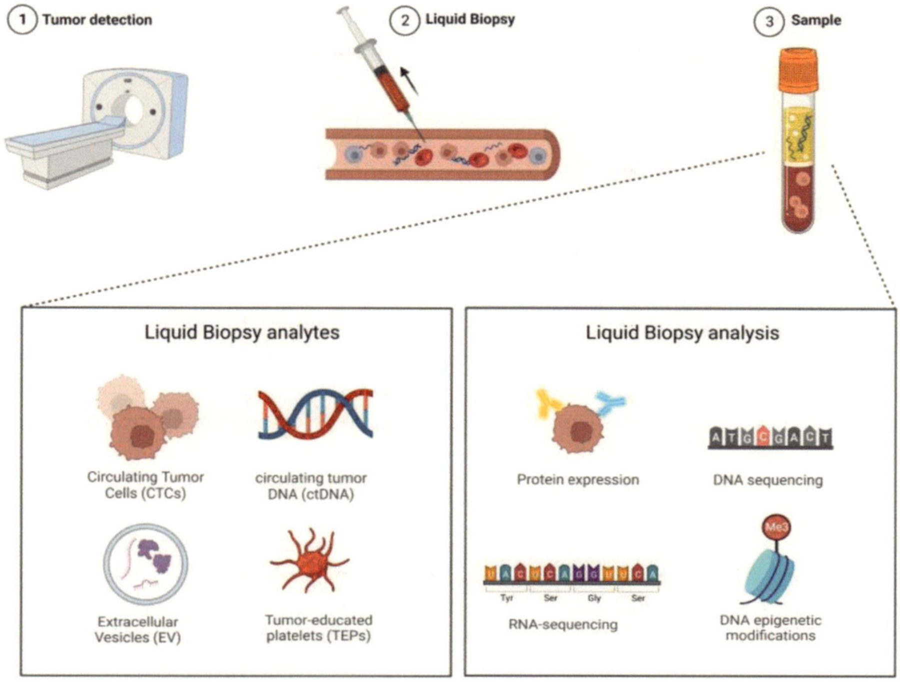

Figure 2.
Liquid biopsy may be taken, for example, after the patient's diagnosis, from a venipuncture, and after sample processing, allowing the analysis of their analytes with different technical approaches. In the same way, this type of sample can be studied during follow-up, especially in case of resistance to the treatment ("created with BioRender.com").

microvesicles, and platelets (**Figure 2**). The ctDNA and CTCs are the only one's components with a clinical application approved by the US Food and Drug Administration (FDA) [8].

2. Cell-free DNA

DNA was discovered in 1869 by a Swiss physician, Friedrich Miescher, who obtained the first crude purification of "nuclein" due to its occurrence in the cells' nuclei, and the double helix structure of DNA was discovered in 1953 [9, 10].

Although it is believed that free circulating nucleic acids are a recent finding, as early as 1948, before determining the structure of DNA, Mandel et al. found nucleic acids in the blood of healthy individuals, unknowingly that it would be the first step toward "liquid biopsy" [11].

The cfDNA is usually a double-stranded DNA whose length ranges between 100 and 300 base pairs. On many occasions, the length of cfDNA corresponds to the characteristic pattern of the process of apoptosis of multiples of 180 base pairs. There are at least two potential, but not mutually exclusive, mechanisms by which DNA can enter the bloodstream. These mechanisms can be classified into passive and active mechanisms [12]:

- The passive mechanism, the primary cause of the presence of cfDNA in the blood, is due to release when normal cell damage occurs during the process of apoptosis or in situations of necrosis, where cells release nuclear DNA and mitochondrial DNA into circulation during cell destruction.

- The active release of DNA has been identified in studies with cultured cell lines of different origins, raising the hypothesis of the spontaneous release of DNA fragments into circulation.

Multiple theories have been formulated to explain why cancer cells actively release DNA into circulation, including the possibility that cancer cells release oncogenic DNA to affect the transformation of susceptible cells at distant sites and thus generate invasion in other organs [13].

It has been observed that in cancer patients, cfDNA levels are much higher than those in healthy individuals because as the tumor increases in size, it induces both adjacent healthy cells and tumor cells to be apoptotic and necrotic processes. Considering this event, cfDNA belonging to tumor cells called circulating tumor DNA (ctDNA) can also be found in the blood. The amount of cfDNA that comes from tumor cells (ctDNA) depends on the characteristics of each tumor such as its size, the stage in which it is or its ability to invade the vascular endothelium [14].

Blood ctDNA analysis offers a novel clinical application to detect tumor-specific genetic aberrations in patients. This approach has a more excellent dynamic range than cfDNA, is more specific, and has many potential clinical applications. However, it is also technically more challenging due to high levels of cfDNA originating from the initial nontumor tissue. High analytical sensitivity and specialized equipment for ctDNA detection are required because the quantity and quality of tumor-derived DNA can vary dramatically. Techniques allow reliable monitoring of tumor-associated genetic aberrations, including somatic mutations, loss of heterozygosity, and chromosomal aberrations in the blood at frequencies as low as 0.01% [15].

In addition, ctDNA can also be detected in biological fluids other than blood, such as urine, cerebrospinal fluid, or pleural fluid, which further increases its diagnostic possibilities [16].

2.1 Cell-free DNA analysis

The success of Liquid Biopsy analysis is strictly related to the preanalytical steps, including blood, sampling, storage, and processing. Delays between plasma extraction and isolation may increase background levels due to DNA derived from the lysis of peripheral blood cells. The primary source of cfDNA is plasma that is isolated in peripheral blood. Plasma is preferred to serum because normal DNA can be released during coagulation, resulting in a more significant dilution of ctDNA. EDTA tubes or tubes containing formaldehyde-free preservative reagents should be used to prevent clotting and DNAase activity for blood collection. When EDTA-containing tubes are used to collect blood, plasma separation should be performed within 4 hours of removal to prevent lysis of leukocytes [16, 17].

The ctDNA generally represents between 0.01 and 10% of cfDNA, so its detection requires high analytical capacity and sensitivity [16]. In this context, next-generation sequencing (NGS) allows cancer diagnosis and improves the prognosis and the monitoring of the efficacy of therapies. Several different NGS platforms use different sequencing technologies, but all these platforms sequence millions of small DNA fragments in parallel. Bioinformatics analyses aim to piece together these fragments by mapping the individual reads to the human reference genome (pipelines). Each of the three billion bases in the human genome is sequenced several times to provide accurate data and insight into unexpected DNA variation. NGS can sequence whole genomes or specific genomic areas of interest, including all 22,000 coding genes, whole-genome sequencing (WGS), and whole-exome sequencing (WES), which is a genomic technique for sequencing all of the protein-coding regions of genes in a genome, known as the exome; or small numbers of individual genes (NGS panels) [18].

Figure 3 shows the mathematical relationship between the kb covered by the sequencing and the depth of readings obtained, which is inversely proportional. In a ctDNA, as input is scarce, panels of a few genes up to approximately 300 genes are the most used technique, with a desired depth of more than 1000X. Although WGS has been used with ctDNA, the depth used is 0.1 x (Tumor Fraction).

Emphasis will be placed in Liquid Biopsy on the following:

- Tumor Mutation Burden (TMB) is the number of mutations per megabase of DNA (Mut/Mb). It indirectly measures the neoantigens needed to boost the immune response. This measure correlates with response to immunotherapy [19].

- Tumor Burden (ctDNA/cfDNA ratio) is the quantity of ctDNA related to the total amount of cfDNA and has been suggested as a tool for prognostication and follow-up in patients. The ctDNA generally represents between 0.01 and 10% of cfDNA, so its detection requires high analytical capacity and sensitivity.

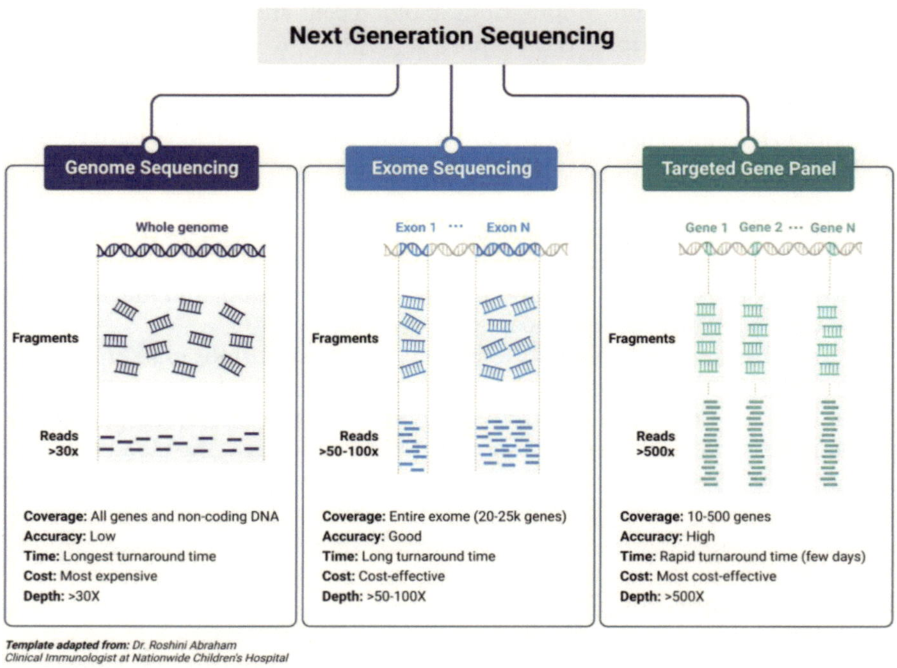

Figure 3.
Next-generation sequence approaches according to the properties of each method ("created with BioRender.com").

However, the prognostic value of ctDNA and its relation to tumor burden has yet to be substantiated [20].

- Fragmentomic is the pattern in length of cfDNA originating in different types of cells. Neoplasms result in altered fragmentomic profiles of cfDNA that could help identify tumors in early stages since they vary according to the stage, localization, and tissue origin [21].

- Methylomic is the study of the addition of a methyl group (-CH3) to a cytokine base (C) of DNA located before, continuously, to a guanine (G). It is the principal epigenetic mechanism and can cause alterations in transcription without the need for an alteration in the DNA sequence. It plays a critical regulatory role in the onset and progression of cancer. Methylation signatures are encoded in cfDNA, and this information is helpful for diagnosis but can also be harnessed to identify the location of tumors, especially those of unknown primary [22].

- Tumor Fraction (TFx) is an estimate using computational tools of the fraction of tumors in cell-free DNA from ultra-low-pass whole-genome sequencing (ULP-WGS, 0.1x coverage). Different algorithms exist for calculating TFx from cfDNA data, such as ichorCNA and ACE. TFx could correlate with clinical features associated with overall survival, and decreased TFx could be a promising biomarker for initial therapeutic response. Quantification of transcription factors (TF) in ctDNA has the potential to serve as a pragmatic, tumor-independent prognostic tool [23].

- Clonal Hematopoiesis of Indeterminate Potential (CHIP) is defined as the age-related accumulation of somatic mutations in hematopoietic stem cells, which leads to clonal expansion of mutations in blood cells and is a primary source of false-positive results from ctDNA analysis [24].

- MicroSatellite Instability (MSI) is genetic hypermutability resulting from impaired DNA mismatch repair (MMR). This measure correlates with response to immunotherapy [25].

Research on cfDNA has recently increased thanks to new digital genomic technologies that allow us to find rare variants of different mutations in DNA, such as digital PCR (dPCR), BEAMing (beads, emulsion, amplification, and magnetics), and polymerization activated by pyrophosphorolysis [18].

In all cases, Liquid Biopsy allows the study of druggable tumor markers, the follow-up of the patient throughout the treatment, and the detection of resistance to it. With a single sample and over time using only a blood sample, it is possible to detect and identify in real-time the tumor analytes drained into the bloodstream that characterizes the tumor and its metastases with high sensitivity and specificity (**Figure 4**).

3. Circulating tumor cell (CTC)

Circulating Tumor Cells (CTCs) are, by definition, epithelial cells, which means they present an epithelial phenotype characterized by the expression of markers such as E-cadherin, Cytokeratins family (CKs), Epithelial splicing regulator1

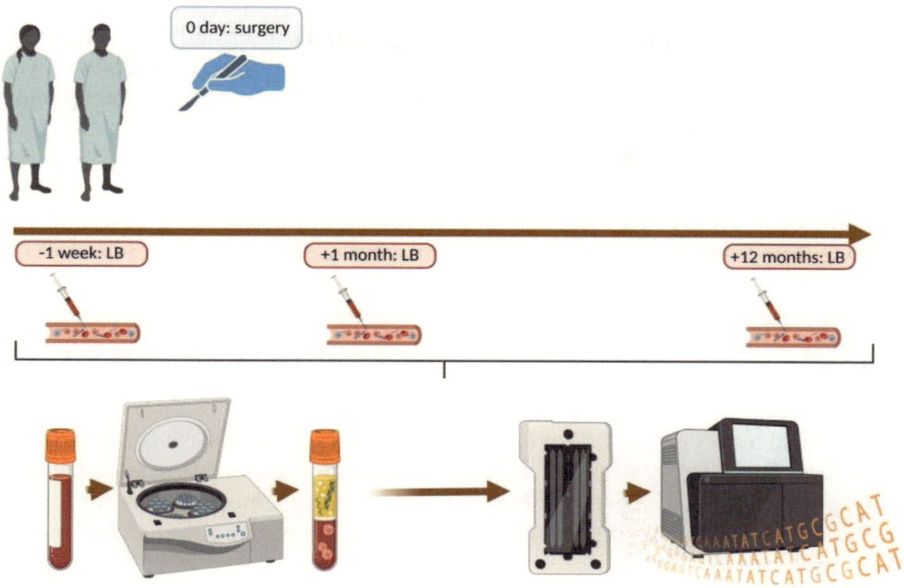

Figure 4.
Throughout the patient's follow-up, serial liquid biopsies can be taken to be evaluated, and therapeutic decisions can be made based on their results ("created with BioRender.com").

(ESPR1), Zonula occludens (ZO), and Epithelial cellular adhesion molecule (EpCAM). These epithelial markers are crucial for maintaining the architectural integrity of cells [26–28].

E-cadherin, in particular, plays a significant role in supporting epithelial tissue architecture and is a critical component of adherens junctions [29]. The downregulation of E-cadherin during tumoral processes is associated with increased dissemination ability of tumor cells (TCs) and the progression of Epithelial-Mesenchymal Transition (EMT) [30].

CKs are intermediate filaments forming a complex network extending from the nucleus's surface to the periphery of epithelial cells [31]. They are essential cytoskeleton components and include a large protein family with up to 20 types found in various epithelial tissues. Among the principal CKs are CK7, CK8, CK18, and CK19. Like E-cadherin, CKs' expression is associated with the disease's evolution and dissemination ability.

ESPR1 is a protein that exhibits high expression associated with the epithelial phenotype under pathophysiological conditions like cancer. It specifically regulates the expression of FGFR2-IIIb, an epithelial cell-specific isoform of FGFR2. Its downregulation is linked to the EMT process [32].

ZO refers to cytological structures in epithelium and endothelium cells, creating an impenetrable barrier preventing the free flow of substances between cells. These structures consist of a protein network that approximates the lipid membranes of adjacent cells, including Claudins and Ocludins. The downregulation of these proteins is involved in the initial steps of the EMT process [33].

EpCAM is a cell surface glycoprotein highly expressed in epithelial cancer cells, mediating cell-cell adhesion in epithelia [34, 35]. The expression of this protein depends on the stage of EMT. CTCs face various pressures as they circulate through the bloodstream and encounter different microenvironments in the body [36]. Blood flow shear stress affects the physical properties of CTCs, potentially altering their shape, size, and adhesion properties. Additionally, they navigate through narrow capillaries and small vessels, which may influence their ability to establish secondary tumors in distant organs.

Furthermore, CTCs encounter immune system pressure since the immune system recognizes them as foreign entities [37]. Like natural killer (NK) cells and cytotoxic T cells, immune cells exert pressure on CTCs to eliminate them from circulation. CTCs may evade immune surveillance by downregulating surface antigens and immune checkpoint proteins [38]. Upon reaching distant organs, CTCs encounter unique microenvironments with varying nutrient availability, oxygen levels, and interactions with the extracellular matrix. Adapting to these microenvironments is essential for CTC survival and metastatic formation.

CTCs acquire new biological features in response to these pressures, leading to morphological heterogeneity. This heterogeneity is associated with EMT, where CTCs can exhibit different cellular characteristics, such as retaining an epithelial phenotype resembling the original tumor cells, showing a more mesenchymal phenotype, or even displaying hybrid phenotypes with both epithelial and mesenchymal markers [39, 40].

EMT is a complex biological process through which epithelial cells undergo molecular changes resulting in acquiring mesenchymal characteristics and losing the epithelial phenotype. EMT involves a loss of cell-cell adhesion, cytoskeleton rearrangement, and gene expression changes. N-cadherin and other factors play a significant role in promoting the mesenchymal characteristics of transitioning cells [41, 42]. While EMT is necessary for CTC survival, its persistence may inhibit tumor cell proliferation. The process is reversible, and it is thought that CTCs may acquire an epithelial phenotype after undergoing EMT. However, the reversion may not be complete, leading to differences between tumor cells from the primary tumor and those found in metastases [43].

3.1 Molecular dynamics of CTCs induced by interaction with the microenvironment

The phenotypic and morphological heterogeneity is a result of genetic and epigenetic changes. As a critical survival mechanism for these CTCs, the EMT process activation involves the regulation of different gene pathways, biochemical pathways, and metabolic reprogramming [39].

The regulation and activation of EMT are complex processes involving numerous gene pathways. The activation of N-cadherin, a canonical gene in this process, is governed by p120 catenin, which localizes N-cadherin at cholesterol-rich microdomains [44]. When N-cadherin's extracellular domains initially bind, it triggers the activation of Rac, a member of the Rho GTPase family. This activation promotes localized actin filament assembly and the formation of membrane protrusions at cell-cell contact points [45]. Subsequently, RhoA, another member of the Rho GTPase family, becomes activated, displacing Rac's function. RhoA facilitates the maturation of N-cadherin-based cell-cell junctions by causing β-catenin to be sequestered into the cadherin intracellular domain [46]. β-catenin plays a crucial role by linking to α-catenin, which accumulates at newly formed cell-cell junctions and suppresses actin branching.

Furthermore, α-catenin anchors the N-cadherin-catenin complex to the actin cytoskeleton through actin-binding proteins like cortactin and α-actinin, thus promoting the maturation of cell-cell contacts [47]. Notably, the adhesive function of N-cadherin is regulated by posttranslational modifications of the N-cadherin-catenin complex. For instance, the stability of the N-cadherin-catenin complex heavily relies on the phosphorylation status of N-cadherin and the associated catenins, which are under the control of tyrosine kinases such as Fer and Src, as well as the tyrosine phosphatase PTP1B. These posttranslational modifications can influence the strength and dynamics of cell–cell adhesion mediated by N-cadherin, ultimately affecting various cellular processes, including EMT [48]. Therefore, the Upregulation of N-cadherin identifies an aggressive phenotype associated with an increased ability of CTCs to migrate [49]. CTCs can migrate as single cells or clusters, a "collective cell migration" [50, 51]. Collective cell migration facilitates the invasion of epithelial cells through the localized tumor-host microenvironment, thereby promoting metastasis [52]. Additionally, this process allows the maintenance of physical interconnectivity, collective cell polarity, and coordinated cytoskeletal activity and facilitates a more efficient directional migration in response to a chemotactic gradient than individual migrating cells. This is an interesting point since the ability of CTCs to survive is higher when they travel in clusters [53]. Circulating tumor cells (CTCs) and their clusters, known as circulating tumor microemboli (CTM), are related to tumor heterogeneity and clonal evolution [54]. These CTM exhibit distinct phenotypic and molecular characteristics compared to single CTCs and demonstrate higher metastatic potential and resistance to apoptosis compared to their single-cell counterparts [55]. The microemboli are composed of different cell types, including immune cells such as neutrophils or platelets [56]. CTM exhibits a different molecular profile compared to single cells. In this way, it has been demonstrated that CTM's epigenetic profile differs from single CTCs. Similarly, single-cell RNA sequencing revealed very little difference in expression patterns among single CTCs and CTM [57]. Recent works have demonstrated that the association of tumor cells with immune cells, such as platelets, can modify the expression of pathway genes correlated with EMT and promote the expression of stemness [58, 59]. Platelets have also been shown to decrease NK cell antitumor activity through a TGF-β-mediated decrease in NKG2D [60]. An exciting aspect of these interactions with platelets is the exchange of biological information between CTCs and platelets through direct interaction, making this transference of biomolecules a bidirectional process [61]. The transfer of biomolecules from platelets to tumor cells involves an increase in proliferation pathways, inhibition of antiapoptotic pathways, and even modification of lipid composition of the nuclear and cell membranes. The main consequence of this exchange is the modification at functional, genetic, and phenotypic levels [59].

Regarding the interaction with other immune cells, neutrophils play a significant role [62]. Neutrophils promote cell cycle progression [63]. Like platelets, CTCs can interact indirectly by secreting soluble factors, and they can also directly interact with neutrophils through different receptors, including VCAM1, ICAM-1, and β1 integrin. Interestingly, there is a strong alliance between platelets, neutrophils, and CTCs, as releasing soluble mediators, such as CXCL5 or CXCL7, by activated platelets promotes the recruitment of neutrophils [64]. The interaction with neutrophils, thus, favors the formation and arrest of tumor cell/neutrophil complexes on the endothelium wall, which supports the survival of CTCs in the blood system [65].

All this evidence suggests that the association of CTCs with different nontumor cells, such as platelets or neutrophils, is an essential process in the dissemination, migration, and survival of CTCs. These interactions can induce the expression of transcription factors (TFs) that allow the activation of the EMT process [66]. It has been demonstrated that these interactions with different immune cells promote the activation of the TFs Twist1 and Snail, both of which are associated with the EMT process [67]. Twist1 is an essential helix–loop–helix transcription factor involved in embryogenesis and tumor development and progression through the activation of EMT [68]. This transcription factor negatively acts on the E-box of E-cadherin. Its role in metastasis and CTC diffusion implicates complex relationships with oncogenic and antioncogenic proteins.

Additionally, these interactions induce the activation of the AKT2 and PI3K pathways. AKT2 is a member of the protein kinase B (PKB) family, which are serine/threonine protein kinases [69, 70]. The oncogenic serine/threonine kinase AKT, a downstream effector of the phosphatidylinositol 3′ kinase (PI3K), has been described as a transcriptional repressor of the E-cadherin gene. Both elements are associated with EMT and are used to classify the presence of CTCs with EMT phenotype [71]. They are part of the PI3K/AKT/mTOR pathway, which plays a significant role in the motility of cancer cells. The AKT pathway is pivotal in EMT and has a nodal function for extracellular and intracellular signaling pathways. Furthermore, the regulation of AKT depends on the Upregulation of PI3K expression and the downregulation of the phosphatase PTEN expression.

The Phosphatase and Tensin Homolog (PTEN) gene is a critical tumor suppressor gene that significantly regulates cell growth, survival, and proliferation. It encodes a protein called PTEN, which functions primarily as a lipid phosphatase, modulating the levels of phosphatidylinositol (3,4,5)-trisphosphate (PIP3) within cells. Additionally, EMT can induce several receptors that mediate interactions between neutrophils and CTCs, or between CTCs and platelets/fibrin, including CD44, ICAM-1, $\alpha v\beta 3$, and VCAM1 [72].

One of the significant consequences of EMT in CTCs is its impact on antiapoptotic pathways [73]. Epithelial cells usually have strong cell–cell adhesion, which provides a protective environment and promotes cell survival. However, CTCs lose these tight cell-cell adhesions during EMT, making them more vulnerable to apoptosis or programmed cell death. Nevertheless, acquiring mesenchymal characteristics during EMT helps CTCs escape apoptosis signals and gain a survival advantage. These interactions can promote, in the same way, the Upregulation of antiapoptotic proteins, such as Bcl-2 and Bcl-xL, which inhibit the intrinsic pathway of apoptosis [74]. These proteins prevent mitochondrial outer membrane permeabilization and the release of pro-apoptotic factors, thereby protecting CTCs from apoptosis. Additionally, EMT can also downregulate pro-apoptotic proteins, like Bax and Bak, which are involved in promoting apoptosis. The reduction of these proteins further contributes to the resistance of CTCs to apoptosis signals [75].

The survival and capacity of CTCs have also been correlated with the acquisition of characteristics of CSCs (Cancer Stem Cells) [76]. Different hypotheses have been proposed to understand the presence of a subpopulation of CTCs with stem cell properties. One of them is based on the fact that tumor somatic cells undergoing EMT migrate from the primary tumor into the blood. The second hypothesis suggests that fully differentiated cancer cells can acquire these stem cell properties due to the induction of EMT pathways [77, 78]. As mentioned in previous works, the interaction of CTCs (somatic cells) with platelets could induce the expression of genes associated with stem cell markers. Among these markers are REX1, OCT4, and NANOG. OCT4 and NANOG have been found to activate and regulate REX-1 (Zfp-42) cooperatively. REX-1 is a pluripotency marker usually found in undifferentiated embryonic stem cells [34]. OCT4, NANOG, SOX-2, and REX-1 are essential elements of self-regulation, and substantial evidence shows these transcription factors' epigenetic role in regulating stem cells [79].

4. Conclusions

Precision Medicine aims to eliminate the "one-size-fits-all" patient management model but needs tissue biopsies to identify druggable biomarkers. Nevertheless, tissues may be scarce or inaccessible for molecular studies. Liquid Biopsy is an effective alternative to select patients who may benefit from specific treatments, constituting a diagnostic, prognostic, and predictive tool. The Liquid Biopsy allows for diagnosing the disease by detecting ctDNA or CTCs in the blood, checking if a person has resolved their disease or if, on the contrary, they suffer from a minimal residual disease that can increase. Liquid Biopsy evaluates the result of the treatment by measuring in real time the fluctuations of the tumor analytes and detecting genetic alterations that determine resistance to the drugs used. The ctDNA and CTCs are the only components of Liquid Biopsy with a clinical application approved.

One of the main benefits of ctDNA is that it allows it to preserve the molecular characteristics of the tumor tissue from which it comes, including mutations, epigenetic changes, and copy number variations. This property makes the blood acquire a potential utility as a surrogate of the tumor, which can identify actionable or druggable alterations in circulating tumor-derived DNA.

CTCs' morphological heterogeneity reflects the genetic and phenotypic diversity they acquire during EMT. This cellular plasticity allows CTCs to adapt to different microenvironments and survive, contributing to cancer metastasis. It is only possible to fully understand the biology of CTCs by analyzing their microenvironment. The ability of CTCs to survive, inhibit apoptosis pathways, and induce stemness could depend on direct and indirect interactions with other cell populations that coexist with them.

Conflict of interest

The authors declare no conflict of interest.

Author details

Valeria Denninghoff[1,2]* and Maria Jose Serrano[2,3,4]

1 Molecular Oncology Clinical Lab, University of Buenos Aires (UBA)—National Council for Scientific and Technical Research (CONICET), Buenos Aires, Argentina

2 Liquid Biopsy and Cancer Interception Unit, GENYO, Centre for Genomics and Oncological Research (Pfizer/University of Granada/Andalusian Regional Government), Granada, Spain

3 Integral Oncology Division, University Hospital Virgen de las Nieves, Granada, Spain

4 Instituto Biosanitario Granada (iBS-Granada), Granada, Spain

*Address all correspondence to: vdenninghoff@conicet.gov.ar

IntechOpen

References

[1] Sholl LM, Aisner DL, Varella-Garcia M, Berry LD, Dias-Santagata D, Wistuba II, et al. Multi-institutional oncogenic driver mutation analysis in lung adenocarcinoma: The lung cancer mutation consortium experience. Journal of Thoracic Oncology. 2015;**10**:768-777. DOI: 10.1097/JTO.0000000000000516

[2] Crowley E, Di Nicolantonio F, Loupakis F, Bardelli A. Liquid biopsy: Monitoring cancer-genetics in the blood. Nature Reviews. Clinical Oncology. 2013;**10**:472-484. DOI: 10.1038/nrclinonc.2013.110

[3] Gerlinger M, Rowan AJ, Horswell S, Math M, Larkin J, Endesfelder D, Gronroos E, Martinez P, Matthews N, Stewart A, Tarpey P, Varela I, Phillimore B, Begum S, McDonald NQ, Butler A, Jones D, Raine K, Latimer C, Santos CR, Nohadani M, Eklund AC, Spencer-Dene B, Clark G, Pickering L, Stamp G, Gore M, Szallasi Z, Downward J, Futreal PA, Swanton Cet al. Intratumor heterogeneity and branched evolution revealed by multiregion sequencing. The New England Journal of Medicine 2012;**366**:883-892. DOI: 10.1056/NEJMoa1113205

[4] Bettegowda C, Sausen M, Leary RJ, Kinde I, Wang Y, Agrawal N, et al. Detection of circulating tumor DNA in early- and late-stage human malignancies. Science Translational Medicine. 2014;**6**:224ra24. DOI: 10.1126/scitranslmed.3007094

[5] Jamal-Hanjani M, Quezada SA, Larkin J, Swanton C. Translational implications of tumor heterogeneity. Clinical Cancer Research. 2015;**21**:1258-1266. DOI: 10.1158/1078-0432.CCR-14-1429

[6] Serrano MJ, Garrido-Navas MC, Diaz Mochon JJ, Cristofanilli M, Gil-Bazo I, Pauwels P, et al. International society of liquid biopsy. Precision prevention and cancer interception: The new challenges of liquid biopsy. Cancer Discovery. 2020;**10**:1635-1644. DOI: 10.1158/2159-8290.CD-20-0466

[7] Rolfo C, Mack PC, Scagliotti GV, Baas P, Barlesi F, Bivona TG, Herbst RS, Mok TS, Peled N, Pirker R, Raez LE, Reck M, Riess JW, Sequist LV, Shepherd FA, Sholl LM, Tan DSW, Wakelee HA, Wistuba II, Wynes MW, Carbone DP, Hirsch FR, Gandara DR. Liquid biopsy for advanced non-small cell lung cancer (NSCLC): A statement paper from the IASLC. Journal of Thoracic Oncology 2018;13:1248-1268. DOU: 10.1016/j.jtho.2018.05.030

[8] de Rubis G, Rajeev Krishnan S, Bebawy M. Liquid biopsies in cancer diagnosis, monitoring, and prognosis. Trends in Pharmacological Sciences. 2019;**40**:172-186. DOI: 10.1016/j.tips.2019.01.006

[9] Dahm R. Friedrich Miescher and the discovery of DNA. Developmental Biology. 2005;**278**:274-288. DOI: 10.1016/j.ydbio.2004.11.028

[10] Watson JD, Crick FH. Molecular structure of nucleic acids; a structure for deoxyribose nucleic acid. Nature. 1953;**171**(4356):737-738. DOI: 10.1038/171737a0

[11] Mandel P, Metais P. Les acides nucléiques du plasma sanguin chez l'homme [Nuclear Acids In Human Blood Plasma]. Comptes Rendus des Seances de la Societe de Biologie et de Ses Filiales. 1948;**142**:241-243

[12] Bohers E, Viailly PJ, Jardin F. cfDNA sequencing: Technological approaches and Bioinformatic issues. Pharmaceuticals (Basel). 2021;**14**:596. DOI: 10.3390/ph14060596

[13] Fares J, Fares MY, Khachfe HH, Salhab HA, Fares Y. Molecular principles of metastasis: A hallmark of cancer revisited. Signal Transduction and Targeted Therapy. 2020;**5**:28. DOI: 10.1038/s41392-020-0134-x

[14] Volik S, Alcaide M, Morin RD, Collins C. Cell-free DNA (cfDNA): Clinical significance and utility in cancer shaped by emerging technologies. Molecular Cancer Research. 2016;**14**:898-908. DOI: 10.1158/1541-7786.MCR-16-0044

[15] Xia L, Li Z, Zhou B, Tian G, Zeng L, Dai H, et al. Statistical analysis of mutant allele frequency level of circulating cell-free DNA and blood cells in healthy individuals. Scientific Reports. 2017;**7**:7526. DOI: 10.1038/s41598-017-06106-1

[16] Malapelle U, Pisapia P, Addeo A, Arrieta O, Bellosillo B, Cardona AF, et al. Liquid biopsy from research to clinical practice: Focus on non-small cell lung cancer. Expert Review of Molecular Diagnostics. 2021;**21**:1165-1178. DOI: 10.1080/14737159.2021.1985468

[17] Pisapia P, Luis Costa JL, Pepe F, Russo G, Gragnano G, Russo A, et al. Next generation sequencing for liquid biopsy-based testing in non-small cell lung cancer in 2021. Critical Reviews in Oncology/Hematology. 2021;**161**:103311. DOI: 10.1016/j.critrevonc.2021.103311

[18] Denninghoff VC. Molecular pathology in the new age of personalized medicine [internet]. In: Pathology - from Classics to Innovations. London, UK, London, UK: IntechOpen; 2021. DOI: 10.5772/intechopen.94927

[19] Lawlor RT, Mattiolo P, Mafficini A, Hong SM, Piredda ML, Taormina SV, et al. Tumor mutational burden as a potential biomarker for immunotherapy in pancreatic cancer: Systematic review and still-open questions. Cancers (Basel). 2021;**13**:3119. DOI: 10.3390/cancers13133119

[20] Arisi MF, Dotan E, Fernandez SV. Circulating tumor DNA in precision oncology and its applications in colorectal cancer. International Journal of Molecular Sciences. 2022;**23**:4441. DOI: 10.3390/ijms23084441

[21] Ding SC, Lo YMD. Cell-free DNA Fragmentomics in liquid biopsy. Diagnostics (Basel). 2022;**12**:978. DOI: 10.3390/diagnostics12040978

[22] Shimizu D, Taniue K, Matsui Y, Haeno H, Araki H, Miura F, et al. Pan-cancer methylome analysis for cancer diagnosis and classification of cancer cell of origin. Cancer Gene Therapy. 2022;**29**:428-436. DOI: 10.1038/s41417-021-00401-w

[23] Husain H, Pavlick DC, Fendler BJ, Madison RW, Decker B, Gjoerup O, et al. Tukachinsky H tumor fraction correlates with detection of actionable variants across > 23,000 circulating tumor DNA samples. JCO Precision Oncology. 2022;**6**:e2200261. DOI: 10.1200/PO.22.00261

[24] Chan HT, Chin YM, Nakamura Y, Low SK. Clonal Hematopoiesis in liquid biopsy: From biological noise to valuable clinical implications. Cancers (Basel). 2020;**12**:2277. DOI: 10.3390/cancers12082277

[25] Tieng FYF, Abu N, Lee LH, Ab Mutalib NS. Microsatellite instability in colorectal cancer liquid biopsy-current updates on its potential in non-invasive detection, prognosis and as a predictive

marker. Diagnostics (Basel). 2021;**11**:544. DOI: 10.3390/diagnostics11030544

[26] Mocellin S, Keilholz U, Rossi CR, Nitti D. Circulating tumor cells: The 'leukemic phase' of solid cancers. Trends in Molecular Medicine. 2006;**12**:130-139. DOI: 10.1016/j.molmed.2006.01.006

[27] Warzecha CC, Shen S, Xing Y, Carstens RP. The epithelial splicing factors ESRP1 and ESRP2 positively and negatively regulate diverse types of alternative splicing events. RNA Biology. 2009;**6**:546-562. DOI: 10.4161/rna.6.5.9606

[28] Lindley LE, Briegel KJ. Molecular characterization of TGFbeta-induced epithelial-mesenchymal transition in normal finite lifespan human mammary epithelial cells. Biochemical and Biophysical Research Communications. 2010;**399**:659-664. DOI: 10.1016/j.bbrc.2010.07.138

[29] Gall TM, Frampton AE. Gene of the month: E-cadherin (CDH1). Journal of Clinical Pathology. 2013;**66**:928-932. DOI: 10.1136/jclinpath-2013-201768

[30] Thiery JP, Sleeman JP. Complex networks orchestrate epithelial-mesenchymal transitions. Nature Reviews. Molecular Cell Biology. 2006;**7**:131-142. DOI: 10.1038/nrm1835

[31] Serrano MJ, Lorente JA, Delgado Rodríguez M, Fernández A, Fernández M, de la Torre C, et al. Circulating tumour cells in peripheral blood: Potential impact on breast cancer outcome. Clinical & Translational Oncology. 2011;**13**:204-208. DOI: 10.1007/s12094-011-0641-x

[32] Warzecha CC, Jiang P, Amirikian K, Dittmar KA, Lu H, Shen S, et al. An ESRP-regulated splicing programme is abrogated during the epithelial-mesenchymal transition. The EMBO Journal. 2010;**29**:3286-3300. DOI: 10.1038/emboj.2010.195

[33] Umeda K, Matsui T, Nakayama M, Furuse K, Sasaki H, Furuse M, et al. Establishment and characterization of cultured epithelial cells lacking expression of ZO-1. The Journal of Biological Chemistry. 2004;**279**:44785-44794. DOI: 10.1074/jbc.M406563200

[34] Rao CG, Chianese D, Doyle GV, Miller MC, Russell T, Sanders RA Jr, et al. Expression of epithelial cell adhesion molecule in carcinoma cells present in blood and primary and metastatic tumors. International Journal of Oncology. 2005;**27**:49-57

[35] de Wit S, van Dalum G, Lenferink AT, Tibbe AG, Hiltermann TJ, Groen HJ, et al. The detection of EpCAM(+) and EpCAM(−) circulating tumor cells. Scientific Reports. 2015;**5**:12270. DOI: 10.1038/srep12270

[36] Heeke S, Mograbi B, Alix-Panabières C, Hofman P. Never travel alone: The crosstalk of circulating tumor cells and the blood microenvironment. Cell. 2019;**8**:714. DOI: 10.3390/cells8070714

[37] Garrido-Navas C, de Miguel-Perez D, Exposito-Hernandez J, Bayarri C, Amezcua V, Ortigosa A, et al. Cooperative and escaping mechanisms between circulating tumor cells and blood constituents. Cell. 2019;**8**:1382. DOI: 10.3390/cells8111382

[38] Liu X, Song J, Zhang H, Liu X, Zuo F, Zhao Y, et al. Immune checkpoint HLA-E:CD94-NKG2A mediates evasion of circulating tumor cells from NK cell surveillance. Cancer Cell. 2023;**41**:272-287.e9. DOI: 10.1016/j.ccell.2023.01.001

[39] Genna A, Vanwynsberghe AM, Villard AV, Pottier C, Ancel J, Polette M,

et al. EMT-associated heterogeneity in circulating tumor cells: Sticky friends on the road to metastasis. Cancers (Basel). 2020;**12**:1632. DOI: 10.3390/cancers12061632

[40] Francart ME, Lambert J, Vanwynsberghe AM, Thompson EW, Bourcy M, Polette M, et al. Epithelial-mesenchymal plasticity and circulating tumor cells: Travel companions to metastases. Developmental Dynamics. 2018;**247**:432-450. DOI: 10.1002/dvdy.24506

[41] Bonnomet A, Brysse A, Tachsidis A, Waltham M, Thompson EW, Polette M, et al. Epithelial-to-mesenchymal transitions and circulating tumor cells. Journal of Mammary Gland Biology and Neoplasia. 2010;**15**:261-273. DOI: 10.1007/s10911-010-9174-0

[42] Jie XX, Zhang XY, Xu CJ. Epithelial-to-mesenchymal transition, circulating tumor cells and cancer metastasis: Mechanisms and clinical applications. Oncotarget. 2017;**8**:81558-81571. DOI: 10.18632/oncotarget.18277

[43] Jolly MK, Ware KE, Gilja S, Somarelli JA, Levine H. EMT and MET: Necessary or permissive for metastasis? Molecular Oncology. 2017;**11**:755-769. DOI: 10.1002/1878-0261.12083

[44] Taulet N, Comunale F, Favard C, Charrasse S, Bodin S, Gauthier-Rouviere C. N-cadherin/p120 catenin association at cell-cell contacts occurs in cholesterol-rich membrane domains and is required for RhoA activation and myogenesis. The Journal of Biological Chemistry. 2009;**284**:23137-23145. DOI: 10.1074/jbc.M109.017665

[45] Spiering D, Hodgson L. Dynamics of the rho-family small GTPases in actin regulation and motility. Cell Adhesion & Migration. 2011;**5**:170-180. DOI: 10.4161/cam.5.2.14403

[46] Huber AH, Weis WI. The structure of the β-catenin/E-cadherin complex and the molecular basis of diverse ligand recognition by β-catenin. Cell. 2001;**105**:391-402. DOI: 10.1016/s0092-8674(01)00330-0

[47] Desai R, Sarpal R, Ishiyama N, Pellikka M, Ikura M, Tepass U. Monomeric α-catenin links cadherin to the actin cytoskeleton. Nature Cell Biology. 2013;**15**:261-273. DOI: 10.1038/ncb2685

[48] Loh CY, Chai JY, Tang TF, Wong WF, Sethi G, Shanmugam MK, et al. The E-cadherin and N-cadherin switch in epithelial-to-mesenchymal transition: Signaling, therapeutic implications, and challenges. Cell. 2019;**8**:1118. DOI: 10.3390/cells8101118

[49] Mrozik KM, Blaschuk OW, Cheong CM, Zannettino ACW, Vandyke K. N-cadherin in cancer metastasis, its emerging role in haematological malignancies and potential as a therapeutic target in cancer. BMC Cancer. 2018;**18**:939. DOI: 10.1186/s12885-018-4845-0

[50] Friedl P, Gilmour D. Collective cell migration in morphogenesis, regeneration and cancer. Nature Reviews. Molecular Cell Biology. 2009;**10**:445-457. DOI: 10.1038/nrm2720

[51] Visal TH, den Hollander P, Cristofanilli M, Mani SA. Circulating tumour cells in the -omics era: How far are we from achieving the 'singularity'? British Journal of Cancer. 2022;**127**:173-184. DOI: 10.1038/s41416-022-01768-9

[52] Wu S, Liu S, Liu Z, Huang J, Pu X, Li J, et al. Classification of circulating tumor cells by epithelial-mesenchymal transition markers. PLoS One.

2015;**10**:e0123976. DOI: 10.1371/journal.pone.0123976

[53] Perea Paizal J, Au SH, Bakal C. Squeezing through the microcirculation: Survival adaptations of circulating tumour cells to seed metastasis. British Journal of Cancer. 2021;**124**:58-65. DOI: 10.1038/s41416-020-01176-x

[54] Zhang D, Zhao L, Zhou P, Ma H, Huang F, Jin M, et al. Circulating tumor microemboli (CTM) and vimentin+ circulating tumor cells (CTCs) detected by a size-based platform predict worse prognosis in advanced colorectal cancer patients during chemotherapy. Cancer Cell International. 2017;**17**:6. DOI: 10.1186/s12935-016-0373-7

[55] Menyailo ME, Tretyakova MS, Denisov EV. Heterogeneity of circulating tumor cells in breast cancer: Identifying metastatic seeds. International Journal of Molecular Sciences. 2020;**21**:1696. DOI: 10.3390/ijms21051696

[56] Kurma K, Alix-Panabières C. Mechanobiology and survival strategies of circulating tumor cells: A process towards the invasive and metastatic phenotype. Frontiers in Cell and Development Biology. 2023;**11**:1188499. DOI: 10.3389/fcell.2023.1188499

[57] Castro-Giner F, Aceto N. Tracking cancer progression: From circulating tumor cells to metastasis. Genome Medicine. 2020;**12**:31. DOI: 10.1186/s13073-020-00728-3

[58] Pereira-Veiga T, Schneegans S, Pantel K, Wikman H. Circulating tumor cell-blood cell crosstalk: Biology and clinical relevance. Cell Reports. 2022;**40**:111298. DOI: 10.1016/j.celrep.2022.111298

[59] Rodriguez-Martinez A, Simon-Saez I, Perales S, Garrido-Navas C, Russo A, de Miguel-Perez D, et al. Exchange of cellular components between platelets and tumor cells: Impact on tumor cells behavior. Theranostics. 2022;**12**:2150-2161. DOI: 10.7150/thno.64252

[60] Kopp HG, Placke T, Salih HR. Platelet-derived transforming growth factor-β Down-regulates NKG2D thereby inhibiting natural killer cell antitumor reactivity. Cancer Research. 2009;**69**:7775-7783. DOI: 10.1158/0008-5472.CAN-09-2123

[61] Labelle M, Begum S, Hynes RO. Direct signaling between platelets and cancer cells induces an epithelial-mesenchymal-like transition and promotes metastasis. Cancer Cell. 2011;**20**:576-590. DOI: 10.1016/j.ccr.2011.09.009

[62] Man Y, Minying Z, Rui N, Xiaohui Y, Shifeng T, Linlin F, et al. Roles of tumor-associated neutrophils in tumor metastasis and its clinical applications. Front Cell Developmental Biology. 2022;**10**:938289. DOI: 10.3389/fcell.2022.938289

[63] Leone K, Poggiana C, Zamarchi R. The interplay between circulating tumor cells and the immune system: From immune escape to cancer immunotherapy. Diagnostics (Basel). 2018;**8**:59. DOI: 10.3390/diagnostics8030059

[64] Braun A, Anders HJ, Gudermann T, Mammadova-Bach E. Platelet-cancer interplay: Molecular mechanisms and new therapeutic avenues. Frontiers in Oncology. 2021;**11**:665534. DOI: 10.3389/fonc.2021.665534

[65] Peralta M, Osmani N, Goetz JG. Circulating tumor cells: Towards mechanical phenotyping of metastasis. iScience. 2022;**25**:103969. DOI: 10.1016/j.isci.2022.103969

[66] Wang X, Zhao S, Wang Z, Gao T. Platelets involved tumor cell EMT during circulation: Communications and interventions. Cell Communication and Signaling: CCS. 2022;**20**:82. DOI: 10.1186/s12964-022-00887-3

[67] Pandolfi L, Bozzini S, Frangipane V, Percivalle E, De Luigi A, Violatto MB, et al. Neutrophil extracellular traps induce the epithelial-mesenchymal transition: Implications in post-COVID-19 fibrosis. Frontiers in Immunology. 2021;**12**:663303. DOI: 10.3389/fimmu.2021.663303

[68] Qin Q, Xu Y, He T, Qin C, Xu. Normal and disease-related biological functions of Twist1 and underlying molecular mechanisms. Journal of Cell Research. 2012;**22**:90-106. DOI: 10.1038/cr.2011.144

[69] Ward MP, E Kane L, A Norris L, Mohamed BM, Kelly T, Bates M, et al. Platelets, immune cells and the coagulation cascade; friend or foe of the circulating tumour cell? Molecular Cancer. 2021;**20**:59. DOI: 10.1186/s12943-021-01347-1

[70] Charles Jacob HK, Charles Richard JL, Signorelli R, Kashuv T, Lavania S, Vaish U, et al. Modulation of early neutrophil granulation: The circulating tumor cell-Extravesicular connection in pancreatic ductal adenocarcinoma. Cancers (Basel). 2021;**13**:2727. DOI: 10.3390/cancers13112727

[71] Smit DJ, Cayrefourcq L, Haider MT, Hinz N, Pantel K, Alix-Panabières C, et al. High sensitivity of circulating tumor cells derived from a colorectal cancer patient for dual inhibition with AKT and mTOR inhibitors. Cell. 2020;**9**:2129. DOI: 10.3390/cells9092129

[72] Ring A, Nguyen-Sträuli BD, Wicki A, Aceto N. Biology, vulnerabilities and clinical applications of circulating tumour cells. Nature Reviews. Cancer. 2023;**23**:95-111. DOI: 10.1038/s41568-022-00536-4

[73] Pang S, Xu S, Wang L, Wu H, Chu Y, Ma X, et al. Molecular profiles of single circulating tumor cells from early breast cancer patients with different lymph node statuses. Thorac Cancer. 2023;**14**:156-167. DOI: 10.1111/1759-7714.14728

[74] Kapoor I, Bodo J, Hill BT, Hsi ED, Almasan A. Targeting BCL-2 in B-cell malignancies and overcoming therapeutic resistance. Cell Death & Disease. 2020;**11**:941. DOI: 10.1038/s41419-020-03144-y

[75] Carberry S, D'Orsi B, Monsefi N, Salvucci M, Bacon O, Fay J, et al. The BAX/BAK-like protein BOK is a prognostic marker in colorectal cancer. Cell Death & Disease. 2018;**9**:125. DOI: 10.1038/s41419-017-0140-2

[76] Aramini B, Masciale V, Arienti C, Dominici M, Stella F, Martinelli G, et al. Cancer stem cells (CSCs), circulating tumor cells (CTCs) and their interplay with cancer associated fibroblasts (CAFs): A New World of targets and treatments. Cancers (Basel). 2022;**14**:2408. DOI: 10.3390/cancers14102408

[77] Toloudi M, Apostolou P, Chatziioannou M, Papasotiriou I. Correlation between cancer stem cells and circulating tumor cells and their value. Case Reports in Oncology. 2011;**4**:44-54. DOI: 10.1159/000324403

[78] Laplane L. "the CSC Theory". Cancer Stem Cells: Philosophy and Therapies. Cambridge, MA and London, England: Harvard University Press; 2016. pp. 27-44. DOI: 10.4159/9780674969582-004

[79] Shariati F, Favaedi R, Ramazanali F, Ghoraeian P, Afsharian P, Aflatoonian B, et al. Increased expression of stemness genes REX-1, OCT-4, NANOG, and SOX-2 in women with ovarian endometriosis versus normal endometrium: A case-control study. International Journal of Reproductive Biomedicine. 2019;**16**:ijrm.v16i12.3684. DOI: 10.18502/ijrm.v16i12.3684

Chapter 14

Companion Animals as Models for Human Mammary Cancer Research

Pamela Cruz

Abstract

In both humans and companion animals, cancer is one of the leading causes of death worldwide. Given the increasing incidence in humans and dogs, there is an urgent need to find or improve strategies for diagnosis, treatment and prognosis. Hence, the importance of having very similar study models. Both canine and feline models have advantages over their murine counterparts in the study of breast cancer and cancer in general. Among other things, at the molecular and genetic levels, in terms of risk factors, spontaneous disease onset and tumour heterogeneity, domestic animals share greater similarities with the human species than the murine model. In addition, they share environmental and socioeconomic factors. Another advantage is their similar response to chemotherapy treatment, and rapid imaging results can be obtained with the same screening techniques used in humans. Finally, this chapter discusses the main features that make the canine and feline model the main source for the study of breast cancer *in vitro* and *in vivo*.

Keywords: breast cancer, companion animals, oestrogen receptor, EGFR, signalling pathways

1. Introduction

Breast cancer is one of the most common cancers in women worldwide. The disease is often hormonally regulated, with estradiol and some selective oestrogen receptor modulators (SERMs) influencing the development and/or progression of many breast tumours due to their association with nuclear and cytoplasmic oestrogen receptors (ERs). Binding of SERMs to these receptors leads to genomic and "non-genomic" effects (rapid activation of cellular phenomena, e.g., signalling cascades) and affects the development of some tumours in different ways. Treatment of breast cancer with anti-oestrogens or aromatase inhibitors (AIs) is often effective in patients with "ER -positive" breast cancer; unfortunately, not all cancers respond to such treatments. In addition, some treated tumours often develop resistance to these therapies.

Importantly, breast cancer can be classified into the following subtypes according to the presence and/or absence of various receptors: luminal A (ER+ and/or progesterone receptor (PR)+, EGFR2-), luminal B (ER+ and/or PR+, EGFR2+), EGFR2 over-expressed (ER-, PR-, EGFR2+), basal-like or triple negative (ER-, PR-, EGFR2-, cytokeratin (CK) 5/6 positive and/or epidermal growth factor receptor/EGFR positive) and normal breast-like tumours [1]. Luminal tumours have been associated with the most favourable prognoses, while EGFR2-overexpressing and basal-like tumours have been associated with the worst prognoses [1]. Approximately two out of three women with the disease have a tumour characterised by ER ("ER-positive") [2].

In other species, spontaneous tumours in cats and dogs are similar to human cancer. These animals share the same lifestyle as humans, and their tumours are genetically heterogeneous, as are randomly selected groups of cancer patients [3].

For research purposes, both the canine and feline models of breast cancer are of great importance for the study of this pathology due to a number of similarities at the molecular, histological and etiological levels.

2. Breast cancer in women

Worldwide, the number of women with breast cancer is steadily increasing. In 2019, 2,002,350 million new cases were found, resulting in 700,660 deaths from the disease [4]. As a result, it has become one of the most common cancers affecting women. In developed countries, the disease affects one in eight women, with an average age at diagnosis of 61 years. Approximately 2% of breast tumours occur in young women aged 20–34, 11% between the ages of 35–44 and 87% in patients aged 45 and older. Most tumours are diagnosed at an early stage, without spread to the contralateral breast or axillary lymph nodes (i.e. ductal carcinomas in situ and stages I, IIA, IIB and IIIA) and are considered potentially curable. It is encouraging to note that the survival of those patients is improving, reaching a survival rate of around 88% in the following five years of treatment. The prognosis appears to be worse in women aged ≤35 years at diagnosis [5]. Although characterised by cellular, molecular and clinical heterogeneity [1], it is accepted that reproductive endocrine factors, especially those related to increased exposure to oestrogens and/or progestogens, are among the major risk factors for this disease [6].

3. Canine mammary cancer

Within veterinary clinical practice, it is common to have patients presenting with mammary cancer. Canine bitches have a high percentage of mammary tumours, with malignant neoplasms accounting for 30–50%, of which 50–75% recur or metastasise within one to two years [7]. Most malignant breast tumours are classified as epithelial tumours or carcinomas. Pure sarcomas represent a minority. Benign tumours include simple/complex adenomas, fibroadenomas and benign mixed tumour [8].

Comparatively, some prognostic factors are similar for human and canine species, although regional lymph node metastasis does not seem to be of major importance in canines. Metastatic spread is similar in both species, except that liver and bone metastases are not common in canines as they are in humans [9].

As in humans, the risk of canine mammary neoplasia is affected by oestrogen exposure during early mammary development [10]. Factors influencing females such as advanced age, treatment with progesterone or synthetic progestins, obesity at an early age, nulliparity, breed (heredity) and diet also increase the predisposition to develop mammary tumours in bitches [11]. Epidemiological studies in humans have shown that a high-fat diet and obesity increase the risk of mammary cancer. A study conducted in the United States showed that among neutered canines, the risk of developing mammary cancer was reduced if the dogs were lean (determined by body condition score) at nine to twelve months of age [12]. Consumption of homemade diets (compared to commercial foods) was also associated with an increased risk [13].

Several international studies have estimated that the incidence of obesity in the canine population varies between 22% and 40% [14], with the incidence of feline obesity being of similar frequency [15]. Several researchers agree that, similar to the trend in humans, the incidence of obesity in the pet population is increasing [16, 17].

Obesity is known to be a risk factor for mammary cancer as adipocytes have a high capacity to produce oestrogen from androgens, so cells in a mammary gland with a large amount of adipose tissue will be exposed to high concentrations of oestrogen. In animal models, biomarkers such as increased concentrations of IGF-1, leptin and sex hormones, as well as decreased concentrations of adiponectin, have been shown to promote tumour development. The same has been observed in humans [17].

The average age of presentation of mammary tumours is from ten to eleven years, with rare occurrence in canines younger than four years. Several spaniel breeds and, according to some studies, poodles and dachshunds seem to be predisposed to this condition [18]. Studies have reported that 25% of small breed dogs manifest histologically malignant tumours compared to 58% of medium to large breed patients [19]. A higher predisposition to mammary tumours has also been found in purebred dogs compared to mongrels [20].

One in four non-ovariohysterectomised bitches over four years of age is expected to develop mammary neoplasia [20]. Therefore, one of the control measures would be to perform ovariohysterectomies before the first, second or third oestrous cycle, as they are known to have a positive effect in decreasing the relative risk of developing mammary tumours to 0.5%, 8% or 26%, respectively [21]. In support of the above, a positive effect of ovariectomy in females is recognised, and its performance is recommended before the age of forty years [22].

The presence of oestrogen receptors (ERs), progesterone receptors (PRs) and epidermal growth factor receptors (EGFR) in both normal mammary tissue and mammary tumour tissue has been described in all species, including the canine species. The amount of steroid receptors in healthy tissue varies significantly with age (older canines have more ERs), location (posterior glands have higher concentrations of ERs) and the stage of the cycle (the highest number of ERs is found in the mid-luteal phase and the lowest concentrations of ERs in the early luteal phase). The EGFR content in the normal gland varies according to proliferative (oestrus, early and mid-luteal phase) and non-proliferative (early pro-estrus and anestrus) status. Most benign tumours contain ERs and PRs, the latter existing at levels similar to the normal gland [23]. In contrast, carcinomas, devoid of remnants of normal mammary epithelium, contain ERs and PRs in decreased numbers, with rare occurrence of metastases [24]. In a study by Millanta and colleagues, no significant differences in quantitative ER expression were found between normal, dysplastic, benign and carcinoma in situ tissue, while ER expression in invasive carcinomas was significantly lower [25].

Other research has revealed overexpression of messenger ribonucleic acid (mRNA) for the oncogene epidermal growth factor receptor 2 (also called EGFR2, HER2, erbB-2 or neu) in most malignant breast tumours (not so in benign ones) although without local invasion or regional metastatic disease. This suggests that EGFR2 overexpression may play a role in favouring the malignant process [26]. However, another study indicates that these proteins were more often expressed in benign tumours (50%) than in malignant tumours (19%) [27]. Dutra *et al.* detected EGFR2 protein expression in 35.4% of the malignant tumours analysed, while none of the benign tumours contained EGFR2 [28]. All these results show the heterogeneity of breast tumours and that, despite so much research, the importance of this receptor in the pathogenesis of this disease has not yet been fully elucidated.

Antuofermo *et al.* found that the canine model of intraepithelial mammary lesions, which is histologically and in the expression pattern of REα and HER-2 very similar to the human species, is ideally suited for the study of RE-negative (HER-2 + or -) human breast cancer [10].

The p53 tumour suppressor gene is the most frequently mutated gene in human cancer. Trials in canine mammary cancer found that 17% of carcinomas tested had mutations in p53 [29]. The p53 gene could contribute to prognostic assessment in canine mammary carcinomas, as it does in human tumours. Alterations of a second tumour suppressor gene, BRCA2, which is partly responsible for human hereditary mammary tumours, have been described in canine mammary neoplasms. These mutations appear to affect the interaction with RAD51 and thus DNA repair [30].

4. Feline mammary cancer

Mammary tumours are the third most common tumour in felines, after haematopoietic neoplasms and skin tumours [20].

The incidence of mammary tumours is less than half that seen in humans and dogs, accounting for 12% of all tumours affecting felines and 17% of neoplasms in cats [20]. Mammary tumours have also been reported in males, although less frequently (1–5% of feline mammary tumours) [31]. In contrast to humans and canines, 85–93% of feline mammary tumours are malignant [32]. Invasion of the lymphatic system and lymph nodes is common. In several studies, more than 80% of cats with mammary malignancy had metastases to one or more of the following organs at the time of death: lymph nodes, lungs, liver, adrenal glands and kidneys [33].

More than 80% of feline mammary tumours are histologically classified as adenocarcinomas, the same predominant type of human mammary cancer [7]. Sarcomas, squamous cell carcinomas and mucinous carcinomas are less common malignancies. Approximately 15% of breast masses are benign neoplasms or dysplasias, including simple/complex adenomas and fibroadenomas. In addition, there are three types of non-inflammatory hyperplasia of the feline mammary gland: ductular hyperplasia, lobular hyperplasia and fibroepithelial hyperplasia [34].

There is evidence associating the presentation of mammary tumours with breed; domestic shorthair and Siamese cats appear to have higher incidence rates [32].

The mean age of presentation for feline mammary tumours is 10–12 years, with cases occurring from 9 months to 23 years of age [32].

Dorn *et al.* described that female cats spayed at 6 months of age had an approximately seven times lower risk of mammary cancer than intact female cats [20]. A case–control study by Overly and colleagues showed that cats spayed before 6 months of age had a 91% reduced risk of mammary carcinoma compared to intact cats, and those spayed before 1 year of age had an 86% reduced risk [35].

A strong association has also been documented between prior use of drugs containing synthetic progestins or oestrogen-progestin combinations and the development of benign or malignant mammary tumours in female cats. In both cases, the risk was three times higher in treated than in untreated cats [36].

Both normal tissue and benign proliferative lesions express low levels of ERs and moderate levels of PRs. Comparison of steroid receptor expression in human and feline mammary cancer indicates that the levels of ERs and PRs are decreased in feline mammary carcinoma. This could signify a loss of steroid hormone dependence during malignant progression, which would occur at earlier stages in feline mammary cancer than in human [37].

Feline mammary carcinoma has been proposed as a useful model for comparison with hormone-independent human mammary carcinomas because they share similar features such as equivalent age of incidence, histopathology and patterns of metastasis [3]. To this end, molecular studies have evaluated the overexpression of epidermal growth factor receptor 2 (also called EGFR2, HER2, erbB2 or neu) in feline mammary carcinomas. When this oncogene is amplified and overexpressed in human mammary cancer, EGFR2 is associated with clinically aggressive tumours and a poor overall prognosis [3] and may also predict poor response to hormone therapy and standard chemotherapy regimens [38]. This overexpression is reported to occur in 10–40% of human mammary carcinomas [3]. Millanta and colleagues described the same overexpression in 59% of feline mammary carcinoma cases studied and found that it was associated with shorter overall survival [25]. A second study showed that the feline EGFR2 gene domain had 92% homology with its human counterpart and found EGFR2 overexpression in 39% of the mammary carcinomas tested [3].

5. Oestrogen receptor

The response of target cells to oestrogen, primarily 17β-estradiol E2, is primarily determined by their oestrogen receptor (ER) content, proteins belonging to the steroid, thyroid and vitamin D receptor superfamily. Oestradiol (E2) diffuses across the plasma membrane of target cells and signals through hormone-specific oestrogen receptors. Two types of signalling can result from such binding, a genomic or classical pathway and a non-genomic or non-genotropic pathway (represented by rapidly activating cellular phenomena, e.g. signalling cascades). In the genomic pathway, oestrogens bind to the ER, inducing a conformational change of the ER that causes its dissociation from chaperones, followed by receptor dimerisation and activation of the transcriptional domain of the receptor [39]. Therefore, these receptors are considered ligand-inducible transcription factors [40]. The normal or canonical model for ER-mediated regulation of gene expression involves direct binding of the dimerised ER to DNA sequences known as "oestrogen response elements" (EREs) [41]. In either case, ER interaction with E2 leads to transcriptional activation of associated genes by recruiting co-activators and components of the basal transcriptional machinery [42].

Initially thought to be found only at the nuclear level, several studies have revealed the existence of these receptors at the plasma membrane, in the cytoplasm and even in the mitochondrion. The plasma membrane-associated ER is involved in the non-genomic oestrogen signalling pathway, which can lead to cytoplasmic alterations and/or regulation of gene expression [43].

For many years, it was believed that there was a single ER. However, in 1995, a second ER, REβ (so named to differentiate it from REα, an ER previously cloned from rat uterus), was cloned from rat prostate complementary DNA (cDNA) [44]. These two isoforms, ER alpha (REα) and ER beta (REβ), have similarities in size, estradiol affinity constants and structure but are encoded in different genes [45].

Despite the beneficial effects of oestrogens at the bone, cardiovascular and nervous system levels [40], several studies have demonstrated their involvement in the development of the breast cancer due to the effects of their signalling pathways and on the selective expression of REα and REβ during tumour genesis and progression [6].

6. Treatments for ER-positive breast cancer

The most commonly employed breast cancer treatments consist of anti-oestrogen and/or aromatase inhibitors (AIs), which are usually effective only in patients with ER-positive breast cancer [46]. Anti-oestrogen agents were called selective oestrogen receptor modulators (SERMs) some years ago because they manifested variable biochar properties: agonist and antagonist in terms of responses triggered in different tissues [45]. Oestradiol and SERMs are now known to influence the establishment and/or progression of many mammary tumours through association with oestrogen receptors. Binding of SERMs to ER regulates genomic and/or non-genomic effects and differentially influences the development of some tumours. For more than two decades, the anti-oestrogen tamoxifen was the treatment of choice for ER-positive female breast cancer, due to its antagonistic action in the mammary gland, where it inhibits transcription of target genes [46]. While this compound exerts an antagonistic effect on oestradiol in the breast, it exerts agonist activity in other tissues such as bone and endometrial [47]. This is demonstrated by the increased risk of endometrial cancer observed with prolonged tamoxifen treatment [48].

ICI 182,780 (also known as fulvestrant) is a "pure" steroidal anti-oestrogen, which differs from tamoxifen in its mechanism of action and in the lack of agonist activity in ER-containing tissues other than the breast. At the cellular level, apart from binding to the ER and increasing its degradation, ICI 182,780 would recruit cancer cells in G0/G1 by inducing the expression of a cyclin-dependent kinase inhibitor, p21kip1 [49]. Fulvestrant is also known as the first SERD (selective oestrogen receptor degrader) [50].

Several non-steroidal aromatase inhibitors, including anastrozole and letrozole, have been available for almost two decades and are efficient alternatives for the management of anti-oestrogen-resistant breast cancer in post-menopausal women [46]. It is worth mentioning that not all ER-positive breast tumours react to these treatments, and in many cases, resistance can develop; this can be "intrinsic" (never responds to treatment) or acquired (initially remits, but then progresses again) [2]. The development of resistance appears to be related to the activation of ER-dependent signalling pathways by agents not considered to date as conventional ligands [51]. Other mechanisms associated with the resistance phenomenon include the epidermal growth factor receptor (EGFR), which is overexpressed in many tumours that are unresponsive to the aforementioned therapies. Amplification of the epidermal growth factor receptor 2 (EGFR2/HER2/erbB2/neu) gene, resulting in overexpression of EGFR2, has been found in 15–25% of human breast cancers, a frequency of genetic alteration second only to p53 mutations [52]. EGFR2 overexpression is an important predictive marker as its presentation generally represents an aggressive cancer with poor prognosis, as well as a unique target for molecular targeted therapy. Resistance is driven by intense signalling that activates the "downstream" cascade of kinases, which in turn stimulate the ER, increasing its transcriptional activity. This is known as "crosstalk" between ER and EGFR tyrosine kinases [53].

7. Mammary cancer signalling pathways

The main signalling pathways linked to mammary cancer, and shared by human and canine species, are those related to oestrogen, MAPK, PI3K/AKT, KRAS, PTEN and Wnt/β-catenin [54].

Cyclins are a family of proteins that control the progression of cells through the cell cycle by activating cyclin-dependent kinase (Cdk) enzymes. The cell cycle is promoted by the activation of these cyclin-dependent kinases, which are positively regulated by cyclins and negatively regulated by Cdk inhibitors (CKIs). This well-controlled expression is altered in tumour cells [55]. D-type cyclins (D1, D2, D3), regulatory subunits of Cdk4/6 kinases, function as critical mitogenic sensors that integrate growth factor-initiated signals with G1 phase progression. Mitogenic stimulus triggers the accumulation of active cyclin D1-Cdk4 complexes through increased cyclin expression, decreased cyclin proteolysis and promotion of cyclin D1-Cdk4 assembly. Mitogen-dependent expression of cyclin D1 requires growth factor-mediated activation of a transductional signalling cascade involving Ras, Raf-1 and extracellular signal-regulated protein kinases (ERK1 and 2) [56].

Overexpression of cyclin D1 has been linked to breast cancer progression and growth, as well as to the development of resistance to hormone therapy. Several hormones are involved in the proliferation of breast cancer cells, with cyclin D1 being an important target of the intracellular signalling pathways of these hormones [57].

Overexpression of cyclins A and E has been associated with poor prognosis [58] and overexpression of cyclin B1 with tumour grade (related to the fact that the higher the presence of the Ki-67 antigen, the more aggressive the tumour), mitosis and adverse clinical outcomes [59]. Cyclin D1 is overexpressed in more than 50% of human breast cancers [60]. Some studies show that cyclin D1 expression is positively correlated with ER status and negatively correlated with tumour grade and size, suggesting that cyclin D1 overexpression is a good prognostic marker, particularly when co-expressed with ER [61]. There are reports showing that cyclin D1 overexpression predicts resistance to tamoxifen treatment in breast cancer patients [58].

The importance of cyclin D1 nuclear localisation is critical for the cell cycle regulatory functions of cyclin D1-dependent kinase during the G1 phase and for the inhibition of proteolytic degradation of cyclin D1 [56]. Cyclin D1 degradation is regulated through the 26S proteosome, and efficient proteolysis requires phosphorylation of threonine-286. The ability of targeted phosphorylation of nuclear exported cyclin D1 leads to the hypothesis that cyclin D1 destruction occurs preferentially in the cytoplasm [62]. The ability of the CKIs, p27kip1 and p21cip1 to reduce the range of cyclin D1 passing into the cytoplasm is consistent with this observation [63].

Reinforcing this, a duality of CKIs has recently been described in that they are required as potent inhibitors of Cdk2 kinase and as a positive regulator of the cyclin D1-Cdk4 complex. Studies showed that inhibition of cyclin D1 nuclear export by CKIs is required for nuclear accumulation of the cyclin D1-Cdk4 complex during the G1 phase of the cell cycle [56].

Overexpression of EGFR2 has been linked to aggressive breast cancers with high metastasis and chemoresistance. For example, its presence has been shown to lead to increased resistance to tamoxifen. EGFR2 has also been shown to generate resistance to another compound used in breast cancer treatment, paclitaxel (Taxol®). Some findings have described that the mechanism of resistance is based on EGFR2 directly phosphorylating the cyclin-dependent kinase, Cdk2, and generating a transcriptional upregulation of p21cip1; however, the mechanism by which EGFR2 induces this transcriptional upregulation is not yet defined [64].

Among the classical function of p21cip1, a CKI that regulates progression through the G1 phase of the cell cycle, is to act as an effector of tumour suppressor proteins such as p53, BRCA1, WT1 and TGFβ [65]. Another important role, recently attributed, is that of attenuating epithelial-mesenchymal transition (EMT) cell characteristics in human mammary cancer cells. For example, p21cip1 antagonises the repression exerted by Twist on E-cadherin promoter activity [65].

Cadherins are glycoproteins with calcium-dependent transmembrane domains that mediate cell–cell adhesion. The cadherin family includes many different types. E-cadherin is the most studied. It is located on the surface of epithelial cells in regions of cell–cell contact known as adherens junctions. To perform their adhesive function, cadherins must form complexes with proteins of the cytoplasmic plate, called catenins, and with the actin cytoskeleton [66]. The development of malignant tumours, in particular the transition to invasive metastatic cancer, is characterised by the ability of tumour cells to overcome cell–cell adhesion and invade surrounding tissue [67]. This phenomenon is known as epithelial-mesenchymal transition (EMT). Studies in ovarian cancer have revealed that cells with low E-cadherin expression are more invasive [67, 68], and the absence of E-cadherin expression in ovarian cancer may predict short survival [69]. Several studies have shown that restoration of E-cadherin expression results in a reversion from an invasive phenotype to a sessile epithelial tumour cell phenotype, providing evidence that E-cadherin may act as an invasion suppressor molecule [70].

Factors that may play a role in the progression of canine mammary tumours include the expression of adherens junction and gap junction proteins such as E-cadherin, connexins and paxillin. In general, the most invasive, proliferative and aggressive tumour is, histologically, the one with the lowest expression of the protein in a localised and intense form, indicating a change that favours increased cell motility [71]. E-cadherin expression has been reported to be reduced or absent in 70% of feline mammary carcinomas compared to normal tissue [72].

The ability of β-catenin to act as part of the adhesive and transcriptional machinery is due to its modulation through phosphorylated serine/threonine and tyrosine residues: reduced serine/threonine phosphorylation destabilises the adhesion complex formed with cadherins and facilitates nuclear translocation of β-catenin and subsequent gene transcription. On the other hand, tyrosine phosphorylation results in its dissociation from E-cadherin and loss of association with the cytoskeleton, promoting reduced cell–cell adhesion and cell spreading. It is suggested that tyrosine phosphorylation would be promoted by EGFR2 [73]. Furthermore, the levels of complexes formed between β-catenin and EGFR2 are elevated in the most aggressive and metastatic tumour types in humans [74].

On the other hand, it is known that the amount of ERα is higher than that of ERβ in breast cancer cells. Oestrogens have a paradoxical role in human cancer as a promoter of carcinoma progression in some cases and inhibitor of cancer cell invasion in others. This could be explained by the antagonistic effect of ligand-bound ERα and ERβ on cancer pathogenesis. Studies in breast and gynaecological cancer have shown a positive effect of ERα on tumour cell proliferation and growth, while ERβ would promote apoptosis and inhibition of tumour growth [75].

One study showed that ERβ expression correlated positively with β-catenin expression at the cell membrane and negatively with β-catenin translocation to the nucleus [76]. This would imply a crosstalk between ER signalling and the Wnt/β-catenin pathway [77]. In addition, ERβ was positively correlated with the maintenance of E-cadherin in the plasma membrane of mammary tumour cells [76]. Another study using a prostate cancer cell line endogenously expressing REα and REβ showed that induction of EMT with TGFβ or exposure to hypoxia concomitantly led to a reduction in the number of REβ, suggesting that loss of REβ promotes EMT in prostate cancer cells [78].

8. Conclusion

The increasing incidence of mammary cancer in humans and dogs has forced the search for better diagnostic, treatment and/or prognostic strategies. Alternatively, several authors compare and highlight the similarities that allow postulating the canine and feline species as models for the study of such cancer and thus replace the murine model. Thus, important advances have been made in this area with promising results. However, given the complex nature of malignant mammary tumours, much remains to be studied.

Conflict of interest

The author declares no conflict of interest.

Nomenclature

ER	oestrogen receptor
ERα	oestrogen receptor alpha
ERβ	oestrogen receptor beta
SERMs	selective oestrogen receptor modulators
AIs	aromatase inhibitors
PR	progesterone receptor
EGFR	epidermal growth factor receptor
CK	cytokeratin
EGFR2/HER2/erbB2/neu	epidermal growth factor receptor 2
ICI 182,780	fulvestrant
SERD	selective oestrogen receptor degrader
Cdk	cyclin-dependent kinase
CKIs	Cdk inhibitors
EMT	Epithelial-mesenchymal transition

Author details

Pamela Cruz
University of Chile, Santiago, Chile

*Address all correspondence to: pamela.cruz.espinoza@gmail.com

References

[1] Kwan ML, Kushi LH, Weltzien E, Maring B, Kutner SE, Fulton RS, et al. Epidemiology of breast cancer subtypes in two prospective cohort studies of breast cancer survivors. Breast Cancer Research. 2009;**11**(3):R31. DOI: 10.1186/bcr2261

[2] Leary AF, Sirohi B, Johnston SR. Clinical trials update: Endocrine and biological therapy combinations in the treatment of breast cancer. Breast Cancer Research. 2007;**9**(5):112. DOI: 10.1186/bcr1763

[3] De María R, Olivero M, Iussich S, Nakaichi M, Murata T, Biolatti B, et al. Spontaneous feline mammary carcinoma is a model of HER2 overexpressing poor prognosis human breast cancer. Cancer Research. 2005;**65**:907-912. DOI: 10.1158/0008-5472.907.65.3

[4] Xu Y, Gong M, Wang Y, Yang Y, Liu S, Zeng Q. Global trends and forecasts of breast cancer incidence and deaths. Scientific Data. 2023;**10**:334. DOI: 10.1038/s41597-023-02253-5

[5] Hickey M, Peate M, Saunders CM, Friedlander M. Breast cancer in young women and its impact reproductive function. Human Reproduction Update. 2009;**15**(3):323-339. DOI: 10.1093/humupd/dmn064

[6] Conway K, Parrish E, Edmiston SN, Tolbert D, Tse CK, Moorman P, et al. Risk factors for breast cancer characterized by the estrogen receptor alpha A908G (K303R) mutation. Breast Cancer Research. 2007;**9**(3):R36. DOI: 10.1186/bcr1731

[7] Misdorp W. Tumors of the mammary gland. In: Meuten DJ, editor. Tumors in Domestic Animals. 4th ed. Iowa: Iowa State Press; 2002. pp. 575-606. DOI: 10.1002/9780470376928

[8] Hellmén E. The pathogenesis of canine mammary tumours. Cancer Journal. 1996;**9**(6):282-286

[9] Owen LN. A comparative study of canine and human breast cancer. Investigative & Cell Pathology. 1979;**2**(4):257-275

[10] Antuofermo E, Miller MA, Pirino S, Xie J, Badve S, Mohammed SI. Spontaneous mammary intraepithelial lesions in dogs – A model of breast cancer. Cancer Epidemiology, Biomarkers & Prevention. 2007;**16**(11):2247-2256. DOI: 10.1158/1055-9965.EPI-06-0932

[11] Pérez Alenza MD, Peña L, Del Castillo N, Nieto AI. Factors influencing the incidence and prognosis of canine mammary tumours. The Journal of Small Animal Practice. 2000;**41**(7):287-291. DOI: 10.1111/j.1748-5827.2000.tb03203.x

[12] Sonnenschein EG, Glickman LT, Goldschmidt MH, Mckee LJ. Body conformation, diet and risk of breast cancer in pet dogs: A case-control study. American Journal of Epidemiology. 1991;**133**:694-703. DOI: 10.1093/oxfordjournals.aje.a115944

[13] Pérez Alenza MD, Rutteman GR, Peña L, Beynen AC, Cuesta P. Relation between habitual diet and canine mammary tumors in a case-control study. Journal of Veterinary Internal Medicine. 1998;**12**(3):132-139. DOI: 10.1111/j.1939-1676.1998.tb02108.x

[14] McGreevy PD, Thomson PC, Pride C, Fawcett A, Grassi T, Jones B. Prevalence of obesity in dogs examined by Australian veterinary practices and

the risk factors involved. The Veterinary Record. 2005;**156**(22):695-702. DOI: 10.1136/vr.156.22.695

[15] German AJ. The growing problem of obesity in dogs and cats. The Journal of Nutrition. 2006;**136**(7 Suppl):1940S-1946S. DOI: 10.1093/jn/136.7.1940S

[16] Linder DE, Santiago S, Halbreich ED. Is there a correlation between dog obesity and human obesity? Preliminary findings of overweight status among dog owners and their dogs. Frontiers in Veterinary Science. 2021;**8**:654617. DOI: 10.3389/fvets.2021.654617

[17] Marchi PH, Vendramini THA, Perini MP, Zafalon RVA, Amaral AR, Ochamotto VA, et al. Obesity, inflammation, and cancer in dogs: Review and perspectives. Frontiers in Veterinary Science. 2022;**9**:1004122. DOI: 10.3389/fvets.2022.1004122

[18] Zatloukal J, Lorenzová J, Tichý F, NecaS A, Kecová H, Kohout P. Breed and age as risk factors for canine mammary tumours. Acta Veterinaria. 2005;**74**:103-109. DOI: 10.2754/avb200574010103

[19] Itoh T, Uchida K, Ishikawa K, Kushima K, Kushima E, Tamada H, et al. Clinicopathological survey of 101 canine mammary gland tumors: Differences between small-breed dogs and others. The Journal of Veterinary Medical Science. 2005;**67**(3):345-347. DOI: 10.1292/jvms.67.345

[20] Dorn CR, Taylor DO, Schneider R, Hibbard HH, Klauber MR. Survey of animal neoplasms in alameda and contra costa counties, California. II. Cancer morbidity in dogs and cats from Alameda County. Journal of the National Cancer Institute. 1968;**40**(2):307-318

[21] Schneider R, Dorn CR, Taylor DO. Factors influencing canine mammary cancer development and postsurgical survival. Journal of the National Cancer Institute. 1969;**43**(6):1249-1261

[22] Mulligan RM. Mammary cancer in the dog: A study of 120 cases. American Journal of Veterinary Research. 1975;**36**(9):1391-1396

[23] Donnay I, Rauïs J, Wouters-Ballman P, Devleeschouwer N, Leclercq G, Verstegen JP. Receptors for oestrogen, progesterone and epidermal growth factor in normal and tumorous canine mammary tissues. Journal of Reproduction and Fertility. Supplement. 1993;**47**:501-512

[24] Donnay I, Rauïs J, Devleeschouwer N, Wouters-Ballman P, Leclercq G, Verstegen J. Comparison of estrogen and progesterone receptor expression in normal and tumor mammary tissues from dogs. American Journal of Veterinary Research. 1995;**56**(9):1188-1194

[25] Millanta F, Calandrella M, Bari G, Niccolini M, Vannozzi I, Poli A. Comparison of steroid receptor expression in normal, dysplastic, and neoplastic canine and feline mammary tissues. Research in Veterinary Science. 2005;**79**(3):225-232. DOI: 10.1016/j.rvsc.2005.02.002

[26] Ahern TE, Bird RC, Bird AE, Wolfe LG. Expression of the oncogene c-erbB-2 in canine mammary cancers and tumor-derived cell lines. American Journal of Veterinary Research. 1996;**57**(5):693-696

[27] Rungsipipat A, Tateyama S, Yamaguchi R, Uchida K, Miyoshi N, Hayashi T. Immunohistochemical analysis of c-yes and c-erbB-2 oncogene products and p53 tumor suppressor protein in canine mammary tumors. The Journal of Veterinary Medical

Science. 1999;**61**(1):27-32. DOI: 10.1292/jvms.61.27

[28] Dutra AP, Granja NV, Schmitt FC, Cassali GD. c-erbB-2 expression and nuclear pleomorphism in canine mammary tumors. Brazilian Journal of Medical and Biological Research. 2004;**37**(11):1673-1681. DOI: 10.1590/s0100-879x2004001100013

[29] Wakui S, Muto T, Yokoo K, Yokoo R, Takahashi H, Masaoka T, et al. Prognostic status of p53 gene mutation in canine mammary carcinoma. Anticancer Research. 2001;**21**(1B):611-616

[30] Thumser-Henner P, Nytko KJ, Rohrer BC. Mutations of BRCA2 in canine mammary tumors and their targeting potential in clinical therapy. BMC Veterinary Research. 2020;**16**(1):30. DOI: 10.1186/s12917-020-2247-4

[31] Skorupski KA, Overley B, Shofer FS, Goldschmidt MH, Miller CA, Sørenmo KU. Clinical characteristics of mammary carcinoma in male cats. Journal of Veterinary Internal Medicine. 2005;**19**(1):52-55. DOI: 10.1892/0891-6640(2005)19<52:cco mci>2.0.co;2

[32] Burrai GP, Mohammed SI, Miller MA, Marras V, Pirino S, Addis MF, et al. Spontaneous feline mammary intraepithelial lesions as a model for human estrogen receptor- and progesterone receptor-negative breast lesions. BMC Cancer. 2010;**10**:156. DOI: 10.1186/1471-2407-10-156

[33] Hassan BB, Elshafae SM, Supsavhad W, Simmons JK, Dirksen WP, Sokkar SM, et al. Feline mammary cancer: Novel nude mouse model and molecular characterization of invasion and metastasis genes. Veterinary Pathology. 2017;**54**(1):32-43. DOI: 10.1177/0300985816650243

[34] Carpenter JL, Andrews LK, Holzworth J. Tumors and tumor-like lesions. In: Holzworth J, editor. Diseases of the Cat: Medicine and Surgery. Philadelphia: WB Saunders; 1987. pp. 408-416

[35] OverleyB, ShoferFS, GoldschmidtMH, Sherer D, Sorenmo KU. Association between ovarihysterectomy and feline mammary carcinoma. Journal of Veterinary Internal Medicine. 2005;**19**(4):560-563. DOI: 10.1892/0891-6640(2005)19 [560:aboafm]2.0.co;2

[36] Misdorp W, Romijn A, Hart AA. Feline mammary tumors: A case-control study of hormonal factors. Anticancer Research. 1991;**11**(5):1793-1797

[37] Rutteman GR, Blankenstein MA, Minke J, Misdorp W. Steroid receptors in mammary tumours of the cat. Acta Endocrinologica. 1991;**125**(Suppl 1):32-37

[38] Ross JS, Fletcher JA. The HER-2/neu oncogene: Prognostic factor, predictive factor and target for therapy. Seminars in Cancer Biology. 1999;**9**(2):125-138. DOI: 10.1006/scbi.1998.0083

[39] Marino M, Galluzzo P, Ascenzi P. Estrogen signaling multiple pathways to impact gene transcription. Current Genomics. 2006;**7**(8):497-508. DOI: 10.2174/138920206779315737

[40] Lewis JS, Jordan VC. Selective estrogen receptor modulators (SERMs): Mechanisms of anticarcinogenesis and drug resistance. Mutation Research. 2005;**591**(1-2):247-263. DOI: 10.1016/j.mrfmmm.2005.02.028

[41] Klinge CM. Estrogen receptor interaction with estrogen response elements. Nucleic Acids Research. 2001;**29**(14):2905-2919. DOI: 10.1093/nar/29.14.2905

[42] Glass CK, Rosenfeld MG. The coregulator exchange in transcriptional functions of nuclear receptors. Genes & Development. 2000;**14**(2):121-141

[43] Levin ER. Integration of the extranuclear and nuclear actions of estrogen. Molecular Endocrinology. 2005;**19**(8):1951-1959. DOI: 10.1210/me.2004-0390

[44] Kuiper GG, Enmark E, Pelto-Huikko M, Nilsson S, Gustafsson JA. Cloning of a novel receptor expressed in rat prostate and ovary. Proceedings of the National Academy of Sciences of the United States of America. 1996;**93**(12):5925-5930. DOI: 10.1073/pnas.93.12.5925

[45] Dutertre M, Smith CL. Molecular mechanisms of selective estrogen receptor modulator (SERM) action. The Journal of Pharmacology and Experimental Therapeutics. 2000;**295**(2):431-437

[46] Schiff R, Chamness GC, Brown PH. Advances in breast cancer treatment and prevention: Preclinical studies on aromatase inhibitors and new selective estrogen receptor modulators (SERMs). Breast Cancer Research. 2003;**5**(5):228-231. DOI: 10.1186/bcr626

[47] Deroo BJ, Korach KS. Estrogen receptors and human disease. The Journal of Clinical Investigation. 2006;**116**(3):561-570. DOI: 10.1172/JCI27987

[48] Fisher B, Costantino JP, Wickerham DL, Cecchini RS, Cronin WM, Robidoux A, et al. Tamoxifen for the prevention of breast cancer: Current status of the National Surgical Adjuvant Breast and bowel project P-1 study. Journal of the National Cancer Institute. 2005;**97**(22):1652-1662. DOI: 10.1093/jnci/dji372

[49] Varshochi R, Halim F, Sunters A, Alao JP, Madureira PA, Hart SM, et al. ICI182,780 induces p21Waf1 gene transcription through releasing histone deacetylase 1 and estrogen receptor alpha from Sp1 sites to induce cell cycle arrest in MCF-7 breast cancer cell line. The Journal of Biological Chemistry. 2005;**280**(5):3185-3196. DOI: 10.1074/jbc.m408063200

[50] Downton T, Zhou F, Segara D, Jeselsohn R, Lim E. Oral selective Estrogen receptor degraders (SERDs) in breast cancer: Advances, challenges, and current status. Drug Design, Development and Therapy. 2022;**16**:2933-2948. DOI: 10.2147/DDDT.S380925

[51] Riggins RB, Schrecengost RS, Guerrero MS, Bouton AH. Pathways to tamoxifen resistance. Cancer Letters. 2007;**256**(1):1-24. DOI: 10.1016/j.canlet.2007.03.016

[52] Slamon DJ, Godolphin W, Jones LA, Holt JA, Wong SG, Keith DE, et al. Studies of the HER-2/neu proto-oncogene in human breast and ovarian cancer. Science. 1989;**244**(4905):707-712. DOI: 10.1126/science.2470152

[53] Arpino G, Wiechmann L, Osborne CK, Schiff R. Crosstalk between the estrogen receptor and the HER tyrosine kinase receptor family: Molecular mechanism and clinical implications for endocrine therapy resistance. Endocrine Reviews. 2008;**29**(2):217-233. DOI: 10.1210/er.2006-0045

[54] Pinho SS, Carvalho S, Cabral J, Reis CA, Gärtner F. Canine tumors: A spontaneous animal model of human carcinogenesis. Translational Research. 2012;**159**(3):165-172. DOI: 10.1016/j.trsl.2011.11.005

[55] Malumbres M, Barbacid M. Cell cycle, CDKs and cancer: A changing paradigm. Nature Reviews. Cancer. 2009;**9**(3):153-166. DOI: 10.1038/nrc2602

[56] Alt JR, Gladden AB, Diehl JA. p21(Cip1) promotes cyclin D1 nuclear accumulation via direct inhibition of nuclear export. The Journal of Biological Chemistry. 2002;**277**(10):8517-8523. DOI: 10.1074/jbc.M108867200

[57] Lanzino M, Sisci D, Morelli C, Garofalo C, Catalano S, Casaburi I, et al. Inhibition of cyclin D1 expression by androgen receptor in breast cancer cells–identification of a novel androgen response element. Nucleic Acids Research. 2010;**38**(16):5351-5365. DOI: 10.1093/nar/gkq278

[58] Boström P, Söderström M, Palokangas T, Vahlberg T, Collan Y, Carpen O, et al. Analysis of cyclins A, B1, D1 and E in breast cancer in relation to tumour grade and other prognostic factors. BMC Research Notes. 2009;**2**:140. DOI: 10.1186/1756-0500-2-140

[59] Suzuki T, Urano T, Miki Y, Moriya T, Akahira J, Ishida T, et al. Nuclear cyclin B1 in human breast carcinoma as a potent prognostic factor. Cancer Science. 2007;**98**(5):644-651. DOI: 10.1111/j.1349-7006.2007.00444.x

[60] Arnold A, Papanikolaou A. Cyclin D1 in breast cancer pathogenesis. Journal of Clinical Oncology. 2005;**23**(18):4215-4224. DOI: 10.1200/JCO.2005.05.064

[61] Hwang TS, Han HS, Hong YC, Lee HJ, Paik NS. Prognostic value of combined analysis of cyclin D1 and estrogen receptor status in breast cancer patients. Pathology International. 2003;**53**(2):74-80. DOI: 10.1046/j.1440-1827.2003.01441.x

[62] Diehl JA, Cheng M, Roussel MF, Sherr CJ. Glycogen synthase kinase-3beta regulates cyclin D1 proteolysis and subcellular localization. Genes & Development. 1998;**12**(22):3499-3511. DOI: 10.1101/gad.12.22.3499

[63] Cheng M, Olivier P, Diehl JA, Fero M, Roussel MF, Roberts JM, et al. The p21(Cip1) and p27(Kip1) CDK 'inhibitors' are essential activators of cyclin D-dependent kinases in murine fibroblasts. The EMBO Journal. 1999;**18**(6):1571-1583. DOI: 10.1093/emboj/18.6.1571

[64] Hawthorne VS, Huang WC, Neal CL, Tseng LM, Hung MC, Yu D. ErbB2-mediated Src and signal transducer and activator of transcription 3 activation leads to transcriptional up-regulation of p21Cip1 and chemoresistance in breast cancer cells. Molecular Cancer Research. 2009;**7**(4):592-600. DOI: 10.1158/1541-7786.MCR-08-0316

[65] Liu M, Casimiro MC, Wang C, Shirley LA, Jiao X, Katiyar S, et al. p21CIP1 attenuates Ras- and c-Myc-dependent breast tumor epithelial mesenchymal transition and cancer stem cell-like gene expression in vivo. Proceedings of the National Academy of Sciences of the United States of America. 2009;**106**(45):19035-19039. DOI: 10.1073/pnas.0910009106

[66] Gumbiner BM. Cell adhesion: The molecular basis of tissue architecture and morphogenesis. Cell. 1996;**84**(3):345-357. DOI: 10.1016/s0092-8674(00)81279-9

[67] Martin TA, Ye L, Sanders AJ, et al. Cancer invasion and metastasis: Molecular and cellular perspective. In: Madame Curie Bioscience Database. [Internet]. Austin (TX): Landes Bioscience; 2000-2013 Available from: https://www.ncbi.nlm.nih.gov/books/NBK164700/

[68] Veatch AL, Carson LF, Ramakrishnan S. Differential expression of the cell-cell adhesion molecule E-cadherin in ascites and solid human ovarian tumor cells. International Journal of Cancer. 1994;**58**(3):393-399. DOI: 10.1002/ijc.2910580315

[69] Kielbik M, Szulc-Kielbik I, Klink M. E-cadherin expression in relation to clinicopathological parameters and survival of patients with epithelial ovarian cancer. International Journal of Molecular Sciences. 2022;**23**(22):14383. DOI: 10.3390/ijms232214383

[70] Vleminckx K, Vakaet L Jr, Mareel M, Fiers W, van Roy F. Genetic manipulation of E-cadherin expression by epithelial tumor cells reveals an invasion suppressor role. Cell. 1991;**66**(1):107-119. DOI: 10.1016/0092-8674(91)90143-m

[71] Torres LN, Matera JM, Vasconcellos CH, Avanzo JL, Hernandez-Blazquez FJ, Dagli ML. Expression of connexins 26 and 43 in canine hyperplastic and neoplastic mammary glands. Veterinary Pathology. 2005;**42**(5):633-641. DOI: 10.1354/vp.42-5-633

[72] Dias Pereira P, Gärtner F. Expression of E-cadherin in normal, hyperplastic and neoplastic feline mammary tissue. The Veterinary Record. 2003;**153**(10):297-302. DOI: 10.1136/vr.153.10.297

[73] Hiscox S, Jiang WG, Obermeier K, Taylor K, Morgan L, Burmi R, et al. Tamoxifen resistance in MCF7 cells promotes EMT-like behaviour and involves modulation of beta-catenin phosphorylation. International Journal of Cancer. 2006;**118**(2):290-301. DOI: 10.1002/ijc.21355

[74] Schroeder JA, Adriance MC, McConnell EJ, Thompson MC, Pockaj B, Gendler SJ. ErbB-beta-catenin complexes are associated with human infiltrating ductal breast and murine mammary tumor virus (MMTV)-Wnt-1 and MMTV-c-Neu transgenic carcinomas. The Journal of Biological Chemistry. 2002;**277**(25):22692-22698. DOI: 10.1074/jbc.M201975200

[75] Koehler KF, Helguero LA, Haldosén LA, Warner M, Gustafsson JA. Reflections on the discovery and significance of estrogen receptor beta. Endocrine Reviews. 2005;**26**(3):465-478. DOI: 10.1210/er.2004-0027

[76] Su Y, Simmen RC. Soy isoflavone genistein upregulates epithelial adhesion molecule E-cadherin expression and attenuates beta-catenin signaling in mammary epithelial cells. Carcinogenesis. 2009;**30**(2):331-339. DOI: 10.1093/carcin/bgn279

[77] Goulioumis AK, Fuxe J, Varakis J, Repanti M, Goumas P, Papadaki H. Estrogen receptor-beta expression in human laryngeal carcinoma: Correlation with the expression of epithelial-mesenchymal transition specific biomarkers. Oncology Reports. 2009;**22**(5):1063-1068. DOI: 10.3892/or_00000537

[78] Zhao C, Dahlman-Wright K, Gustafsson JÅ. Estrogen signaling via estrogen receptor {beta}. The Journal of Biological Chemistry. 2010;**285**(51):39575-39579. DOI: 10.1074/jbc.R110.180109